CLINICAL INTERPRETATION OF ACID-BASE AND ELECTROLYTE DISORDERS

CASE STUDIES

Ivo Casagranda
Mario Tarantino

CLINICAL INTERPRETATION OF ACID-BASE AND ELECTROLYTE DISORDERS

CASE STUDIES

In collaboration with
Rodolfo Sbrojavacca, Michele Santoro

edra

Original title
I. Casagranda, M. Tarantino – Acqua e sale. Interpretazione dei disordini acido-base e idroelettrolitici attraverso i casi clinici

ISBN: 978-88-214-5113-3

Book Publishing Manager: Costanza Smeraldi
Paper, Printing and Binding Manager: Michele Ribatti

Cover: Paolo Ballerini

ISBN: 978-88-214-5115-7
eISBN: 978-88-214-5116-4

Edra S.p.A.
Via G. Spadolini 7, 20141 Milano (Italy)
Tel. 02 881841
www.edizioniedra.it

Printed by "Koninska Drukarnia Dziełowa", Konin (Polonia) - March 2020

(*) Edra S.p.A. is part of LSWR GROUP

Editors

Ivo Casagranda
Adjunct Professor, Emergency Medicine, at the School of Internal Medicine, University of Pavia. Italy
Former Director of Emergency Department, General Hospital, Alessandria, Italy

Mario Tarantino
Former Director of Laboratory of Clinical Biochemistry and Microbiology
General Hospital, Saronno, Varese, Italy

Authors

Rodolfo Sbrojavacca
Former Director of Emergency Department, University Hospital, Udine. Italy

Michele Santoro
Emergency Department, Agostino Gemelli University Hospital, Roma, Italy

Contributors

Gaetano Esposito
Emergency Department, University Hospital, Udine. Italy

Andrea Bellone
Emergency Department, Niguarda General Hospital , Milano, Italy

Nicolò Capsoni
School of Emergency Medicine, University of Milano – Bicocca, Italy

Giulio Cassano
School of Emergency Medicine, University of Milano - Bicocca, Italy

Preface

This textbook, the result of years of clinical and teaching activity by me and fellow authors, as well as the continuous and valuable feedback obtained from students, is organized into three parts.
The first part, focused on the study of acid-base disorders, begins with the history of blood gas analysis: with this narrative we wanted to retrace years of brilliant discoveries by paying tribute to the scientists who allowed us to take advantage of their work. Two chapters include the fundamentals of physiological acid-base biochemistry and the contributions given by three major schools in diagnostic interpretation. The "core" consists of the two chapters that take the reader by the hand along the path of clinical interpretation with the use of case studies, placing them in the position of the doctor, as if they were beside the patient's bed. This sections ends with the treatment which includes a general part and a more specific one, focused on the most frequent pathological conditions in clinical activity.
The second part deals with sodium and water and begins with their history in physiology and in clinical practice that is full of eminent scientists. It then continues with the fundamentals of physiology to arrive at the alterations of the sodium-water relationship (hypo- and hypernatremia); even in this case the approach to interpretation and therapy is conducted by clinical cases. Finally, the section ends with the chapter regarding the use of fluids in medical practice.
The third part deals with those electrolytes that we could define as "membrane electrolytes", because they determine and condition the electrophysiological aspects: potassium, calcium and magnesium ions. Even these elements are discussed starting with homeostasis and arriving at the pathological conditions caused by their concentration alterations and their treatment. Also in this presentation the clinical case is the fundamental didactic tool.

Finally, we have to present the cover: the sea (salt and water) and pink flamingos, symbols of life born from sea, that live in brackish water, preferably alkaline, are depicted.

I close this preface with thanks to my travelling companions: Mario Tarantino, with whom I have shared many educational events over the last twenty-five years, whose expertise and experience, for having lived on the field an important part of the history of blood gas analysis, starting from the 1960s (not by chance he wrote the history), remains irreplaceable; Rodolfo Sbrojavacca, to whom I am bound by a common passion for the topics covered; Michele Santoro who followed me with reciprocated confidence in the clinical path and study of this fascinating subject. I also thank Andrea Bellone, Gaetano Esposito, Nicolò Capsoni and Giulio Cassano who contributed to the success of this volume.
A special thanks to Enrico Zucconi for the contribution provided in the drafting of the English edition.
I wish all readers a good read and I apologize in advance for the inevitable slips and shortcomings they may encounter.

Ivo Casagranda

Table of contents

Chapter 5
CLINICAL INTERPRETATION OF MIXED ACID-BASE DISORDERS

Ivo Casagranda

Chapter 6
MANAGEMENT OF ACID-BASE DISORDERS
Gaetano Esposito, Rodolfo Sbrojavacca, Nicolò Capsoni, Giulio Cassano, Andrea Bellone

Section II
SODIUM AND WATER

Chapter 7
SALT AND WATER IN PHYSIOLOGY AND IN CLINICAL MEDICINE
Mario Tarantino

Chapter 8
HOMEOSTASIS OF BODY FLUIDS FUNDAMENTALS OF PHYSIOLOGY

Mario Tarantino

Chapter 9
HYPONATREMIA

Ivo Casagranda

Chapter 10
HYPERNATREMIA

Ivo Casagranda

Chapter 11
THE USE OF FLUIDS IN CLINICAL PRACTICE
Ivo Casagranda

Section III
ELECTROLYTES

Chapter 12
HYPOKALEMIA
Michele Santoro

Chapter 13
HYPERKALEMIA
Michele Santoro

Chapter 14
HYPOCALCEMIA
Michele Santoro

Chapter 15
HYPERCALCEMIA
Michele Santoro

Chapter 16
MAGNESIUM HOMEOSTATIS AND DISORDERS
Michele Santoro

To Nicolò Gentiloni Silveri

SECTION I

ACID-BASE BALANCE

CHAPTER 1

History of blood gas analysis and acid-base balance

Mario Tarantino

The history of the development of knowledge in the field of blood gas analysis and acid-base balance is of particular interest, not only for the acquisitions accumulated over the years, as usually happens in the biological and medical sciences, but above all because – done less frequent – the same principles on which the interpretation of physiological and pathophysiological mechanisms that regulate blood pH and cause its alterations are still constantly evolving, consequently affecting, also substantially, the criteria useful for the diagnosis of acid-base disorders.

The interest in this unusual evolution is supported by substantial literature specifically dedicated to the topic, to which we refer. Here are mentioned the scientists who, between the last decades of the nineteenth century and the first half of the twentieth century, contributed to defining the physiology modern concepts of blood pH homeostasis and the interpretative criteria of the most common acid-base disorders for diagnostic purposes. Their studies and conclusions (to which they arrived at) have subsequently given rise to further developments and controversies that still feed them today. A little over a hundred years ago, in 1908, Lawrence Joseph Henderson (**Figure 1.1**), physiology professor at Harvard University in Boston, published his famous equation that related the concentration of blood hydrogen ions to bicarbonate buffer:

$$[H^+] = k' [H_2CO_3] / [NaHCO_3] \quad (1)$$

giving start to the use of blood gas profile, the foundation of the modern diagnosis of acid-base disorders. It still retains its validity today, despite the criticisms and new interpretative proposals developed from this equation.

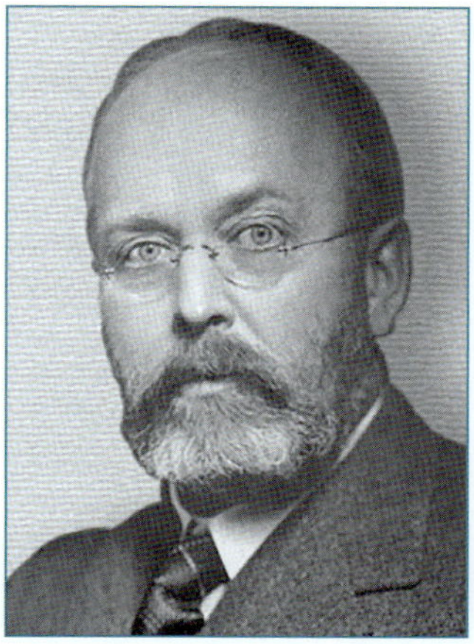

Figure 1.1 Lawrence Joseph Henderson (1878-1942).

However, the principles and concepts that have allowed this definition of physiological biochemistry and acid-base pathophysiology are the fruit of the important and intense preparatory work that numerous scholars on both sides of the Atlantic had accumulated, especially during the nineteenth century, but also in the previous centuries. Referring to the excellent and detailed literature available, here we limit ourselves to recall the most important events and protagonists.

CO_2, HCO_3^-, alkaline reserve

The interest in blood gases manifested itself very soon, following the important discoveries of Antoine-Laurent de Lavoisier (1743-1794) on oxygen, which were not limited to physical and chemical properties of the gas, but extended to the biological meaning, advancing hypotheses of physiological interest on oxygen-carbon dioxide gas exchanges, on respiratory function and also on metabolic processes.

In 1837 the first treatise on blood gases appeared – edited by Heinrich Gustav Magnus (1802-1870) – where, among other things, it was stated that CO_2 was not produced in the lungs, but in other sites where the blood carried the oxygen. Twenty years later, in 1857, another treatise *Die Gase des Blutes* – published by Julius Lothar Meyer (1830-1895) – suggested that blood oxygen should be found not only in the physical form, but partly also chemically bonded. As it is easy to understand, the interest in blood gases was mainly addressed to oxygen, so that the knowledge on its transport and on the respiratory function of hemoglobin advanced more rapidly than those on CO_2. However, once the significance of the elimination products in relation to metabolism, as well as the importance of exchanges with O_2 at the pulmonary level, were ascertained, the physiological interest in CO_2 also progressively established itself. The question that for a long time involved the researchers concerned the nature of the forms in which CO_2 was present in the blood. The difficulty was mainly due to the inadequacy of the investigation means. The existence of blood CO_2 in free form remained long uncertain, and was confirmed only in the 1960s (Gustav Heinrich Wiedemann, 1826-1899; Franz Cornelius Donders, 1818-1889), while only at the end of the nineteenth century the combined form was identified as bicarbonate; the demonstration of the carbamino form linked with hemoglobin (Christian Bohr, **Figure 1.2**), dates back to 1914, as well as the greater affinity of the deoxygenated form with respect to the oxygenated form, a phenomenon known as the Haldane effect (John Scott Haldane, 1860-1936). Also in the same years (1908) Hartog Jacob Hamburger (1859-1924) demonstrated the exchange of bicarbonate with chloride in erythrocytes, thus helping to clarify that CO_2 was transported mainly in blood cells, despite the prevalence of dissociated bicarbonate form in the plasma.

In 1919 Carl Faurholt (1890-1972) showed that the hydration of CO_2 to carbonic acid is an extremely slow process: in fact, under physiological conditions, only one thousandth of the CO_2 physically dissolved in the plasma is in the hydrated form. This discovery involved several physiologists, and in particular Oscar Michael Henriques (1895-1953), because the rapid conversion of CO_2 during the passage through the lungs was difficult to explain. Comparing the kinetics of CO_2 in serum and in the red blood cell lysis, Henriques showed that while in serum the CO_2 content took 1-1½ minutes to halve, the same process in the red blood cells took less than 5 seconds. These observations gave rise to the studies that initially led, in 1930, Donald Dexter Van Slyke (**Figure 1.3**) to indicate the catalytic nature of CO_2 transformation in red blood cells, and later, in 1932, Francis John Worsley Roughton (1899-1972) and Norman Urquhart Meldrum (1907-1933) to identify the responsible enzyme, carbonic anhydrase. As is known, the discovery of this enzyme was very important because its presence was found in many other organs and tissues, also revealing possible defects, such

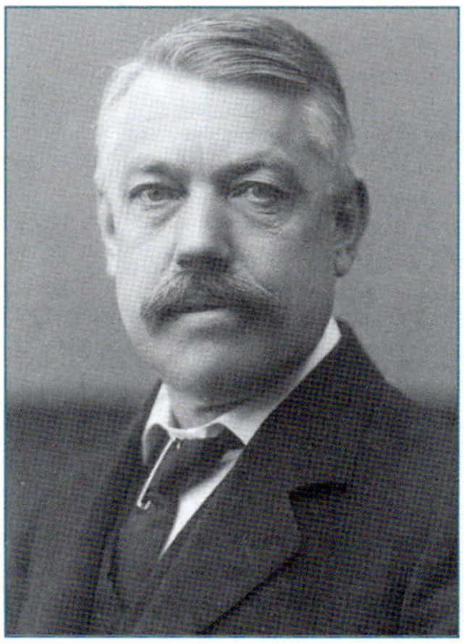

Figure 1.2 Christian Bohr (1855-1911).

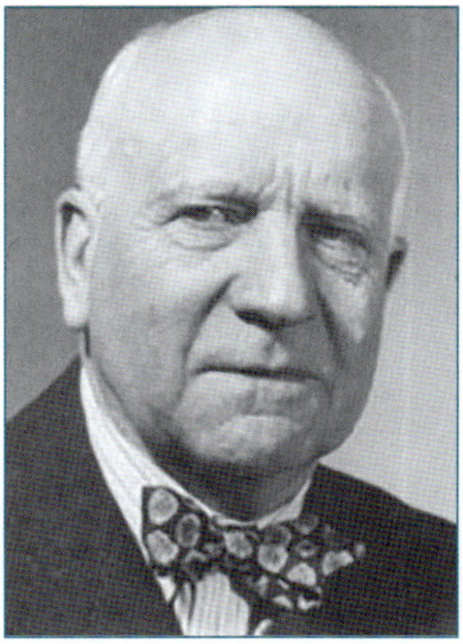

Figure 1.3 Donal Dexter Van Slyke (1883-1971).

as proximal or Type 2 tubular acidosis in the kidneys. Meanwhile, the recognition of the combined form of CO_2 as bicarbonate started to clarify the significance of CO_2 not only as a product of metabolism, but also as an important component of blood pH defense (still generally understood as alkalescence). Friedrich Walter (1850-1905) in 1877 demonstrated a close relationship between carbonic acid and non-carbonic acids; the decrease in CO_2 was detected in various conditions such as strenuous muscle exercise and in loading experiments with acids such as oxalic acid. It was also observed that these conditions were associated with hyperventilation, interpreted as stimulation due to products of muscle metabolism. In 1892 Julius Alfred Jaquet (1865-1937) proposed the term alkaline reserve to indicate the part of CO_2 bound to alkali that was not used in the transport from the tissues to the lungs. The term dominated for a long time among clinical chemistry in acid-base diagnosis, being the acidosis defined as a disorder characterized by the decrease of the alkaline reserve, while the alkalosis as an increase thereof. This was in part due to the slower evolution of technologies for blood pH measurement, but it is also due to the contribution of Van Slyke who, as we will see later, in the early 20th century introduced methods for the determination of CO_2 and bicarbonate in clinical chemistry which, for their analytical reliability and accessibility to clinical routine, dominated for many years in the diagnosis of acid-base disorders. The total CO_2 determination was carried out with a gasometric method using a device designed by Van Slyke himself (**Figure 1.4**): all the CO_2 combined forms were transformed into the gaseous form by adding acid, and the CO_2 was determined manometrically. There was not yet a method to directly measure the free CO_2 portion, the one we

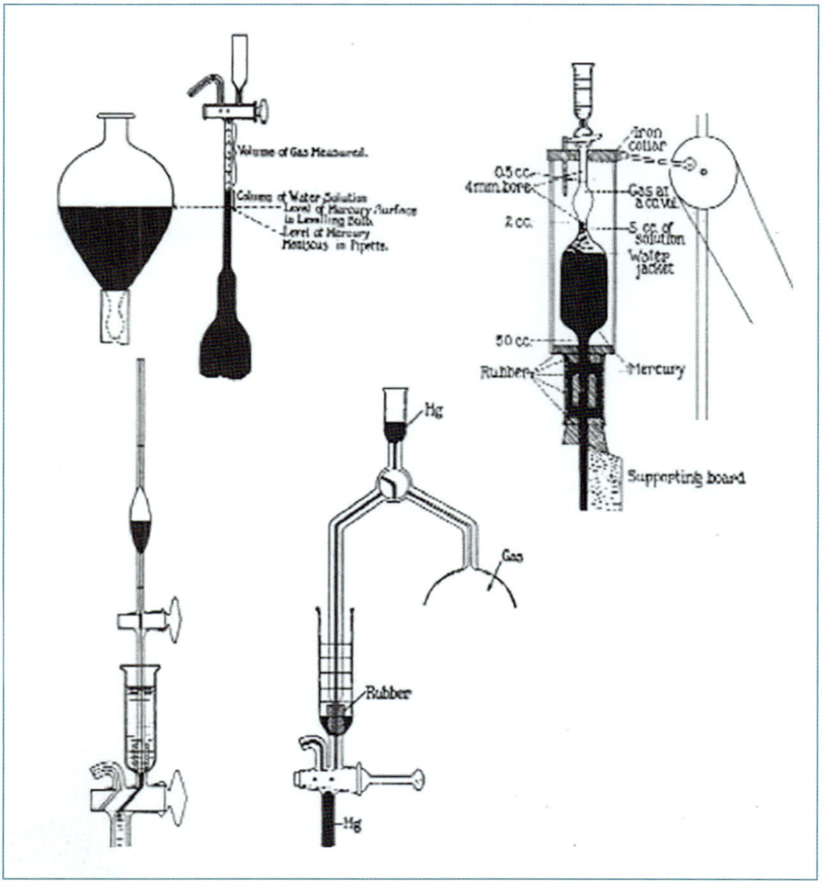

Figure 1.4 Van Slyke device for the manometric determination of CO_2.

refer to as PCO_2, which was indirectly calculated from pH and bicarbonate by a nomogram built on the Henderson equation. This important analytical deficiency greatly influenced the diagnosis of acid-base disorders, in particular the distinction between metabolic and respiratory disorders.

However, although widespread in the clinical chemistry routine, the analytical procedure of the alkaline reserve was not without its difficulties.

In the original procedure, before introducing the sample into the Van Slyke apparatus for the gasometric measurement, it had to be poured into a separating funnel, within which the technician had to blow repeatedly and shake so as to balance the sample to the PCO_2 of 40 mmHg, assuming this was the PCO_2 of the operator technician.

This preliminary operation was necessary to calculate the concentration of bicarbonate, subtracting 1.2 mmoles, the molar equivalent of 40 mmHg, from the total manometrically measured CO_2.

Several variants were proposed, depending on whether it was considered more correct to perform the analysis at 37 °C or at room temperature, at the patient's PCO_2 rather than at 40 mmHg (which required the sample collection in anaerobiosis in oil), or finally, if it was more appropriate to take into account only the plasma or also the cellular buffers, especially hemoglobin, performing the analysis in the so-called separate plasma, that is the plasma on which operations such as titrations or balancing were done after separating the plasma from the blood cells, or on the true plasma, if the same operations were done on the plasma before separating it from the cells.

We will report the most common clinical variants in **Table 1.1**, derived from the treatise of Harry F. Weisberg *Water, Electrolyte and Acid-Base Balance* (The Williams & Wilkins Co. 1953).

Nevertheless, the alkaline reserve determination resisted on the benches of the clinical laboratories for a long time, progressively improved by more accurately standardized and simpler execution methods such as the method of dosing bicarbonate by titration of Van Slyke and Cullen. Those who served in the clinical chemistry laboratory in those years clearly remember this method which, proposed by Van Slyke and Cullen in 1917, remained in the routine until the threshold of the 60s of the twentieth century, while the term alkaline reserve was not used anymore and was replaced, in requests that the wards accompanied the sample to the central laboratory, by the acronym tout court "CO_2".

Theories of acid-base chemistry and the electrometric pH measurement

The prevailing interest we have seen for CO_2 and its products in acid-base physiology and pathology was mainly due to the importance of the studies of Henderson and Van Slyke (to which we have already mentioned above), who had deepened the meaning of the CO_2-bicarbonate system in pH defense of body fluids and had made available methods of investigation ac-

TABLE 1.1 Variants of the alkaline reserve method.

"CO_2"	Measured parameters HCO_3^-	H_2CO_3	CO_2d	Sample	Plasma type	Balancing with CO_2
Content	√	√	√	Anaerobic	True	No, correct results at 37 °C
Capacity	√	√	√	Anaerobic	True	Yes at 40 mmHg environment temp. (20 °C)
Combination capacity	√			Anaerobic	Separated	Yes at 40 mmHg with subtraction for H_2CO_3 and CO_2d
Combination power	√			Aerobic	Separated	Yes at 40 mmHg with subtraction for H_2CO_3 and CO_2d

cessible to the clinical routine. This does not exclude that just as much interest was addressed more generally also to the other aspects of the regulation of neutrality in the animal organism, to use the terms with which Henderson referred to the physiology of the acid-base equilibrium.

The greater slowness in the progress of knowledge, can be attributed, as we shall see, to the difficulty in adapting electrometric methods – which had already arisen in the last decades of the nineteenth century – to the measurement of blood pH and other biological fluids. As can be easily understood, the progress of knowledge on acid-base biochemistry followed that on acid-base chemistry more generally.

In the past, there had been no lack of proposals for theories of acid-base chemistry, starting from de Lavoisier, who had related acids to his interest in oxygen (*oxy-genao*, acid generator), extending it to the field of respiratory and metabolic physiology, to Justus von Liebig (1803-1873), who in 1838 defined acids as substances whose hydrogen content could be replaced by a metal.

But in 1887 an important and particularly interesting theory was proposed by Svante August Arrhenius (**Figure 1.5**), with the contribution of Wilhelm Ostwald (1853-1932) and Jacobus Henricus van 't Hoff (1852-1911). According to the theory of electrolytic dissociation, the electrolytes (salts, acids, bases) in solution dissociate into ions simply because they are in solution, without the need, as Michael Faraday (1791-1867) had previously stated, for intervention using the electric current, which has the sole function of orienting the migration of ions, those positively charged towards the negative pole or cathode (hence the term cations) and those negatively charged towards the positive pole or anode (hence the term anions). The acids and the bases dissociate freeing respectively hydrogen ions H^+ and hydroxyl ions OH^-, being the strength of the acid or of the base measured by the entity of the dissociation, that is the relationship between the dissociated part and the non-dissociated part. A measure of the strength of an acid or a base is its dissociation constant or the equilibrium constant. Another important factor in the dissociation of acids is the degree of dissociation, that is the fraction of acid that dissociates: this factor is not valid for weak acids but mainly for strong acids, which frequently demonstrate important deviations in physicochemical properties by dissociating completely. It is due to the reciprocal influences among the numerous dissociated ions, so that it is necessary to distinguish between the constant of real and apparent dissociation, as demonstrated in 1909 by Niels Bjerrum (1879-1958). Arrhenius's theory has long stood the test of time and its principles remain valid. Its popularity extended to the assimilation of anions with acids and cations with bases (chloride is an acid, sodium is a base), and there are still today those who have remained faithful to this way of seeing the acid-base chemistry.

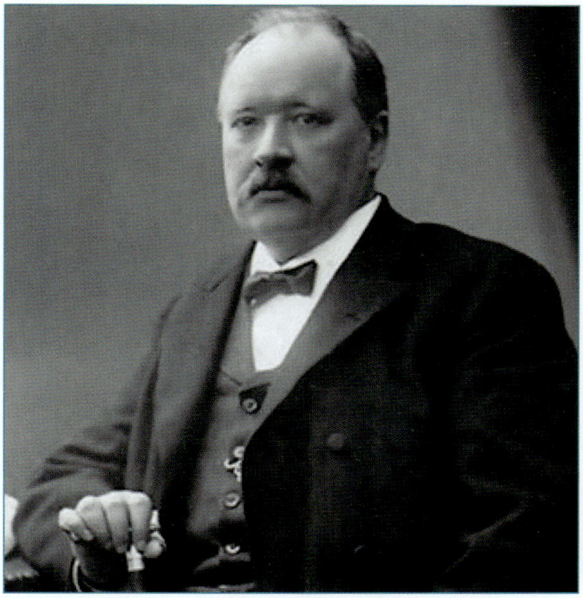

Figure 1.5 Svante August Arrhenius (1859-1927).

However, the definition of acid and base in relation to the ionic composition of water limits the applicability of the Arrhenius-Ostwald theory to aqueous solutions. In 1923, Joannes Nicolaus Brønsted in Denmark and independently Thomas Martin Lowry in the United States (**Figure 1.6**) proposed a new theory that extended the acid-base chemistry beyond the aqueous environment, defining acid as a donor of hydrogen ions – or protons according to the knowledge on atomic structure that

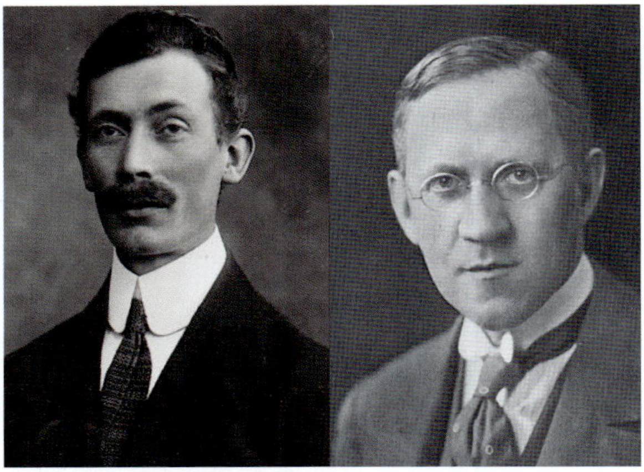

Figure 1.6 Joannes Nicolaus Brønsted (1879-1947) and Thomas Martin Lowry (1874-1936).

in those years were emerging – and base a hydrogen ion acceptor. This theory puts the hydrogen ion at the centre of the acid-base chemistry, and it is still known today as the most widely accepted way of seeing acids and bases, particularly in physiological biochemistry. At the beginning, however, there were difficulties in understanding: it was not easy to convince oneself that a cation is neither an acid nor a base, and that an anion is not an acid but a base. Although the advantages of this interpretative theory were soon established, Arrhenius's concepts did not completely disappear, and even today there are those who do not disdain their use. As we said at the beginning, the history of the acid-base balance is characterized by the continuous evolution of the principles on which it is based.

Later Gilbert Newton Lewis (1875-1946) proposed an even more extensive interpretative theory, based on the atomic structure, which defines acid an acceptor, and base a donor, of a pair of electrons. This theory is of particular interest for organic chemistry, but has not found its way into the medical field like those of Arrhenius and Brønsted-Lowry. On the analytical side, the electrometric pH measurement, already available in the chemical laboratories in the last decades of the nineteenth century, was slow to establish itself in clinical chemistry laboratories due to the technical difficulties of the potentiometric methods then available in blood application. The first electrodes for measuring hydrogen ions were hydrogen electrodes, made in the last decade of the nineteenth century, which for the next thirty years remained the only instrument for potentiometric pH measurement. However, this type of electrode was not suitable for blood, although some measurements were made by several researchers, including Søren Peter Lauritz Sørensen. The results were often completely wrong because the saturation of the sample with hydrogen – preliminary required by the method – caused the loss of CO_2 from the blood sample. Hasselbalch made changes to the method, which however made the process too laborious.

The first glass membrane electrode was devised by Fritz Haber (1868-1934) in 1909 but had no applications in the physiological field, as happened with another glass electrode proposed in 1925 by Phyllis Margaret Tookey Kerridge (1902-1940). The industrial production of the glass membrane electrode began only after 1933.

Alternative methods were based on indicators, or indirect methods of calculation based on the Henderson equation, which nevertheless became reliable only after the Van Slyke apparatus for the gasometric measurement of CO_2 was available.

These difficulties and uncertainties in the pH measurement explain why for a long time the investigations on the acid-base state preferred to rely on CO_2 measurements and alkaline reserve, so as to define acidosis as a decrease in the alkaline reserve, and alkalosis as an increase in the alkaline reserve. No wonder that in 1931 Clyde Lottridge Cummer, in his *Manual of Clinical Laboratory Methods*, stated: "There are two methods that can be applied to the blood to reveal an acidosis: the determination of the carbonate content (so-called alkaline reserve) and the measurement of hydrogen ions concentration (pH). However, this last method does not deserve consideration, because it does only demonstrate minimal variations when the patient is in moribund condition".

Theories of acid-base physiology

The theories of Arrhenius and Brønsted-Lowry were certainly essential for the development of physiological biochemistry. But among the most important studies in the early twentieth century include, as we have already seen, those of Henderson, whose equation opened this "story" not by chance: it still represents the foundation of the blood pH defense today. Henderson long investigated its mechanisms and its regulation in the context of the acid-base balance, extending its research also to respiratory and renal function – always in the acid-base balance –, to the physiology and pathology of other important electrolytes, as well as other aspects of diseases, such as diabetic acidosis. In the study on pH homeostatic defense, Henderson emphasized the centrality of the buffer function, which in the same years had been proposed by Søren Peter Lauritz Sørensen (1868-1939) with the term *buffer*, with which the buffers of railway wagons are named for the purpose to cushion shocks. As already known, Sørensen is also remembered for the proposal of the measurement units of hydrogen ions concentration in logarithmic pH terms.

Henderson emphasized the importance of the dissociation constant, as well as the dependence of the buffer capacity on the relationship between the non-dissociated part and the dissociated part. He also demonstrated the role of the buffer constituted by the CO_2/HCO_3^- system in the extracellular compartment – then still called *milieu interieur* under Claude Bernard's influence –, but also that of phosphates, proteins, hemoglobin in blood pH defense. The magnitude of this protagonist of physiology and pathophysiology of the acid-base equilibrium is illustrated in **Figure 1.7** which shows one of its diagrams for the differentiation of acid-base disorders, and which is surprising for its modernity, anticipating the diagnostic maps that would only appear in literature many years later.

In 1917 Karl Albert Hasselbalch (1874-1962) reworked Henderson's equation in logarithmic terms, in assimilation to the Sørensen pH units, indicating the dissociation constant with the abbreviation pK, immortalizing it as the Henderson-Hasselbalch equation. However, the notoriety of this Danish physiologist is not limited to this reworking. In fact he was also the first to perform reliable measurements of blood pH by using a hydrogen electrode at 38 °C, and to use these measurements to define acid-base disorders, distinguishing them in compensated and decompensated

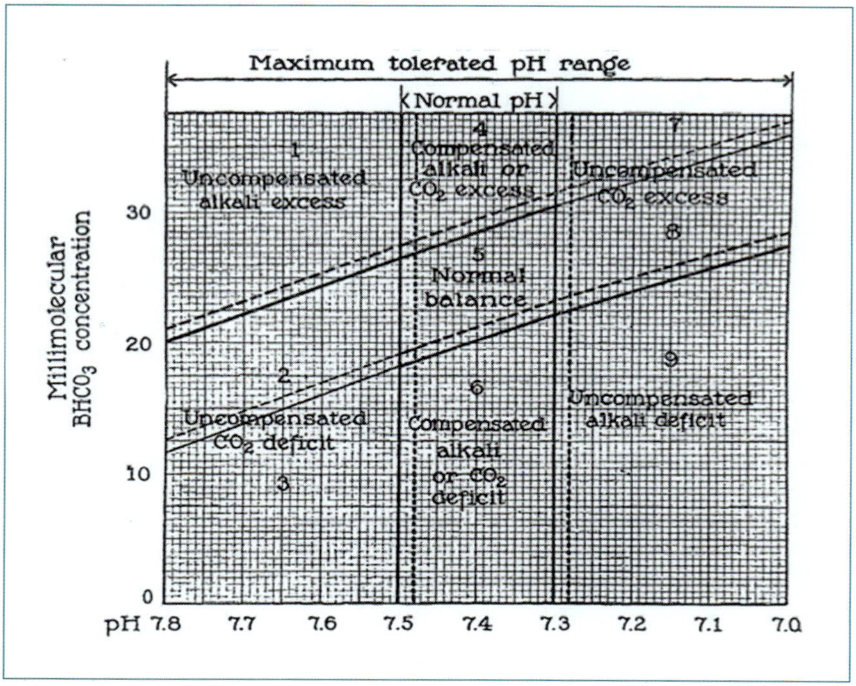

Figure 1.7 Diagram of Henderson-Van Slyke.

based on the real pH, that is the pH measured in the sample without any modification, that Hasselbalch called adjusted pH, or the pH after balancing PCO_2 at 40 mmHg, called the reduced pH (**Figure 1.8**).

No less important was Van Slyke's contribution, of which we have already become acquainted by discussing the alkaline reserve. Precisely following Henderson's studies that highlighted electrolytes contribution in normal and pathological conditions, one of the biggest problems for clinicians was that they did not have simple and accessible methods for investigating this field. In his position as director of the clinical chemistry laboratory of the Rockefeller Institute, and knowing Henderson's studies on bicarbonate, in 1917 Van Slyke conceived, with the collaboration of Walter Palmer and Reginald Heber Fitz, the apparatus for the gasometric determination of CO_2 and of bicarbonate that we have illustrated in Figure 1.4, a method that, as we have already pointed out, remained in the routine of every clinical laboratory for the next fifty years, even though in the simpler variants of the methods for titration that Van Slyke himself prepared later. His scientific production competes for value and extension with that of Henderson. He contributed to the study of alkalosis, both respiratory and metabolic, and no less important were his research on the function of oxygenated and reduced hemoglobin as a buffer, and on the transport of oxygen and CO_2. He also demonstrated the different electrolytic composition between plasma and erythrocytes and deepened the role of the lung and kidney in the acid-base balance. Among his publications, of particular interest is the *Quantitative Clinical Chemistry* treatise which he published in 1931 together with John P. Peters (1887-1955), and that for many years remained the reference textbook for clinical chemists.

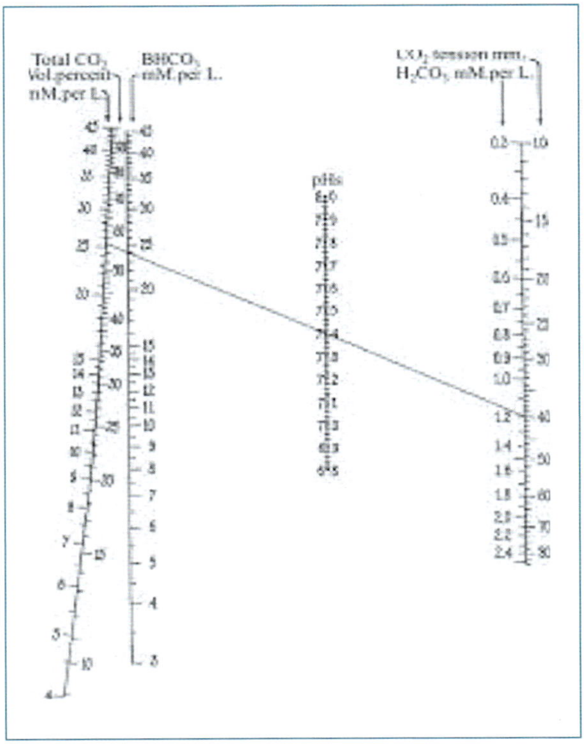

Figure 1.8 Nomogram for PCO_2 calculation from the Henderson's equation.

Progress in knowledge of acid-base disorders

During the nineteenth century, important contributions had accumulated in the field of acid-base pathology. By the middle of the century, Henry Bence-Jones (1813-1878) had shown variations of urine acidity related to meals, stating that these reflect corresponding changes in blood alkalinity, constantly regulated by volatile CO_2 elimination via the lungs. He also demonstrated that the administered sulfuric acid is eliminated quantitatively in the urine, and that patients suffering from vomiting eliminate alkaline urine.

During the cholera epidemic, unfortunately frequent at that time, William Brooke O'Shaughnessy (1809-1889) reported in 1831 the almost complete disappearance of the free alkali in the blood of patients, and Thomas Aitchison Latta (1796-1833) reported the favourable treatment result with sodium bicarbonate and sodium chloride.

Another important contribution was due to Friedrich Walter who confirmed CO_2 significance as an index of blood alkali, relating it to metabolic acids, and demonstrating in animals the decrease after the administration of acids, as well as the corrective effect of the sodium bicarbonate infusion after experimental acidosis. Finally, he demonstrated acidosis as the cause of diabetic coma, without identifying the responsible acid. This was to be found in β-hydroxybutyric acid by Oskar Minkowski (1858-1931) and Bernhard Naunyn (1839-1925) in 1884.

The increase in lactic acid with a decrease in CO_2 and blood alkalinity after strenuous muscular exercise was demonstrated in 1888. Subsequently, the relationship between this acid and hypoxia was identified, while the relationship with anaerobic carbohydrate metabolism was clarified in 1910.

Renal failure acidosis remained unresolved for a long time. Rudolf von Jaksch (1855-1947) had revealed it by blood titration with the litmus indicator, but the results were unreliable. In the following years there is no mention of this acidosis until 1914, when Andrew Watson Sellards (1884-1941) demonstrated the decrease of blood CO_2: a little later a retention of blood phosphates and sulphates was demonstrated.

An impulse of particular importance to the advancement in the pathophysiology knowledge of acid-base disorders, but also more extensively of plasma electrolyte composition and body fluids regulation, came from Pediatrics. Infantile enteritis (*cholera infantum*) severely afflicted this population and was feared by both parents and doctors, due to the limited therapeutic resources available.

The establishment of specialized pediatric departements in European hospitals in the late nineteenth century gave the opportunity for a systematic study.

The anatomopathological findings in deceased children of acute enteritis were almost always negative. It was believed that the causes of the disease were intestinal infection or intoxication, in some cases even a genetic defect. Since a frequent symptom in the acute phase was a breath that was very similar of what Adolf Kussmaul had described in diabetic coma, Adalbert Czerny (1863-1941), professor of Pediatrics in Berlin, in 1897 presented an acidosis as an etiological hypothesis. A few years earlier, in 1880, acidosis caused by keto acids with elimination of β-hydroxybutyric acid had been demonstrated in diabetic coma; an analogous etiopathogenesis in infantile enteritis was therefore a completely plausible hypothesis. To confirm this it seemed at first to contribute to the demonstration of an urine ammonium increase of the small patients; however, the increase was modest, and the hypothesis of an alkali loss with diarrhea could not be substantiated due to the lack of reliable investigation methods. Although urinary ammonium decreased following a bicarbonate supplement, the acidosis hypothesis remained uncertain and caused only bitter disputes for several years among the different German schools of Pediatrics. The initiative to continue the research in practice therefore passed to US schools, also interested in studing this pathology.

However, a problem that hindered investigations was blood sample volume needed for laboratory tests, which in those years was not less than 20-30 mL, even for glycemia alone. These volumes could be supported by an adult, but they were prohibitive and even dangerous for small children. It was thanks to two Scandinavian scientists – the Swedish Otto Knut Olof Folin (1867-1934), the inventor of the method of analysis for glycosuria, and the Norwegian Ivan Christian Bang (1869-1918) – who worked on the elaboration of new methods that used no more than 1-2 mL of blood. The discovery widely opened the doors of the Pediatrics laboratories and caused a veritable revolution in clinical chemistry. US pediatricians interested in infant enteritis problem immediately took advantage, in particular John Howland (1873-1926) who had studied with Czerny in Strasbourg and was therefore aware of the acidosis hypothesis. In order to solve this hypothesis and in any case the problem that afflicted children also in the United States, Howland, who ran Pediatrics Department at the Johns Hopkins Hospital in Baltimore, succeeded in obtaining a laboratory specifically dedicated to research and annexed to the wards, where students from all over the world came to collaborate in research. Thus in 1915 the acidosis was confirmed, based on the decrease of the CO_2 content in the alveolar air and in the blood and on serum pH decrease, as well as the etiopathogenesis of enteric alkali loss was established. However, the treatment aimed solely at correcting acidosis with sodium bicarbonate was disappointing, although with positive effects. When the treatment was extended to fluid loss reintegration, and to electrolyte alterations correction, in particular the invariably associated potassium deficiency, in a short time the mortality of infantile enteritis dropped from over 25% to less than 5%, a true triumph of American Pediatrics.

The main protagonist of this important aspect of body fluids pathophysiology was James Lauder Gamble (**Figure 1.9**), a Harvard pediatrician who had learned the micro-methods of Folin in Boston, Howland's collaborator in Baltimore, and finally professor of Pediatrics at Children's Hospital in Boston. His scientific interest and his activity focused in particular on the physiopathology of water-electrolyte balance and on the relationships between hydro-electrolyte balance and acid-base balance. Of particular importance was the introduction of the expression of the electrolyte concentration in body fluids in moles or in equivalents or submultiples, rather than in grams or submultiples, which highlighted the stoichiometric correspondence between anions and cations, and thus allowed to better understand both the physiological regulation and the pathological alterations of the electrolytes. His column charts known as Gamblegrams (**Figure 1.10**), which illustrate the electrolyte composition of physiological fluids, are widespread and still universally adopted in the medical world, and his text *Chemical Anatomy, Physiology and Pathology of Extracellular Fluid* spread throughout the world and was for many years a reference point for the study of physiology, pathology and therapy of water-electrolyte balance.

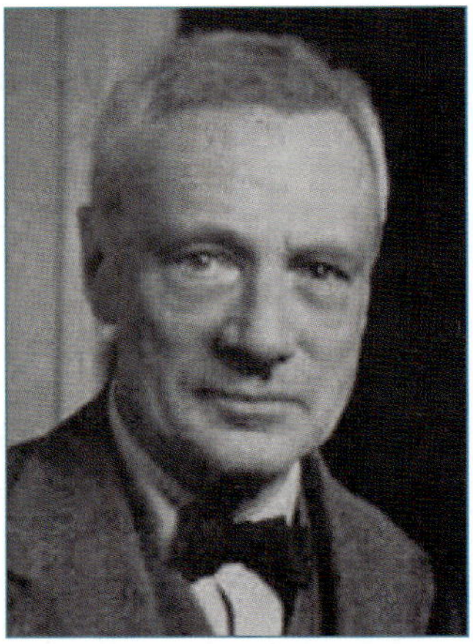

Figure 1.9 James Lauder Gamble (1883-1959).

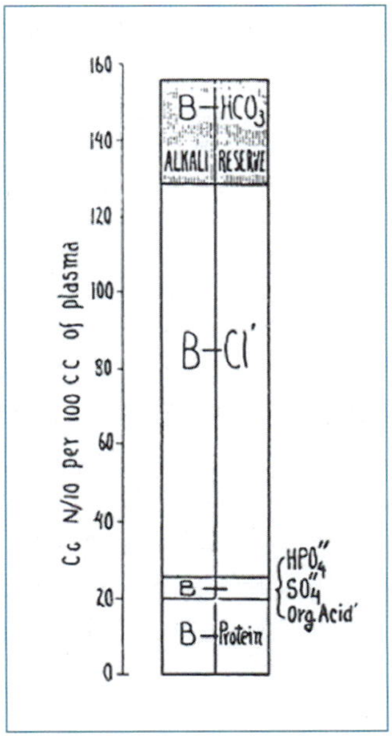

Figure 1.10 Gamblegram.

The expression in molar terms is not only descriptive, but also responds to chemical need to respect stoichiometric equivalence: for example, an important result of this expression was the possibility of measuring the anion gap in the plasma electrolyte composition.

The advantages of this expression were soon appreciated and the specialized literature worked to spread its use, as shown by the illustrations which then appeared in various medical journals (**Figure 1.11**), to overcome the resistance of many clinicians accustomed to expression in mg/100 mL: it was not easy to easily switch from 326.0 mg/100 mL of sodium to 142 mEq/L, from 60.5 vol% of CO_2 to 25 mEq/L of bicarbonate, from 6500 mg/100 mL of protein to 16 mEq/L. Of no less importance was the demonstration of the close relationships existing between electrolyte homeostasis and

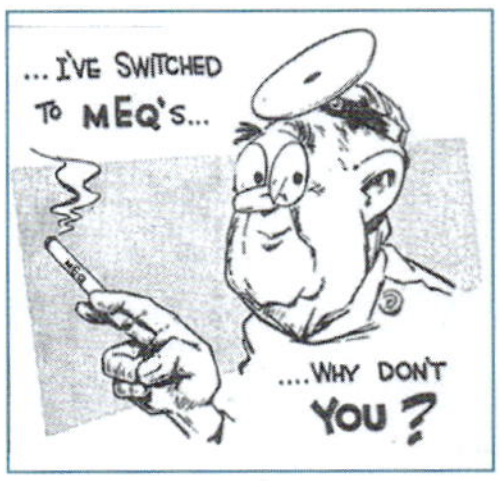

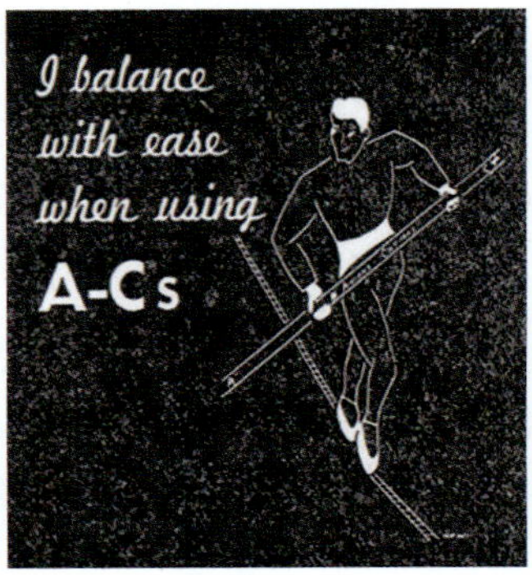

Figure 1.11 Illustrations at 1950s to advertise the notation in mEq/L.

acid-base homeostasis, such as the numerous influences of potassium on acid-base balance and of blood pH on renal elimination of electrolytes. These acquisitions owe the need, which gradually became a rule, to combine the electrolyte profile with blood gas analytical profile in the diagnostic investigation of acid-base disorders which, around the 1930s, was facilitated by the introduction of photometry flame for sodium and potassium dosage in clinical laboratories.

With the Second World War interval, the threshold of the 1950s came with a significant knowledge on acid-base physiology, while the technical difficulties of pH measurement, which limited the diagnosis of acid-base disorders in clinical practice to changes in the alkaline reserve, still left the distinction between metabolic and respiratory disorders confused. As we have already seen above, acidosis was defined as the decrease of the alkaline reserve, the alkalosis as the increase of the alkaline reserve – expressions which we now know to refer to metabolic disorders –, while the characterization of respiratory disorders remained indistinct, although it was known that these were also the cause of alterations in the acid-base balance.

In the same years a further important impulse to knowledge progress on the acid-base balance and its disorders came from the school of Robert Franklin Pitts (**Figure 1.12**) in relation to the mechanisms by which kidney contributes to the regulation of acid-base homeostasis. In previous years three hypotheses had been proposed on urine acidification mechanism: one by Henderson, one by Van Slyke, J. Sendroy and S. Seelig, finally the third by H. Smith but without experimental support.

The first and most popular hypothesis of phosphate reabsorption supported that two forms of phosphate were filtered, the monobasic NaH_2PO_4 and the dibasic Na_2HPO_4, but while the monobasic was eliminated, the dibasic was reabsorbed.

The second hypothesis instead identified carbonic acid as responsible for urine acidification, which is completely impermeable to the tubular nephron and can therefore be eliminated in large quantities.

The third hypothesis sustained that hydrogen ions are secreted in exchange with sodium in the tubular lumen, where they convert phosphate monohydrate into dihydrate.

While the first two hypotheses depend on the glomerular filtrate, the third presented a tubular mechanism that depends only on the quantity of acid that the tubules secrete. As a source of hydrogen ions in the tubular cells the carbonic acid was postulated, formed by the hydration of CO_2 catalyzed by carbonic anhydrase. Pitts confirmed this third hypothesis, demonstrating that the filtered acid was not sufficient to account for the considerably higher amount of eliminated acid, and highlighting the tubular origin of the hydrogen ions by inhibiting acidification with sulfanilamide, a carbonic anhydrase inhibitor. The Pitts school also shed light on bicarbonate reabsorption, demonstrating its threshold at 24 mEq/L, below which its reabsorption is complete, while above reabsorption is proportional to plasma bicarbonate up to a maximal value, and showing that this maximal value is independent of the glomerular filtrate.

These studies constituted the premise to the modern conception of renal regulation physiology of acid-base balance, opening the way to the investigations that lead to the identification of the hydrogen ion and other electrolyte transporters along the nephron, to their molecular identification and to their regulation.

In the same period other discoveries on renal function had remarkable implications on the acid-base balance. The aldosterone discovery, the essential adrenocortical hormone in the regulation of the most important

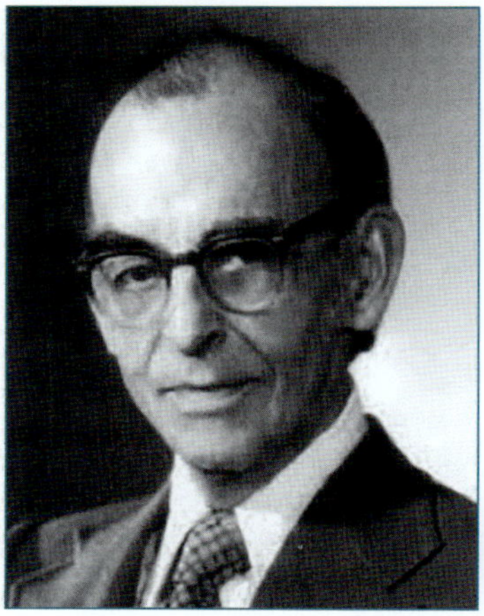

Figure 1.12 Robert Franklin Pitts (1908- 1977)

electrolytes, including the hydrogen ion, dates back to 1952. In 1955 the functional meaning of the loop of Henle was discovered – previously almost unknown – with the proof of Wirz, Hargitay and Kuhn, three physicochemists of Zurich, and also of the mechanism of urine concentration in countercurrent, fundamental, as it is known, for ammonium elimination in the collecting tubule.

The Danish experience: Poul Biørndahal Astrup, Ole Siggaard-Andersen

However, even independently of progress in the nephrological field, the early 1950s were of fundamental importance for knowledge evolution on the acid-base balance, both in its biochemical and physiological aspects and in its pathophysiological and clinical aspects.

Unfortunately, the essential source for this evolution was the polio epidemic which broke out in Copenhagen in 1952 and which frequently caused bulbar paralysis and subsequent respiratory paralysis (**Figure 1.13**). An important alteration was the increase in plasma bicarbonate which, as usual, as we mentioned earlier, was interpreted as an index of an alkalosis of unknown etiology.

However Bjørn Aage Ibsen (**Figure 1.14**) and Poul Biørndahal Astrup (**Figure 1.15**), respectively director of Anesthesiology and Director of the Copenhagen Hospital Laboratory, suggested that this increase was instead a manifestation of CO_2 retention, resorted to the determination of blood pH, whose decrease confirmed the hypothesis of respiratory acidosis, then promptly starting the treatment by tracheotomy and manual ventilation with positive pressure, so as to obtain in a short time the disappearance of the alkalosis.

This Danish experience marked the establishment of intensive care in hospital settings, and decreed the transition of blood gas analysis from research to the clinical-chemical routine, where it highlighted the limits of the sole determination of the alkaline reserve in the diagnosis of acid-base disorders, such as moreover, they revealed the multiple variants of this analysis that were gradually proposed (Table 1.1), even though with almost overlapping diagnostic significance, starting the search for safer and more reliable diagnostic criteria, and at the same time stimulating the processing of new investigation means.

As mentioned at the beginning chapter, this research still continues today; each of the proposed criteria did not stand the time-test without criticism and contro-

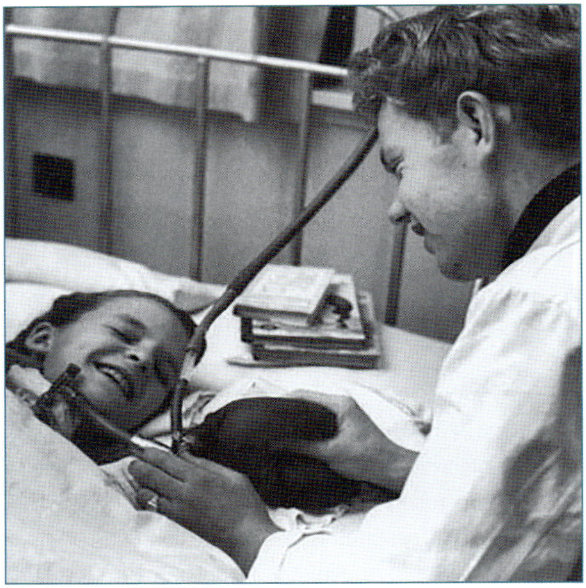

Figure 1.13 Assistance to a small patient admitted during the polio epidemic in Copenhagen in 1952, by a medical student.

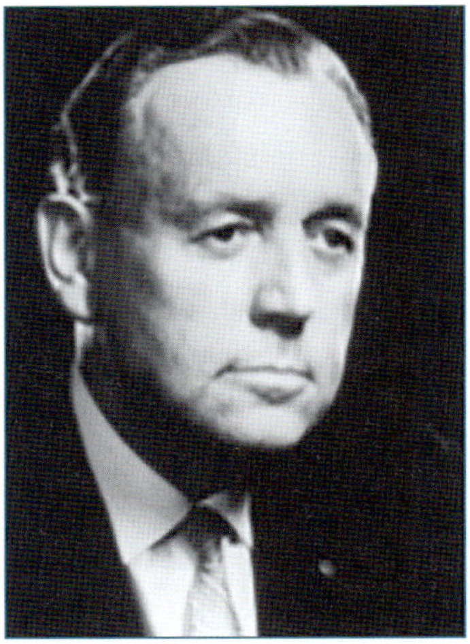

Figure 1.14 Bjørn Aage Ibsen (1915-2007).

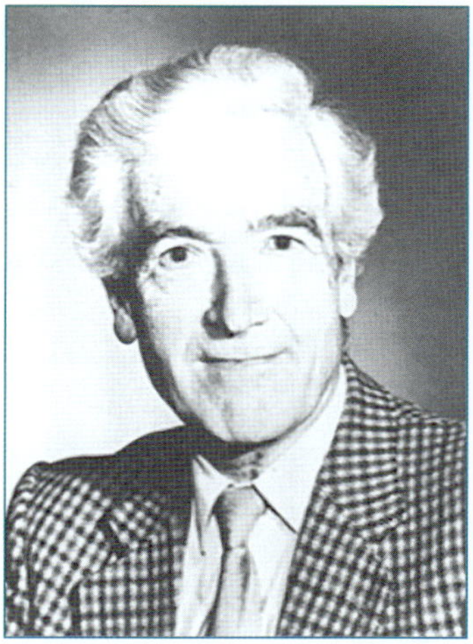

Figure 1.15 Poul Biørndahal Astrup (1915-2000).

versy, with the positive result of the continuous refinement and improvement of the tools and the knowledge evolution.

The need for a reliable blood pH measurement emerged to avoid confusing acidosis with an alkalosis, and even more the need to identify, among the chemical-clinical acid-base parameters, a component capable of expressing specifically the respiratory alterations (respiratory component), and an equally specific component of metabolic alterations (metabolic component), in order to reliably distinguish respiratory-type disorders from metabolic-type disorders. The respiratory component was identifiable in PCO_2, which, however, could only be obtained indirectly by calculating the Henderson-Hasselbalch equation, based on pH and bicarbonate.

The metabolic component was first identified in plasma bicarbonate, but it was soon realized that the interchangeability between PCO_2 and HCO_3^- greatly limited this attribution, as indeed the Copenhagen experience had drastically highlighted.

At the time of the polio epidemic, blood pH determination was rarely performed in clinic, both due to technical difficulties and because it was considered of little clinical interest. PCO_2 determination was possible only indirectly. As we have already said, the diagnostic interpretation of acid-base disorders practically rested solely on the alkaline reserve, or total CO_2 measured with the Van Slyke apparatus.

Some progresses of fundamental importance, both on the analytical-instrumental side, and on the clinical-interpretative side, came from the protagonists of the Danish experience formerly during the epidemic and in the years immediately following. First of all, thanks to Astrup and his students, O. Siggaard-Andersen (**Figure 1.16**), K. Engel (1932), K.E. Jørgensen (1925), G. Kokholm (1931), the electrometric blood pH measurement was perfected and made accessible to pediatric routine also by constructing capillary electrodes which required a sample of 25 μL of blood (**Figure 1.17**). Furthermore, Astrup demonstrated the linear relationship between pH and log PCO_2 (**Figure 1.18**) so that, by measuring pH in the sample such and after balancing at two known PCO_2 values, it was possible to obtain the PCO_2 of the sample under examination from the pH/log PCO_2 chart. Finally, he elaborated an important modification in bicarbonate evaluation, proposing the standard bicarbonate, which for a long time was considered the best index of the metabolic component.

All these technical-analytical and interpretative advances were summarized in a device that at the time appeared futuristic, and that preceded the modern blood gas analyzers. The device, characterized as a balancing method, comprised a glass membrane capillary electrode thermostated at 37 °C together with a reference electrode for measuring blood pH in a sample of 25 μL, and a microtonometer composed of two small glass chambers connected with two cylinders of CO_2 gas at different and known PCO_2, where a drop of the blood sample was subjected to vibration distributing itself in a film on the surface of the chamber and

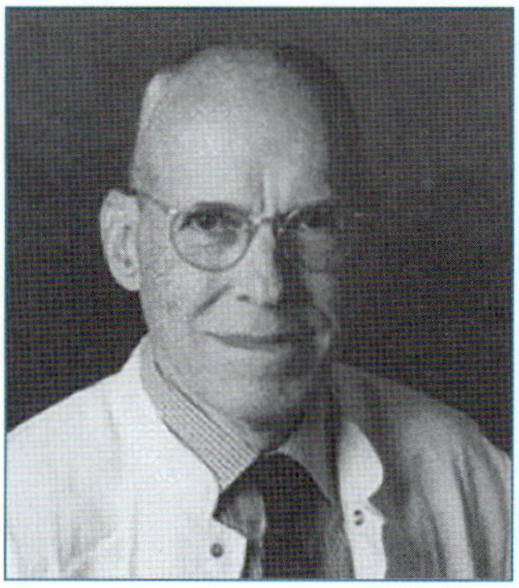

Figure 1.16 Ole Siggaard-Andersen (1932).

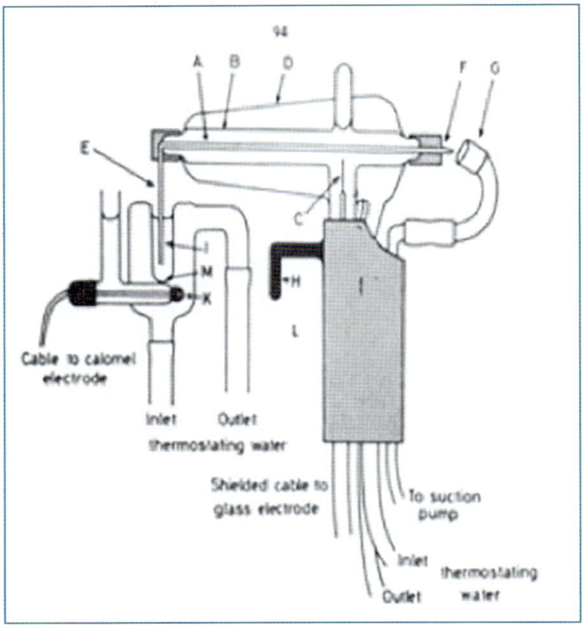

Figure 1.17 Astrup device for blood gas analysis with the balancing method.

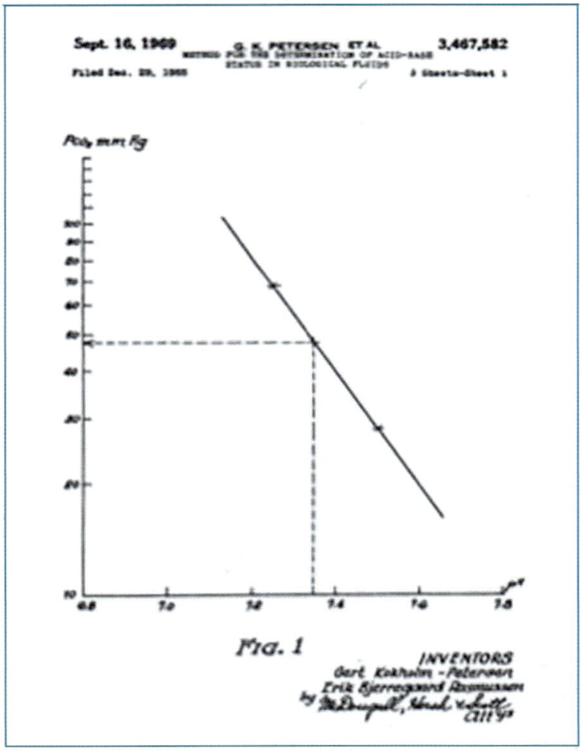

Figure 1.18 pH/log chart.

rapidly balancing with the specific PCO_2. Everything was arranged on a trolley of modest dimensions easily moved around the corridors and rooms of the hospital wards. The data were obtained from specific graphs.

But the Danish school has an even more important analytical contribution, even though in collaboration with the US researchers.

In 1954, Richard Stow (1916), professor of Physical Medicine at the Ohio University, had published the design of an electrode for measuring PCO_2 – actually it was a glass membrane pH electrode, separated from the sample by a membrane selectively permeable to CO_2, and a film of water – which was not further developed, because it was too unstable and too insensitive. The project was taken up by John Wendell Severinghaus (**Figure 1.19**) at the National Health's Institutes in Bethesda which, in addition to important modifications including the choice of membrane and the thermostatic circuit, replaced distilled water with a buffer solution of bicarbonate in sodium chloride.

This solution not only stabilized PCO_2 measurement, but increased its sensitivity, ensuring linearity between 5 and 700 mmHg. The PCO_2 electrode was thus made, immediately meeting widespread interest all over the world. Shortly thereafter, in 1958, Severinghaus, in collaboration with Astrup and other Danish and American researchers, assembled a pH electrode with the PCO_2 electrode, and added an electrode for PO_2 in the meantime made by Leland Clark (1918-2005), and a thermostatic cuvette equipped with a stirrer, made the first modern blood gas analyzer, thus inaugurating the

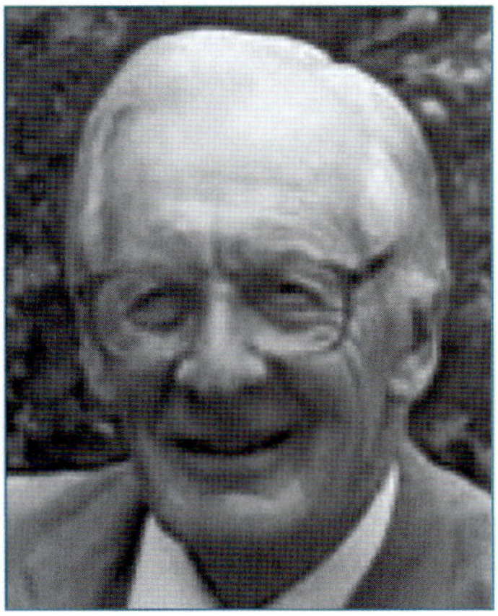

Figure 1.19 John Wendell Severinghaus (1922).

current laboratory diagnosis of acid-base disorders. An equally important contribution of the Danish school concerning the metabolic component was produced by Siggaard-Andersen which, through titration of the whole blood with different acids, bases and CO_2, obtained a measure of blood total bases (buffer base, BB), which he expressed in relative terms, placing the average value of 48 mEq/L = 0, with the term base excess (BE) (**Figure 1.20**).

This indicator of the metabolic component was of great utility because, at least in vitro, it allowed a reliable distinction between metabolic and respiratory disorders. As is known, in fact, since BE is the overall measure of bicarbonate buffer and non-bicarbonate buffers, its variations in metabolic disorders are different from those in respiratory disorders because both categories of buffers are involved in the same direction: therefore BE decreases in metabolic acidosis and increases in metabolic alkalosis.

Instead, in respiratory disorders, BE does not change, because the modifications of bicarbonate buffer are stoichiometrically in the opposite direction to those of non-bicarbonate buffers. The possibility of excluding one or the other category of acid-base disorders was particularly useful for the differentiation of mixed disorders, which in the meantime, with the refinement of the investigation methods, had emerged in clinical diagnostics. It is known to all the importance of these methodological and instrumental advances, which contributed decisively to modern acid-base diagnosis, and which still retain their validity.

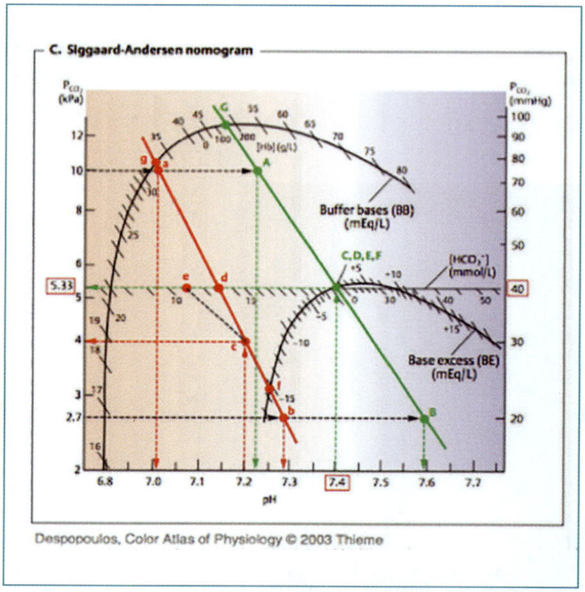

Figure 1.20 Siggaard-Andersen nomogram for BE calculation.

The Boston school and the "in vivo compensation limits"

However, BE as a metabolic component has not stood to time-test.

In 1963 William Benjamin Schwartz (1922-2009) and Arnold Seymour Relman (**Figure 1.21**) of the Nephrology department of Tufts Hospital in Boston published a critique toward BE, arguing that this index is subject to variations regardless of the acid-base cause, because its components, in particular bicarbonate, do not remain confined in the vascular sector, but are distributed throughout the extracellular space, including interstitial space.

A change in BE cannot therefore be interpreted as a specific consequence of an acid-base alteration; in particular even in the respiratory disorders the BE does not remain unchanged, but varies according to the variations of the HCO_3^-. In short, BE is valid in vitro, but not in vivo.

These criticisms provoked an intense controversy between Danish and US researchers, which manifested

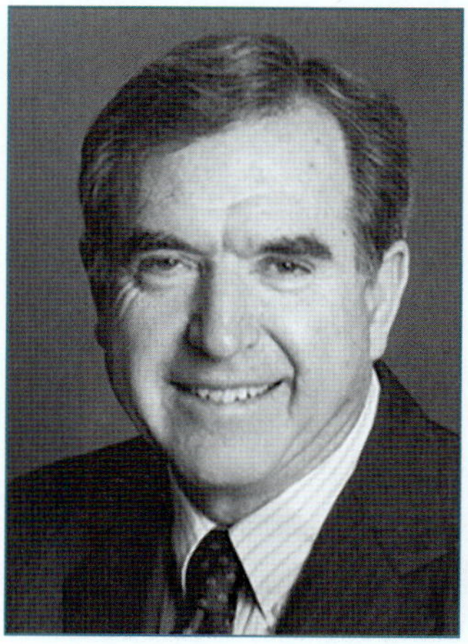

Figure 1.21 Arnold Seymour Relman (1923-2014).

itself with a substantial exchange of publications in the journal "Anesthesiology" between 1965 and 1966 which remains in the history of medical literature under the title *Great Transatlantic Acid-Base Debate*, and which however did not change either opinion to one or the other of the contenders.

The Danish researchers actually made corrections by modifying the BE to take into account the extracellular distribution space, and naming this new index as standard base excess (SBE), an index that is still today supplied with the software of most modern blood gas analyzers.

By contrast, Boston researchers started studies looking for valid indicators in vivo. Thus, both experimenting on animals and examining large series of acid-base disorders certainly not complicated by mixed forms, they investigated, for each of the four fundamental acid-base disorders – respiratory acidosis and alkalosis, metabolic acidosis and alkalosis –, the relationships between the blood gas parameter responsible for the disorder and the parameter responsible for its compensation. They found that these relationships not only exist, but also are predictable with a high probability, so as to allow the formulation, for each of the simple acid-base disorders, of indexes known as "in vivo compensation limits".

For over fifty years these diagnostic indices have stood to time-test and are a valid aid in clinical differentiation of simple and mixed acid-base disorders.

Peter Stewart and the independent variables

However, as we said at the beginning of the chapter, the history of blood gas analysis does not stop here. It is known to all the critical analysis that Peter Arthur Robert Stewart (**Figure 1.22**) made in 1983 contrasting the principles on which the traditional acid-base physiological biochemistry is based. Stewart did not pretend to prepare a new theory, but proposed a revision of the physiological acid-base biochemistry adhering to physico-chemical principles.

According to this view, only the independent variables are determinants of the acid-base balance, and only the alterations of these variables can cause acid-base disorders.

The independent variables are: PCO_2, the difference between the strong ions (strong ion difference, SID), the weak electrolytes of the plasma (Atot), in practice plasmatic inorganic proteins and phosphates; blood pH, or $[H^+]$, and bicarbonate are dependent variables, and as such cannot determine anything in the acid-base balance and its pathology. This last statement greatly affected the medical class "public opinion", in particular the intensivists, who spoke of a "Copernican revolution". Among the independent variables, the greatest interest was obviously directed to SID, which in the previous interpretative theories did not stand out in the foreground, thus focusing the spotlight on the plasmatic gamblegram, in particular on its main components, sodium and chloride.

Since, other things being equal, the decrease in SID is the cause of acidosis, and the increase in SID causes alkalosis, it has been suggested a tendency of the assimilation of anions (chloride) to acids and cations (sodium) to bases, returning then to the Arrhenius theory. Apart from these questionable interpretations, an undoubted progress of Stewart's theory concerns the greater attention paid to residual anions, better known as anion gap (AG) whose variations, as is known, have importance in the diagnosis of metabolic acidosis. The most accurate analysis that Stewart's theory imposes on this unmeasured space, but only calculated

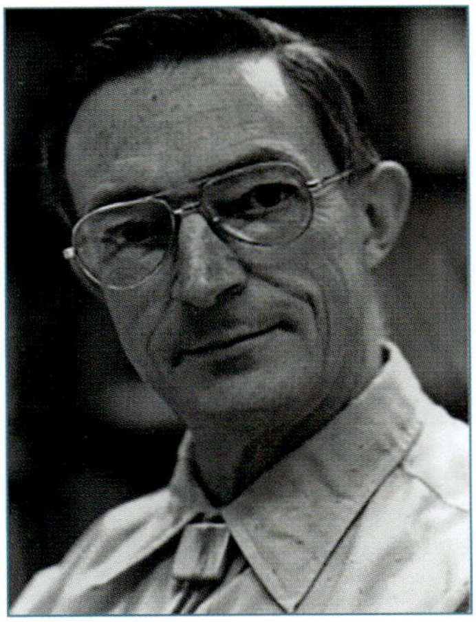

Figure 1.22 Peter Arthur Robert Stewart (1921-1993).

indirectly, has highlighted the importance of already known – and previously neglected – components, such as plasma proteins, especially albumin.

Some collaborators of Stewart who have developed the interpretative theory, have proposed the direct determination of the main non-measured anions present physiologically in plasma, such as bicarbonate, albumin, and inorganic phosphates, naming this complex effective strong ions difference (SIDeff) in order to allow a more precise and accurate indirect evaluation of any pathological residual anions, called strong ions gaps (SIG).

As can be seen, therefore, the story continues. Despite criticisms, controversies, diatribes, every time some new knowledge of physiology or pathophysiology is added, the criteria of diagnostic interpretation of acid-base disorders are improved and the methods or tools of investigation are refined and perfected.

That's why the history of blood gas analysis and acid-base balance is so fascinating.

References

- Arrhenius SA. Über die Dissociation der in Wasser gelösten Stoffe. Z Phys Chem. 1887;1:631-58.
- Astrup PB, Severinghaus JW. The History of Blood Gases, Acids and Bases. Copenhagen, Munksgaard 1986.
- Bohr C, Hasselbalch KA, Krogh A. Über einen in biologischer Beziehung wichtigen Einfluss, den die Kohlensäurespannung des Blutes auf dessen Sauerstoffbindung übt. Skand Arch Physiol. 1904;16:402-12.
- Gamble JL. Chemical Anatomy, Physiology and Pathology of Extracellular Fluid: A Lecture Syllabus. Cambridge, Dept. of Pediatrics, Harvard Medical School 1941.
- Henderson LJ. Blood. A Study in General Physiology. New Haven, Yale University Press 1928.
- Henderson LJ. Das Gleichgewicht zwischen Basen und Säuren im tierischen Organismus. Ergebn Physiol. 1909;8:254-325.
- Henderson LJ. The theory of neutrality regulation in the animal organism. Am J Physiol. 1908;21:427-48.
- Lavoisier AL. Traité élémentaire de chimie. 1. A Paris, chez Cuchet 1789.
- Meyer L. Die Gase des Blutes. Göttingen, Dieterich 1857.
- Ostwald WF. Elektrochemie, ihre Geschichte und Lehre. Leipzig, Veit & Comp. 1896.
- Peters JP, Van Slyke DD. Quantitative Clinical Chemistry. Baltimore, Williams & Wilkins 1931.
- Schwartz WB, Relman AS. A critique of the parameters used in the evaluation of acid-base disorders. N Engl J Med. 1963;268:1383-8.
- Severinghaus JW. Siggaard-Andersen and the "Great Trans-Atlantic Acid-Base Debate". Scand J Clin Lab Invest Suppl. 1993;214:99-104.
- Severinghaus JW, Astrup PB. History of blood gas analysis. Int Anesthesiol Clin. 1987;25(4):1-224.
- Stewart PA. How to Understand Acid-base: A Quantitative Acid-base Primer for Biology and Medicine. New York, Elsevier 1981.
- Van Slyke DD, Neill JM. The determination of gases in blood and other solutions by vacuum extraction and manometric measurement. I. J Biol Chem. 1924;61:523-43.
- Weisberg HF. Water, Electrolyte and Acid-Base Balance. Baltimore, The Williams & Wilkins Co. 1953.

The regulation of blood pH Fundamentals of acid-base physiological biochemistry

Mario Tarantino

Alterations in blood pH can have clinical consequences of not negligible importance (**Tables 2.1 and 2.2**). Since these consequences can be caused not only by an increase, but also by a decrease in the concentration of hydrogen ions ([H^+]), they cannot simply be attributed to toxic effects, but rather they are the expression of the numerous physiological activities that H^+ carry out at cellular level. Just think of the optimal pH of enzymatic activities, such as phosphofructokinase, whose activity in the lactic acid synthesis decreases under acidosis conditions and increases in conditions of alkalosis, performing a sort of metabolic buffer function. Equally important is proteins isoelectric point, which has influence not only on functional activities, but also on their own physical-chemical properties. Hormones, receptors and metabolic processes also depend on pH.

TABLE 2.1 Clinical consequences of severe acidemia.

Cardiovascular
• Decreased cardiac contractility • Arteriolar dilation, venous constriction • Increased pulmonary vascular resistance • Decreased cardiac output, blood pressure, renal and hepatic flow • Sensitivity to arrhythmia due to re-entry, VF threshold reduction • Attenuation of cardiovascular response to catecholamines
Respiratory
• Hyperventilation • Decreased strength of respiratory muscles, muscle fatigue • Dyspnea
Metabolic
• Increased metabolic demand • Insulin resistance • Inhibition of anaerobic glycolysis • Decreased ATP synthesis • Hyperkalemia • Increased protein degradation
Cerebral
• Inhibition of metabolism and regulation of cell volume • Headedness and coma

TABLE 2.2 Clinical consequences of severe alkalemia.

Cardiovascular
• Arteriolar constriction • Decreased coronary flow • Decrease in angina threshold • Predisposition of refractory supraventricular and ventricular arrhythmias
Respiratory
• Hypoventilation with consequent hypercarbia and hypoxemia
Metabolic
• Stimulation of anaerobic glycolysis • Hypokalemia • Ionized calcium decrease • Hypomagnesemia, hypophosphatemia
Cerebral
• Decreased brain flow • Tetany, convulsions, delirium, stupor

Another important aspect is nanomolar size order (10^{-9} Eq/L) to which H^+ act, a million times lower than the millimolar one of almost all the other physiological ions: physiological regulation mechanisms particularly precise and sensitive must therefore be available.
Finally, since this book is mainly dedicated to the presentation of clinical cases, examining the pathophysiological alterations and discussing their diagnostic interpretation, knowledge of the biochemical fundamentals that regulate the pH of the blood in physiological conditions is of essential importance, since the alterations that characterize the acid-base disorders are only quantitative extensions of the same processes that regulate pH in physiological conditions.

The buffer function

Without going into a thorough discussion of acid-base chemistry, we will limit ourselves to the principles that allow us to understand the buffer function, the fundamental mechanism, as we shall see, of the blood pH defense and the physiological acid-base regulation.
The Brönsted-Lowry theory defines acids as H^+ donor, and bases as H^+ acceptor, so that an acid is composed of a base combined with H^+.
A strong acid has a weak base, with little capacity to retain H^+, and therefore in solution it dissociates to a large extent or even completely. A weak acid is formed by a base that, to a greater or lesser extent, can hold H^+, dissociating itself only partially.
The dissociation of an acid depends on the dissociation constant Ka (or ionization constant, or equilibrium constant),

$$Ka = \frac{[H^+]\ [A^-]}{[HA]} \quad (1)$$

which is the relationship between the dissociated part and the non-dissociated part. It is therefore a acid strength measure: the greater the Ka, the stronger the acid. The acid-base reaction is the competition for H^+ between two bases of different strength.

$$\begin{array}{l} HA_1 \rightarrow H^+ + A_1^- \\ \qquad\quad \downarrow \\ HA_2 \leftarrow H^+ + A_2^- \end{array} \quad (2)$$

Even the simple dissociation of an acid in solution is an acid-base reaction between the acid and the solvent.

$$\begin{array}{l} HA \rightarrow H^+ + A^- \\ \qquad\ \downarrow \\ HS \leftarrow H^+ + S^- \end{array} \quad (3)$$

Water is a solvent particularly suited to acid-base chemistry because it has amphoteric properties, reacting both as an acid and as a base: the water ionization constant is 10^{-14}, and since it is dissociated in equal parts in H^+ and OH^-, the concentration of both ions is 10^{-7} Eq/L (100 nEq/L), a concentration which therefore represents neutrality in an aqueous solution at 25 °C. Since often the dissociation of an acid is very limited, especially the weak acids in physiological biochemistry, usually the concentration of the free fraction of the dissociated H^+ is expressed in terms of pH, the negative base 10 logarithm of the concentration in Eq/L: thus for example the average concentration in blood, 0.000.000.040 Eq/L, is more easily expressed as pH 7.40 ($10^{-7.40}$ Eq/L).
However, currently it's also widespread the expression in nanoEquivalents, 10^{-9} Eq/L, equally simple while avoiding the negative logarithmic scale: thus the same average physiological concentration in the blood is 40 nEq/L.
Perhaps the most important aspect to understand the buffer function is that in order to carry out the activities on which the clinical consequences listed in Tables 2.1 and 2.2 depend, the H^+ must be dissociated, in the free form: H^+ combined in the non-dissociated form are functionally silent.
So, for example the pH measurement with the potentiometric method using an ion-selective electrode measures only free H^+, not those combined in the non-dissociated form, because this method measures the activity, proportional to the concentration, of free ions in solution. This property of hydrogen ions already contains in itself the buffer function principle, which in its essence is the transfer of H^+ between the active dissociated form and the inactive non-dissociated form, in order to limit the pH variations after adding or subtracting an acid or a base.

The buffer function exploits the equilibrium of the dissociation of weak acids and bases:

$$HA \underset{k_2v_2}{\overset{k_1v_1}{\rightleftarrows}} H^+ + A^- \quad (4)$$

The weak acid dissociation is the result of two reactions: dissociation of the acid in its ions, which depends on a constant k_1v_1, and re-association of the H^+ and A^- ions in the non-dissociated form HA, which also depends on a constant k_2v_2.
At equilibrium, $v_1 = v_2$. The magnitude of dissociation, or how weak the acid is, that means the acid strength, depends on the relationship between the two constants k_1 and k_2, that is the dissociation constant Ka

$$Ka = \frac{[H^+]\ [A^-]}{[HA]} \quad (5)$$

In analogy with the terminology in pH units, Ka can also be expressed as a negative base 10 logarithm, with the term pK.

The reactions that define the dissociation of a weak acid illustrated in (4) obey the law of mass action.
If we add H^+, the equilibrium of the reaction (4) moves to the left: the association reaction k_2v_2 starts to prevail, so that a part of the added H^+ combines with A^- to form HA up to a new equilibrium: since as we said the activity of H^+ in the non-dissociated form is silent, the increase in the concentration of free H^+, that is the decrease in pH, is partly neutralized, thus limiting the pH change.
A similar result, in the opposite direction of course, follows the subtraction of H^+ with the addition of a base. This is the mechanism of the buffer function, whose purpose is to limit pH variations following the addition or subtraction of an acid or a base to a solution. However, a clarification is needed.
If we examine the titration of a buffer (**Figure 2.1**), we can see that the titration curve is S-shaped: the pH change with the progressive addition of H^+ is reduced, that is the buffer capacity increases, up to a minimum corresponding to the value of pH equal to the pK of the buffer, to then resume increasing.
The buffer capacity is therefore maximum at the pH value equal to the pK of the buffer, and is progressively

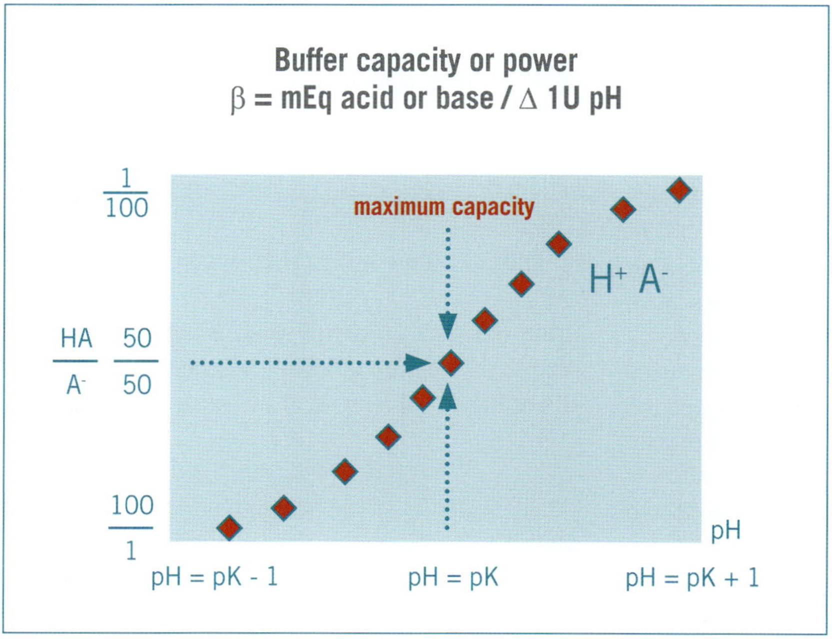

Figure 2.1 Titration curve of a buffer. The buffer capacity or power is maximum at the pH equal to the pK of the buffer, and starts to fade at lower and higher pH values of 1 unit with respect to the pK value: a wide extension, of 100 times, considering the base 10 logarithmic scale.

reduced by fading at pH values of 1 unit above and below the pH equal to the pK of the buffer. This behavior can be explained by reworking equation (5) as a function of $[H^+]$

$$[H^+] = Ka \frac{[HA]}{[A^-]} \quad (6)$$

This equation, known as the Henderson equation, is very important because it shows how pH variations of a solution depend not only and not so much on the amount of acid or base added, but rather on the variations in the ratio between the dissociated part and the non-dissociated part of the buffer.

The version of this equation in logarithmic form is known as the Henderson-Hasselbalch equation:

$$pH = pK + \log \frac{[A^-]}{[HA]} \quad (7)$$

In the following chapters, we will be able to see the usefulness of these equations in the diagnostic interpretation of acid-base disorders.

The physiological production of metabolic acids

In the common western dietary habits the metabolism has a net production of acids: 15,000-20,000 mmol of CO_2, called also volatile acid because it is in equilibrium with its gaseous phase, and 50-70 mmol of other inorganic and organic acids, such as phosphoric acid, sulfuric acid, hydrochloric acid, lactic acid and ketoacids, called fixed acids to differentiate them from the volatile acid. If these quantities are compared with the limits within which blood pH is maintained in physiological conditions, it has understood that very efficient and sensitive mechanisms must be predisposed for the physiological maintenance of the acid-base balance.

The problem does not rely on the elimination of the acids produced, because the capacity of the organs appointed for this purpose – lungs and kidneys – goes far beyond the physiological needs, but rather that of maintaining the pH within vital limits during the transport of these metabolic products from the production sites to the elimination sites.

The fundamental mechanism used to maintain pH in body fluids is the buffer function above described above: there are many components both extra and intracellular that can perform this function, particularly proteins, organic and inorganic phosphates especially intracellular, and in the extracellular the same CO_2 that, as we will see, although being in itself a threat for blood pH, together with bicarbonate can also perform a powerful pH defense function.

"Volatile acid" CO_2d

The CO_2 produced by the metabolism diffuses into the plasma in the physically dissolved form CO_2d, whose concentration is proportional to the partial pressure of its gas phase PCO_2. Since this is maintained under physiological conditions at 40 mmHg, and since the solubility coefficient in blood at 37 °C is 0.03 mMol/mmHg, the average CO_2d concentration in the arterial blood is 1.2 mMol/L (given the proportionality between PCO_2 and CO_2d, the expressions in mMol/L and mmHg are interchangeable). In aqueous solution the CO_2d undergoes hydration to carbonic acid H_2CO_3 which, being a strong acid with pK 3.9, at the physiological pH dissociates readily and completely: therefore the CO_2 affects the acid-base balance. The forms in equilibrium in physiological conditions are therefore:

$$PCO_2 \leftrightarrow CO_2d + H_2O \leftrightarrow H_2CO_3 \leftrightarrow H^+ + HCO_3^- \quad (8)$$

Given the slow CO_2d hydration, which contrasts the prompt dissociation of H_2CO_3, the complex of (8) assumes the characteristics of a weak acid:

$$CO_2d \leftrightarrow H^+ + HCO_3^- \quad (9)$$

where CO_2d plays the role of the non-dissociated acid, whose conjugate base is HCO_3^-. The pK of this "acid-base pair" in the blood at 37 °C is 6.1, so at physiological pH the balance is displaced strongly in the alkaline direction, with the "acid" CO_2 being largely in the dissociated form, with a ratio of 1:20 between the non-dissociated "acid" CO_2d and the conjugate base HCO_3^-. CO_2 is very diffusible through cell membranes and, by flowing into the blood from the tissues where it is produced, more than 95% quickly diffuses into the erythrocytes (**Figure 2.2**).

This diffusion is also favored by two erythrocyte factors: one is carbonic anhydrase (CA), which accelerates the CO_2 hydration to carbonic acid; the other is hemoglobin (Hb), which, by carrying out an important buffer function, while giving up oxygen increases its ability to combine with H^+ that are released by the dissociation of carbonic acid, a phenomenon known as the "Bohr effect".

A minor part of CO_2 is transported in a form directly combined with hemoglobin as a carbamino-compound: this combination also reflects Hb oxygenation state, a phenomenon known as the "Haldane effect". It is worth noting that Hb is a very powerful buffer: the buffering power β is 3 Eq/Mole/1 U pH; in 1 L of blood (hematocrit 45%, hemoglobin 15 g/dL), the buffering power is 27 mEq/1 U pH.

Taking place inside the erythrocyte, these processes help to dispose of the CO_2 facilitating its further diffusion from plasma.

The other product of the dissociation of carbonic acid,

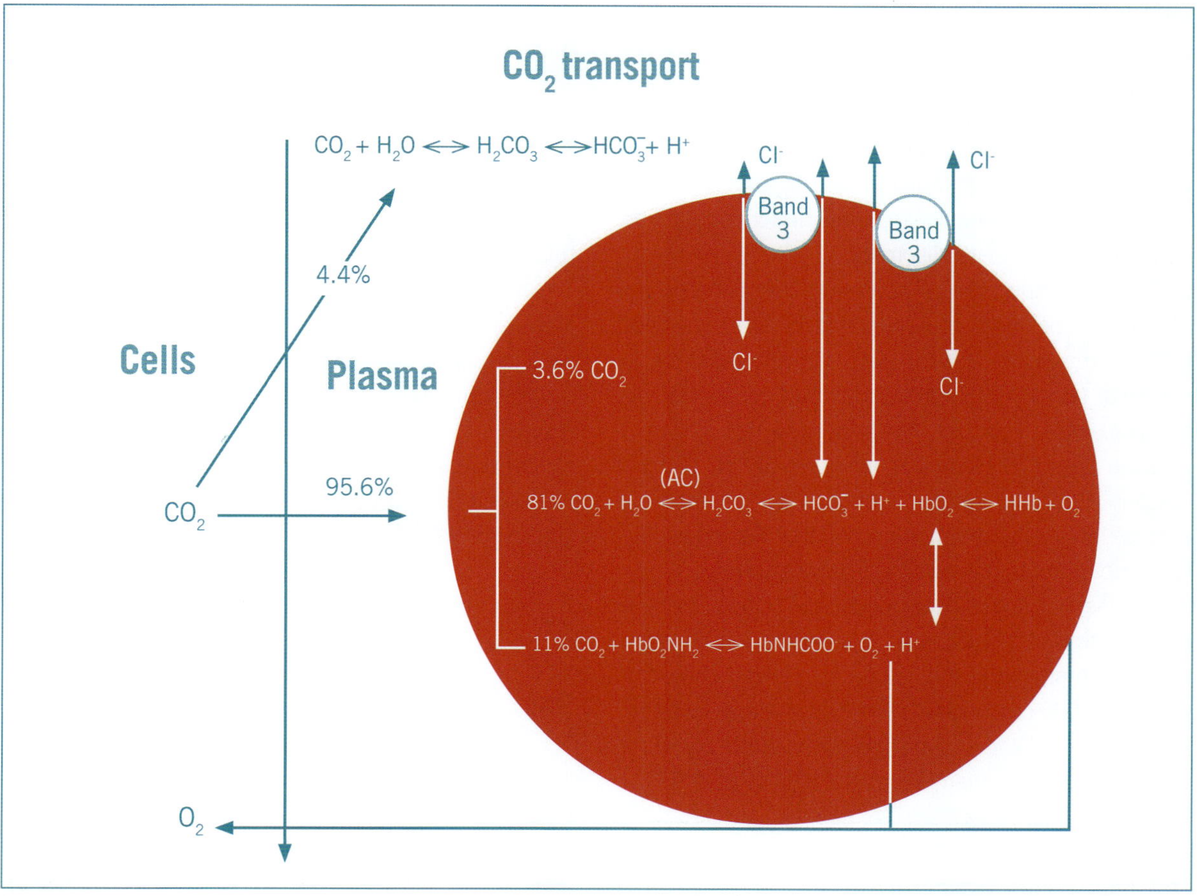

Figure 2.2 The CO_2 that flows from the tissues into the blood diffuses mostly into the erythrocytes, where it is hydrated to carbonic acid and then to bicarbonate, which is transported in the plasma in exchange for chloride. Carbonic anhydrase (CA) has a fundamental importance in this transformation, as well as hemoglobin in the buffer function.

bicarbonate, is transferred into the plasma in exchange with chloride through the exchanger Band 3, located on the erythrocyte membrane ("chlorides exchange" by Hamburger) so that in the end the blood CO_2 resides mainly in plasma as HCO_3^-, although most of it derives from the diffusion in erythrocytes in the form of CO_2d.

The homeostatic maintenance of blood CO_2d is completed by the intervention of the respiratory function, which by regulating the CO_2 elimination depending on the quantity produced, through a direct relationship between PCO_2 in the gaseous phase and CO_2d in the blood, is the fundamental function in maintaining the balance of this metabolic product.

PCO_2 in the gaseous phase, and therefore CO_2d in the blood, is the most effective stimulus for pulmonary ventilation: the increase in PCO_2 of 1 mmHg causes an increase in ventilation of 1-4 L/min. There is therefore a relationship of direct proportionality between PCO_2 and pulmonary ventilation.

Opposite relationship binds blood pH and pulmonary ventilation, which is stimulated directly by a decrease in pH, starting as we will see the respiratory adaptation in metabolic acid-base disorders.

We have examined the CO_2 herein as an acid potential which, together with its conjugated bicarbonate base HCO_3^-, forms an acid-base pair, albeit unorthodox in chemical terms, whose alterations can cause respiratory acid-base disorders. But alongside this role as a possible threat to blood pH, is opposed the primary function of this sui generis acid-base pair in blood pH defense, as the most important buffer in the extracellular compartment known as bicarbonate buffer.

We will discuss about it later, dealing with the protective mechanisms of blood pH; but first we must consider the other products of the metabolism which can compromise the homeostasis of the acid-base balance, and which are known with the term "fixed acids", a term to distinguish them from the "volatile acid" CO_2.

"Fixed acids"

This term brings together the organic and inorganic acids that the metabolism produces and that are not degraded up to the "volatile acid" CO_2. This is not only a physical-chemical but also a physiological distinction because, as we will see, the processes of pH defense aimed at these acids during their blood transport are different and completely independent from those used for the defense against "volatile acid". Also the elimination site is different, since fixed acids, are metabolized by the kidney.

"Fixed acids" are produced by the metabolism of amino acids and organic acids that derive from the degradation of proteins, carbohydrates and fats introduced with food.

Both acid and base are produced, however with the western world eating habits a net production of acids prevails, on average about 50-70 mEq in 24 hours; sulfur amino acids, methionine and cysteine, produce about 70 mEq of H^+ in the 24 hours; the cationic amino acids, lysine, arginine, histidine also produce H^+, in an amount of about 140 mEq in the 24 hours; the metabolism of anionic amino acids, glutamate, aspartate, consumes about 100 mEq of H^+ in 24 hours.

To these must be added the metabolism of organic anions from carbohydrates and fats, such as lactate, acetate, citrate etc., which mainly consume about 60 mEq of H^+ in 24 hours.

The net balance of all these metabolic processes results in the production of about 60 mEq of H^+ in 24 hours. As we shall see, it is precisely with regard to these H^+ producers that bicarbonate buffer has the ability to manifest itself in all its power and efficiency, albeit with the remarkable secondary contribution of the other non-bicarbonate buffers, as well as the kidney whose function goes well beyond the elimination site.

The blood pH defense

Physiological buffers

The fundamental mechanism of the processes that provide homeostatic maintenance of blood pH is the buffer function.

There are many buffers distributed both in the cells and in the extracellular compartment (**Figure 2.3**). Understandably, however, the intracellular distribution prevails, where there are different components with an

isoelectric point suitable for performing the buffer function at physiological pH, especially organic proteins and phosphates (we have already seen, for example, the important function of hemoglobin).
Also in the extracellular, above all in the plasma, proteins and inorganic phosphates contribute to pH defense and particulally in plasma, it is above all important the pH defense function carried out by the acid-base pair CO_2d/HCO_3^-, known by the term "bicarbonate buffer".
Undoubtedly the most fascinating aspect of acid-base physiology, is the phenomenon whereby the same component is on one hand a potential cause of alteration of blood pH and acid-base disorders, and on the other performs at the same time a function that contributes to blood pH defense.
In reality the CO_2d/HCO_3^- pair is not in the best conditions to carry out buffer activity in body fluids because, as we have seen, the pK is 6.1, distant more than one unit from the pH it must protect. At equilibrium

$$Ka = \frac{[H^+]\ [HCO_3^-]}{[CO_2d]\ [H_2O]} \quad (10)$$

and since $[H_2O]$ is constant it can be included in the equilibrium constant that becomes K'a

$$K'a = \frac{[H^+]\ [HCO_3^-]}{[CO_2d]} \quad (11)$$

In the plasma at 37 °C K'a is 8×10^{-7} Eq/L (800 nEq/L): by solving the (11) with respect to $[H^+]$, we have the Henderson equation

$$[H^+] = 800 \frac{[CO_2d]}{[HCO_3^-]} \quad (12)$$

Buffers distribution in water compartments

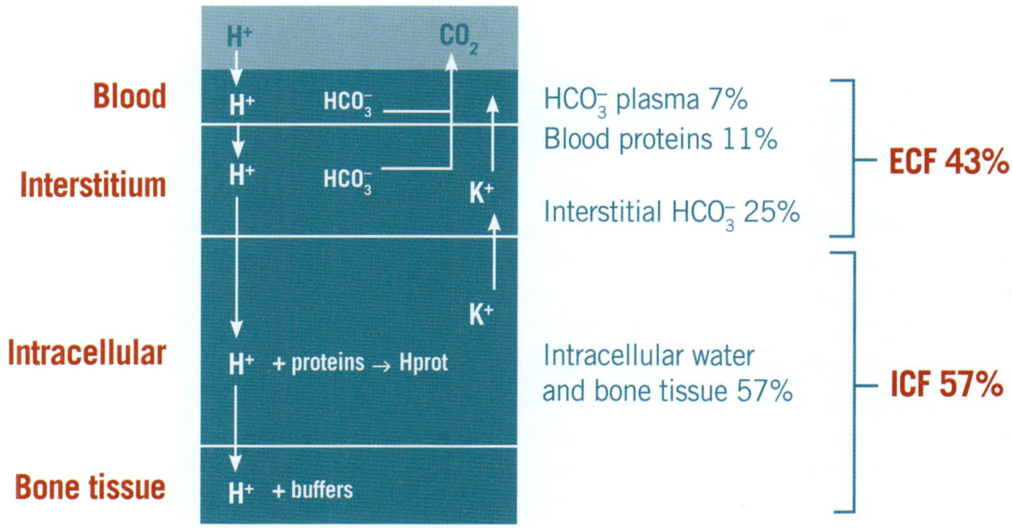

Figure 2.3 Bicarbonate buffer is prevalent in extracellular fluid. The greatest buffer activity is in the intracellular compartment, thanks to the multiplicity of organic proteins and phosphates, and to ion exchange in bone tissue.
ECF: extracellular fluid; ICF: intracellular fluid

which in the logarithmic form becomes the Henderson-Hasselbalch equation

$$pH = 6.1 + \log \frac{[HCO_3^-]}{[CO_2d]} \quad (13)$$

And since $[CO_2d] = 0.03\ PCO_2$, if we include in the constant also the solubility coefficient 0.03 (800 x 0.03 = 24) and we express $[CO_2d]$ in terms of its partial pressure PCO_2, the Henderson equation becomes the Bleich and Kassirer equation

$$[H^+]\ nEq/L = 24\ \frac{PCO_2\ mmHg}{[HCO_3^-]\ mEq/L} \quad (14)$$

which is the same Henderson equation in a simplified form of useful in clinical practice for checking the blood gas data and facilitating calculations; so for example if the blood gas data have the normal average value, (13) becomes

$$[H^+]\ 40\ nEq/L = 24\ \frac{PCO_2\ 40\ mmHg}{[HCO_3^-]\ 24\ mEq/L} \quad (15)$$

We will see in the following chapters the application and usefulness of this equation in diagnostic interpretation of acid-base disorders.

Physiological adaptations

The bicarbonate buffer with pK more than 1 unit away from pH to be protected, and with a 20/1 ratio between the dissociated and non-dissociated part, very far from the 1:1 ratio optimal for the buffer function, in purely chemical terms cannot certainly be an effective buffer under physiological conditions. But bicarbonate buffer is an open system: both the numerator and the denominator of equation (14) can be quickly adjusted with the intervention, respectively, of the respiratory function and the renal function: because both of these functions are sensitive to pH changes, and because they depend on the $PCO_2/[HCO_3^-]$ ratio, the adjustment takes place in the direction of pH correction towards normal values. Naturally, this adjustment takes place not only with respect to bicarbonate buffer, but also with all the other buffers mentioned above (known as non-bicarbonate buffers).
These corrective interventions are known as respiratory adaptation and renal adaptation, and can take place in any acid-base disorder, unless the cause of the disorder is an alteration of the functions on which the adaptation depends. Thus in respiratory acid-base disorders neither the bicarbonate buffer nor the respiratory adaptation are available. In renal failure and in tubular secretion disorders, acidosis is the manifestation of the importance of the kidney in maintaining acid-base balance. As we shall see while discussing of the clinical cases in the following chapters, the adaptation processes practically never succeed in bringing the blood pH back to normal limits.
However the physiological limits of in vivo adaptation have been studied for each type of acid-base disorder – and calculated with an approximation close to 95% – being of precious utility in the differential diagnosis of acid-base disorders, in particular for the differentiation of mixed acid-base disorders, which we will discuss later.
After examining the role of the respiratory function, the important part played by kidney in maintaining acid-base homeostasis still remains to be examined.

The role of the kidney in the acid-base balance

The kidney is the elimination site of fixed acids, but its function in acid-base homeostasis is far more important, contributing to the maintenance and strengthening of buffer defense processes.
First of all glomerular filtrate bicarbonate is recovered – an operation of vast proportions if we consider that under physiological conditions about 4,500 mEq of this buffer base must be recovered – but the kidney is not limited to this recovery, also providing for the regeneration of the HCO_3^- consumed in the buffering activity towards fixed acids, thus reinstating the reserve of buffer bases of body fluids (including non-bicarbonate buffer bases, by virtue of the isohydric principle).
Of course, these processes take place in exchange with the H^+ elimination of fixed acids.

Bicarbonate recovery

The recovery of filtered bicarbonate occurs almost completely in the proximal tubule (**Figure 2.4**).

The mechanism of this recovery is not a real reabsorption (therefore the term recovery is preferred): filtered HCO_3^- is dehydrated in the tubular lumen in CO_2 and OH^- by carbonic anhydrase of which the cells luminal edge of this nephron tract is rich. While the OH^- combines with the H^+ secreted in exchange with the reabsorption of sodium through a NHE_3 exchanger, forming H_2O (and thus explaining the relatively high pH, 6.8-7.0, in this tubular lumen tract, despite the H^+ secretion to a not insignificant extent), CO_2 diffuses rapidly into the tubular cells, where it is again hydrated to HCO_3^- by cytoplasmic carbonic anhydrase. The reconstituted HCO_3^- is reabsorbed together with sodium by means of a $Na^+HCO_3^-$ co-transporter.

Reabsorbed HCO_3^- is not materially the same as the filtrated, but it is quantitatively equivalent.

Titratable acidity

The same process seen for the recovery of bicarbonate CO_2 hydration catalyzed by carbonic anhydrase also works for the other urine acidification processes of urine that occur in the tubular nephron. These processes are titratable acidity and ammoniagenesis: each of them generates in equivalent measure H^+, which are eliminated, and HCO_3^-, which go to reconstitute the buffer base reserve.

Titratable acidity is so named because it is the process that can be measured by urine titration up to pH 7.40 (**Figure 2.5**). This process consists of the combination of H^+ secreted with urinary compounds that can perform buffer function, especially the inorganic phosphates, but also creatinine, urate, lactate can contribute in certain conditions. At pH 7.40 the phosphate is present in the filtrate in the two forms HPO_4^{--} and $H_2PO_4^-$ in the proportion 4:1, pK 6.8. With the progressive urine acidification proceeding in tubular lumen, HPO_4^{--} is trans-

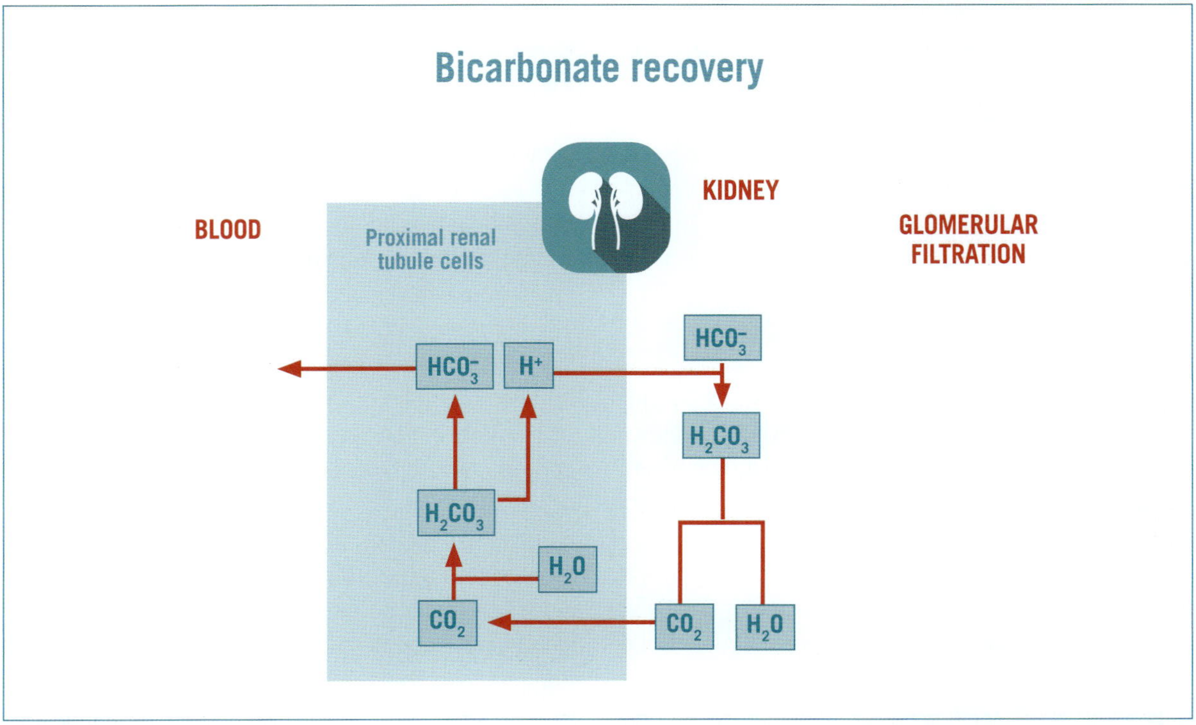

Figure 2.4 Bicarbonate is not reabsorbed as such, but is formed in the tubular cell by CO_2 hydration, catalyzed by carbonic anhydrase.

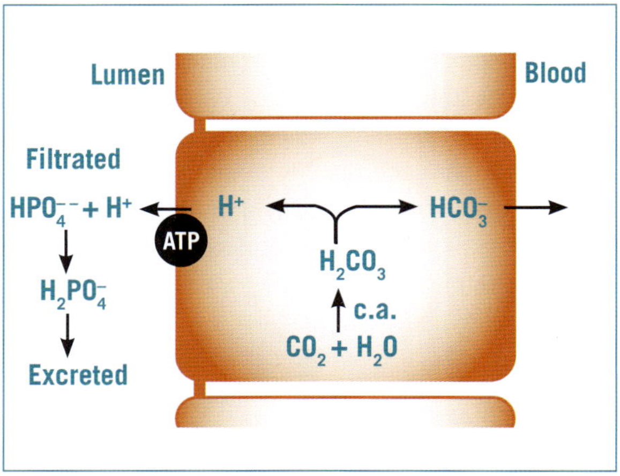

Figure 2.5 Titratable acidity. The H^+ secreted by tubular cells combine in the lumen with buffer substances, such as phosphates, and creatinine, avoiding excessive acidification of the urine.

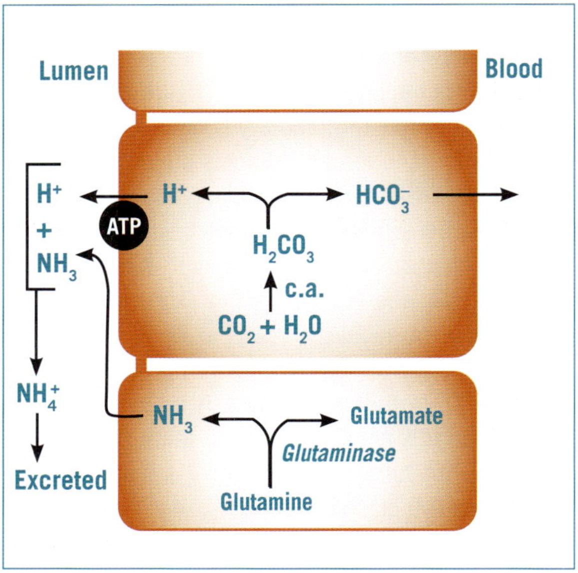

Figure 2.6 Ammoniagenesis. Ammonium is produced by the metabolism of glutamine. For each NH_4^+, molecule, an HCO_3^- molecule is produced, which contributes to the recovery of consumed buffer bases.

formed into $H_2PO_4^-$ by combining with H^+ secreted until everything is in this form at a pH lower than 5.5. This process of H^+ elimination is quantitatively important, being able to reach more than half of the daily acid load to be eliminated, but does not allow for wide extensions, limited both by phosphate availability and urinary pH.

The ammoniagenesis

It is the most important process of urine acidification (**Figure 2.6**), because it is very flexible since it can increase up to ten times in acidemic conditions. The basis of this process is the reaction:

$$NH_3 + H^+ \leftrightarrow NH_4^+ \quad (16)$$

The H^+ elimination as ammonium was once considered a simple buffer mechanism, in which NH_3 ammonia diffuses from the tubular cell into the lumen where it combines with the secreted H^+ to be eliminated as an ammonium ion.

It is now demonstrated that NH_4^+ forms directly in the tubular cell from the metabolism of glutamine, and as such is transported into the tubular lumen to be eliminated. In addition to ammonium, the metabolism of glutamine produces α-ketoglutarate, which is metabolized to HCO_3^-, so that for each H^+ eliminated as ammonium a bicarbonate ion is formed, contributing to the regeneration of the buffer bases consumed in the blood pH defense.

However, ammonium secreted in this way is not directly eliminated, but undergoes a rather complex process. It is reabsorbed in the ascending branch of the loop of Henle replacing the potassium in the $Na^+K^+2Cl^-$ co-transporter and from here it passes into the medullar interstitium where it accumulates in the form of NH_3.

The pre-urine that reaches the distal nephron is therefore almost free of ammonia, favoring its diffusion in the tubular lumen from the medullar interstitium. The high acidity in this sector of the tubular lumen readily converts NH_3 to NH_4^+, which is finally eliminated in the urine.

By means of the described processes, the kidney contributes to a large extent to conservation and regeneration of buffer bases, regulating the denominator of Henderson's equation (12), just as the respiratory system regulates the numerator, in the function of physiological compensation as a complement to buffers biochemical function. Although kidney is the elimination

site of fixed acids, its contribution to acid-base homeostasis also extends to volatile acid CO_2: the variations of blood PCO_2 are in fact followed by parallel changes in renal H^+ elimination and HCO_3^- recovery.
The signal that senses the tubular cells is probably the intracellular pH. As we will see, renal adaptation has a primary role in respiratory acid-base disorders.

Introduction to acid-base disorders

At the conclusion of this chapter dedicated to physiological biochemistry principles of acid-base balance, and to the introduction of the clinical part dedicated to acid-base disorders, we consider useful to illustrate blood gas alterations that characterize the simple ones, both of respiratory and metabolic type, interpreting its pathogenesis and pathophysiology in the light of the concepts we have discussed above.

Respiratory acidosis

This disorder is caused by the increase of blood volatile CO_2d acid as a result of a disorder associated with respiratory failure (**Figure 2.7**).
The increase in the CO_2d/HCO_3^- ratio causes, according to the Henderson equation, an increase in the concentration of H^+ in the blood, that is a decrease in blood pH. Therefore the processes of pH defense are activated, which in this disorder are: 1) the intervention of non-bicarbonate buffers (extra- and intra-cellular proteins, hemoglobin, inorganic and organic phosphates), while obviously the bicarbonate buffer cannot be able to intervene since one of its components is the cause of the disorder; 2) renal adaptation intervenes by increasing the bicarbonate recovery and the H^+ elimination. Since the initiation of renal adaptation is not immediate but takes a few days to manifest itself, the course of respiratory acidosis can be distinguished in an acute phase, in the first 4-5 days, where only the buffer defense is active, followed by a chronic phase where also the renal adaptation is added, with a more important correction of the blood gas analysis alterations.
The in vivo adaptation limits show that in acute phase of respiratory acidosis for every 1 mmHg increase in PCO_2, the increase in $[HCO_3^-]$ is 0.1 mEq/L; in chronic phase the increase in $[HCO_3^-]$ is 0.35 mEq/L for every 1 mmHg increase in PCO_2.
The resulting blood gas profile shows blood pH decrease, PCO_2 increase that caused the disorder and HCO_3^- increase as a result of defense and adaptation processes.

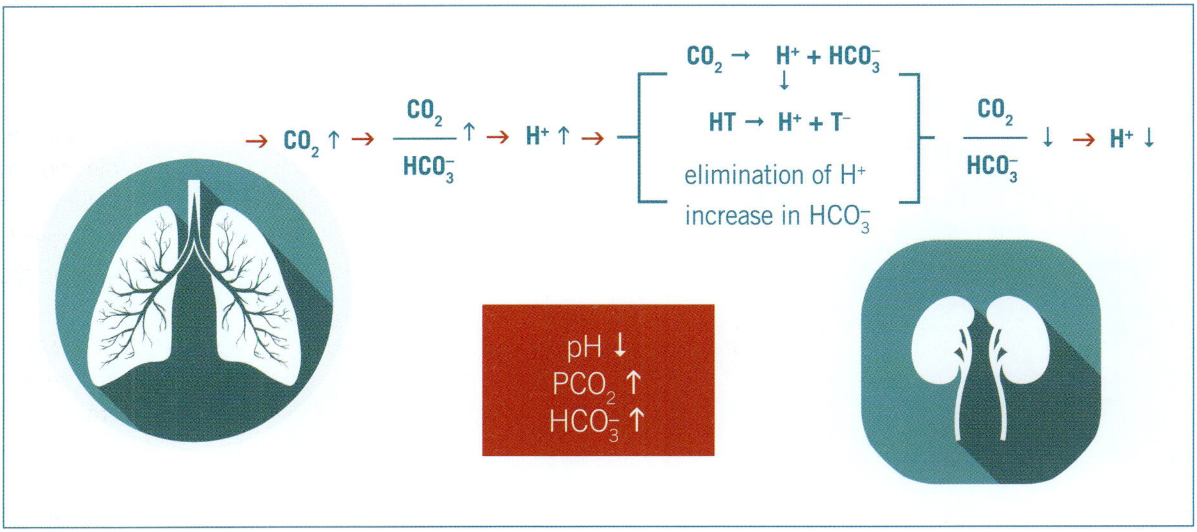

Figure 2.7 Pathological biochemistry of respiratory acidosis.

Respiratory alkalosis

Respiratory alkalosis is due to excessive pulmonary ventilation: the consequent decrease in PCO_2 decreases the CO_2d/HCO_3^- ratio and, according to the Henderson equation, reduces the blood H^+ concentration.

The increase in pH is mitigated by the intervention of non-bicarbonate buffers releasing H^+ which, combining with HCO_3^-, forms CO_2d thus limiting its loss. To this buffer defense is joined, with a certain delay, the kidney that holds back H^+ contributing to the alkalemia correction (**Figure 2.8**).

Like acidosis, respiratory alkalosis also takes place with a biphasic course, in which to a first phase where the disorder is only protected by the biochemical intervention of non-bicarbonate buffers, a second phase follows where the kidney intervention, holding back H^+ and eliminating bicarbonate, contributes to a more effective correction of the acid-base disorder. In the acute phase for every 1 mmHg of PCO_2 decrease there is a reduction of $[HCO_3^-]$ of 0.2 mEq/L; in the chronic form for each reduction of 1 mmHg of the PCO_2 there is a reduction of $[HCO_3^-]$ of 0.4 mEq/L.

Respiratory alkalosis is the only simple acid-base disorder capable, in its chronic form, of spontaneously offset blood pH within physiological limits.

Metabolic acidosis

Unlike respiratory disorders, metabolic disorders have a heterogeneous etiology. Metabolic acidosis in particular may be due to metabolic causes, such as diabetic ketoacidosis, or to causes of renal origin, as it is easy to understand given the important role of this organ in regulating acid-base homeostasis, not just as a site of elimination, as we have already seen. In fact, kidney can cause acid-base disorders even independently of its functionality state, as a possible site of congenital or acquired defects in the transport mechanisms of hydrogen ions or bicarbonate in the tubular cells, in the forms of acidosis that go by the name of renal tubular acidosis (RTA). Finally, a metabolic acidosis can be caused by a loss of buffer bases, such as the just mentioned tubular defects, or enterically through diarrhea.

The buffer defense in metabolic-type disorders can count, in addition to non-bicarbonate buffers, also on bicarbonate buffer which, distributed mainly in the extracellular compartment, as we have seen above, in addition to a quantitatively robust protection in collaboration with non-bicarbonate buffers, ensures an emergency defense, such as to overwhelm the relative slowness of renal adaptation.

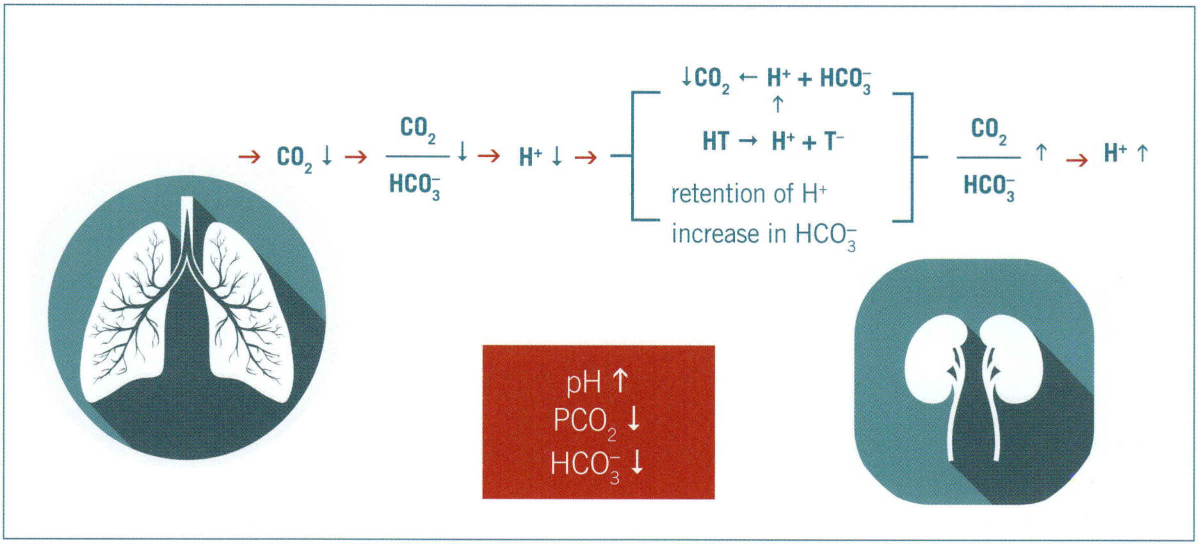

Figure 2.8 Pathological biochemistry of respiratory alkalosis.

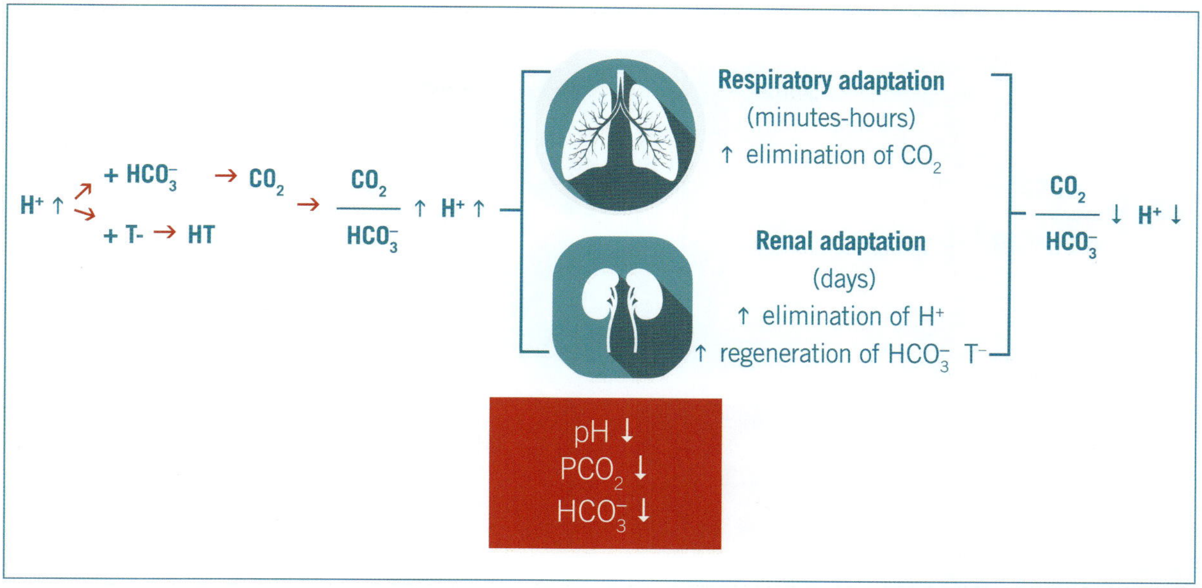

Figure 2.9 Pathological biochemistry of metabolic acidosis.

In addition, metabolic disorders can also rely on respiratory adaptation (**Figure 2.9**).

As shown in the figure, the increase in hydrogen ions that caused the disorder is contrasted both by the bicarbonate buffer and by the non-bicarbonate buffers, whose bases combined with H^+ are transformed into the respective non-dissociated forms CO_2 and HT: the decrease in blood pH that occurs, despite this first defense intervention, is due to the modification of the $CO_2d\backslash HCO_3^-$ ratio according to the Henderson equation, and is nevertheless an expression of a pH defense process, which without the buffer defense intervention it would have precipitated to much more serious values.

The fast intervention of respiratory and renal adaptation processes, respectively with the elimination of pulmonary CO_2, and with the elimination of H^+ and the regeneration of consumed buffer bases, complete the defense processes limiting acidemia.

According to studies on the expected adaptation, in metabolic acidosis, PCO_2 decreases by 1.2 mmHg for every 1 mEq/L decrease in HCO_3^-, as will be shown in more detail in the discussion of clinical cases in the subsequent chapters.

Metabolic alkalosis

In the metabolic alkalosis the pathophysiological processes described for metabolic acidosis take place in the opposite direction (**Figure 2.10**).

It should be kept in mind that the kidney has a great capacity to cope with an alkaline load: the administration of 1000 mEq of bicarbonate a day for two weeks has only a slight shift in the blood pH towards the upper physiological limit values, while there is a massive elimination of bicarbonate in the urine. Therefore, for an alkalosis to be established and maintained over time, the processes that ensure renal efficiency must be altered (see Chapter 4, page 65).

Furthermore, as can be seen in the diagram in the figure, the adaptation processes for the correction of this disorder can only be developed to a limited extent, in particular as regards respiratory adaptation. It is therefore clear that this acid-base disorder, besides being very frequent, is also the most complex in pathophysiological and clinical terms between uncomplicated acid-base disorders.

As well known, in addition to the four simple disorders we have now illustrated, the acid-base clinic is also enriched with mixed disorders, that are the association

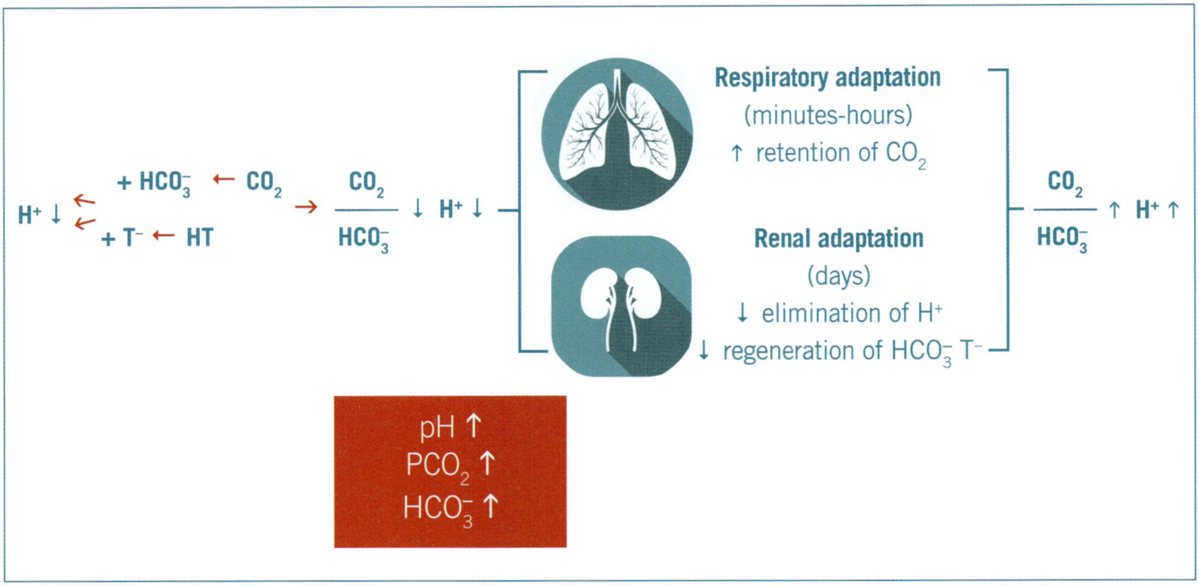

Figure 2.10 Pathological biochemistry of metabolic alkalosis.

of two or even three acid-base disorders. The association of two disorders is more frequent, which can be additive, when it is composed of two acidosis or two alkalosis, or counterbalancing, when an acidosis is associated with an alkalosis; furthermore, the two disorders may be of the same type, that is both metabolic or respiratory, or of both types, for example a respiratory acidosis complicated by a metabolic alkalosis.

A triple disorder occurs when a third mixed acid-base disorder is added to a double mixed disorder.

We leave to the following chapters the treatment of these complex pathologies, limiting ourselves to underline that, as we will see, the diagnostic criteria that allow to investigate and resolve the mixed disorders are based on the precise knowledge of physiology principles and of the physiological limits of adaptation of pH defense and homeostasis of acid-base balance.

References

- Berend K. Diagnostic use of the base excess in acid-base disorders. New Eng J Med. 2018;378(15):1419-28.
- Boron WF, Boulpaep EL. Medical Physiology. 3th ed. Philadelphia, Elsevier 2016.
- Brønsted JN. Einige Bemerkungen über den Begriff der Säuren und Basen. Rec Trav Chim Pays-Bas. 1923;42:718-28.
- Brown D, Wagner CA. Molecular mechanisms of acid-base sensing by the kidney. J Am Soc Nephrol. 2012;23(5):774-80.
- Davenport HW. The ABC of Acid-Base Chemistry. Chicago, University of Chicago Press 1969.
- Dhondup T, Qian Q. Acid-base and electrolyte disorders in patients with and without chronic kidney disease: An update. Kidney Dis. 2017;3(4):136-48.
- Eladari D, Chambrey R, Peti-Peterdi J. A new look at electrolyte transport in the distal tubule. Ann Rev Physiol. 2012;74:325-49.
- Fernandez PC, Cohen RM, Feldman GM. The concept of bicarbonate distribution space: the crucial role of body buffers. Kidney Int. 1989;36(5):747-52.
- Fidkowski C, Helmstrom J. Diagnosing metabolic acidosis in the critically ill: bridging the anion gap, Stewart, and base excess methods. Can J Anaesth. 2009;56(3):247-56.
- Filley GF. Acid-Base and Blood Gas Regulation. Philadelphia, Lea & Febiger 1971.
- Fine LW. Chemistry. 2th ed. Baltimore, William & Wilkins Co. 1978.
- Ganong WF. Review of Medical Physiology. 21th ed. New York. McGraw-Hill 2003.
- Gennari FG, Cohen JJ, Kassirer JP. Measurement of acid-base status. In: Cohen JJ, Kassirer IP. Acid/Base. 8th ed. Boston, Little Brown 1982.
- Halperin ML, Jungas RL. Metabolic production and renal disposal of hydrogen ions. Kidney Int. 1983;24(6):709-13.
- Hasselbalch KA. Die Berechnung der Wasserstoffzahl des

Blutes aus der freien und gebundenen Kohlensäure desselben, und die Sauerstoffbindung des Blutes als Funktion der Wasserstoffzahl. Biochem Z. 1917;78:112-44.

- Henderson LJ. Concerning the relationship between the strength of acids and their capacity to preserve neutrality (Abstract). Am J Physiol. 1908;21:173-79.
- Henderson LJ. The theory of neutrality regulation in the animal organism. Am J Physiol. 1908;21:427-48.
- Hills AG. pH and the Henderson-Hasselbalch equation. Am J Med. 1973;55(2):131-3.
- Kamel KS, Halperin ML. Acid-base problems in diabetic ketoacidosis. New Engl J Med. 2015;372(6):546-54.
- Kassirer JP, Bleich HL. Rapid estimation of plasma carbon dioxide tension from pH and total carbon dioxide content. N Engl J Med. 1965;272:1067-8.
- Kishen R, Honoré PM, Jacobs R et al. Facing acid-base disorders in the third millennium – the Stewart approach revisited. Int J Nephrol Renovasc Dis. 2014;7:209-17.
- Lemann J Jr, Litzow JR, Lennon EJ. The effects of chronic acid loads in normal man: further evidence for the participation of bone mineral in the defense against chronic metabolic acidosis. J Clin Invest. 1966;45(10):1608-14.
- Lloyd P, Freebairn R. Using quantitative acid-base analysis in the ICU. Crit Care Resusc. 2006;8(1):19-30.
- Lowry TM. The uniqueness of hydrogen. J Soc Chem Ind. 1923;42:43-47.
- Madias NE, Cohen JJ. Acid-base chemistry and buffering. In: Cohen JJ, Kassirer IP. Acid/Base. 8th ed. Boston, Little Brown 1982.
- Malnic G, Giebisch G. Symposium on acid-base homeostasis. Mechanism of renal hydrogenion secretion. Kidney Int. 1972;1(5):280-96.
- Narins RG, Emmett M. Simple and mixed acid-base disorders: a practical approach. Medicine. 1980;59(3):161-87.
- Narins RG, Gardner LB. Simple acid-base disturbances. Med Clin North Am. 1981;65(2):321-46.
- Nunn JF. Nunn's Applied Respiratory Physiology. 5th ed. Oxford, Butterworth-Heinemann 1999.
- Rose BD, Post TW. Clinical Physiology of Acid-Base and Electrolyte Disorders. 5th ed. New York. McGraw-Hill 2001.
- Seifter JL, Chang HY. Disorders of acid-base balance: New perspectives. Kidney Dis. 2017;2(4):170-86.
- Trepiccione F, Prosperi F, de la Motte LR et al. New findings on the pathogenesis of distal renal tubular acidosis. Kidney Dis. 2017;3(3):98-105.
- Weiner ID, Verlander JW. Recent advances in understanding renal ammonia metabolism and transport. Curr Opin Nephrol Hypertens. 2016;25(5):436-43.
- West JB. Respiratory Physiology: The essentials. 7th ed. Philadelphia. Lippincott Williams & Wilkins 2005.

Diagnostic interpretation of acid-base disorders Schools comparison

Mario Tarantino

Over the years, especially since the middle of the last century, many criteria for the diagnostic interpretation and the correct therapeutic treatment of acid-base disorders have alternated in the scientific literature.
This is not surprising, considering the clinical importance of acid-base disorders, especially in critically ill patients, where they often become complicated in forms of mixed disorders which, by deceptively presenting themselves with blood gas profile of a simple disorder, require distinctive criteria that guide the correct diagnosis.
Actually, at least until more recent times, it was not a question of proposing new theories opposed to previous ones, but rather of revising concepts in continuous evolution around the same fundamental physiological process, namely pH homeostatic regulation by buffers present in body fluids, assisted by the intervention of respiratory and renal adaptations, as described in the chapter on physiological biochemistry (Chapter 2).
Only in the 80s of the last century, Peter Stewart, a Canadian physiologist, proposed a theory observing acid-base balance from a completely different angle, apparently based on completely new concepts and which has been accepted as a "Copernican revolution", that to a more detailed examination shows, as we will see, not to be so "Copernican".

The metabolic component The Henderson equation

The interpretative criterion based on the modifications of the $PCO_2/[HCO_3^-]$ bicarbonate buffer – which we also follow, and which will be adopted in the clinical cases analysis presented in the following chapters – is the best known and certainly the most widespread today in clinical practice. It is both because it boasts an almost centuries-old time-test, and because together with pH it composes the blood gas profile which, as is known, is the fundamental investigation in the clinical analysis of the acid-base state.
As we explained in the physiology chapter the CO_2/HCO_3^- pair has two contrasting physiological meanings: on one hand it is a potential cause of pH homeostasis alteration, on the other it is one of the most important components of pH defense. These two aspects can be seen in the CO_2 dissociation reaction in aqueous solution:

$$\mathbf{CO_2 + H_2O \leftrightarrow H_2CO_3 \leftrightarrow H^+ + HCO_3^-} \quad (1)$$

The left side of the reaction, that is the hydration of CO_2 to carbonic acid and the subsequent dissociation of this acid with the production of H^+ and HCO_3^-, is the part that plays the role of potential cause of acid-base disorders.
As it depends on the alterations in respiratory function, in the diagnostic interpretation of alterations of the CO_2/HCO_3^- pair in acid-base disorders, this part of the reaction, identifiable as $[CO_2]d$ or PCO_2, is called the "respiratory component".
The reaction runs in the direction of the hydration of CO_2 to carbonic acid when there is an increase in blood $[CO_2]d$ (PCO_2), or in respiratory acidosis, and vice versa, it runs in the opposite direction of dehydration of carbonic acid to CO_2 in respiratory alkalosis.

The right side of the CO_2 dissociation reaction represents instead the pH's defense function that the CO_2/HCO_3^- pair performs as a buffer of robust capacity, being transformed into an open system with the intervention of respiratory and renal function.
Since this buffer function is performed by HCO_3^- towards H^+ that dissociate from the organic and inorganic acids produced by cellular metabolism, in the diagnostic interpretation of the alterations of the CO_2/HCO_3^- pair, this part of the reaction is called the "metabolic component". As already seen in the previous pages, in metabolic acidosis HCO_3^- decreases by consumption in the buffer reaction, while H^+ deficiency in the metabolic alkalosis shifts the dissociation reaction of the carbonic acid to the right with a consequent increase in HCO_3^-.
The relationships between pH homeostasis and the CO_2/HCO_3^- pair are expressed in the Henderson equation, as we saw in Chapter 2, which we report here in its simplified formulation of Bleich-Kassirer:

$$[H^+] = 24 \times PCO_2 / [HCO_3^-] \qquad (2)$$

from which it can be seen that an increase in $[H^+]$ may be due to the increase in the respiratory component (respiratory acidosis) or to the decrease in the metabolic component (metabolic acidosis), while vice versa the decrease in the respiratory component and the increase in the metabolic component are associated respectively with respiratory alkalosis and metabolic alkalosis.
The pathophysiological and pathogenetic mechanisms of acid-base disorders are described in the physiological biochemistry chapter and are extensively discussed in the presentation of clinical cases in subsequent chapters.
Here it is important to underline that the alterations of the Henderson equation make it possible to distinguish a typical blood gas profile for each of the fundamental acid-base disorders, both respiratory and metabolic. To this diagnostic utility we owe the notoriety and the diffusion in literature of the Henderson equation.
However, reaction (1) shows that both components are not free from reciprocal contamination: in particular HCO_3^- always undergoes changes in respiratory disorders, due both to the effect of non-bicarbonate buffers and to the intervention of renal function, as we have seen in Chapter 2.
Therefore HCO_3^- cannot reliably play the role of metabolic component. This unreliability was noticed on the occasion of the polio epidemic in Copenhagen in the 1950s, when the increase in plasma bicarbonate in these patients was interpreted as metabolic alkalosis rather than respiratory acidosis, which in reality it was (at the time it was not easy to resort to measuring the blood pH), thus delaying the appropriate intervention of the tracheotomy.
This dramatic experience stimulated research for more precise and reliable indices and criteria for the diagnostic interpretation of the metabolic component.
It should also be remembered that the interpretation based on the Henderson equation alone does not allow a quantitative assessment of the disorder: it gives descriptive information about the disorder, but cannot explain its pathogenetic mechanism.
Finally, an important aspect, only the alterations of the blood gas profile are not able to reveal mixed acid-base disorders.

The Danish school: standard bicarbonate, buffer base, base excess

Standard bicarbonate (HCO_3^- std) was proposed in the 1950s by Poul Astrup to correct the interpretation deficiencies of the Henderson-Hasselbalch equation. It consists in measuring plasma bicarbonate concentration after balancing the blood sample at PCO_2 of 40 mmHg at 37 °C by tonometry, thus eliminating the HCO_3^- share due to the respiratory component: the average normal value is 24 mEq/L, with physiological limits of 22-26 mEq/L.
Astrup also pointed out the linear relationship between pH and log PCO_2, allowing it to measure blood PCO_2 when the specific Severinghaus electrode was not yet available.
In 1948 R.B. Singer and A.B. Hastings measured the total concentration of blood buffer bases – buffer base (BB)

by titration procedures from physiological values up to neutral values.

They achieved an average normal value of around 40 mEq/L, which includes bicarbonate and non-bicarbonate buffer bases, namely HCO_3^-, plasma proteins (especially albumin), inorganic plasma phosphates, and hemoglobin.

These studies were resumed and further developed by O. Siggaard-Andersen, who defined the measurement of the buffer bases of the whole blood as the amount of acid or base that must be added to the blood to bring the pH to 7.40 while maintaining the PCO_2 at 40 mmHg at 37 °C.

The index thus obtained is expressed not in absolute values but in relative terms with the normal average value equal to zero, normal limits ± 2 mEq/L. In other words, the deficit or excess of bases is measured, therefore the denomination base excess (BE), whose traditional formulation is expressed in the Van Slyke equation:

$$\mathbf{BE = (HCO_3^- - 24.4 + [2.3 \times Hb + 7.7] \times [pH - 7.4]) \times (1 - 0.023 \times Hb)} \quad (3)$$

This equation was then reworked in an "alignment nomogram" where the values calculated at various pH at different hemoglobin concentrations are reported, so that it is easy to detect the BE value simply from the blood gas profile.

In addition to a more accurate quantitative evaluation of the acid-base alteration, the most important aspect of this diagnostic index is the ability to distinguish between respiratory and metabolic disorders. In fact, in respiratory disorders (i.e. acidosis) the buffer response is

$$CO_2d \rightarrow H^+ + HCO_3^-$$
$$\downarrow$$
$$HT \leftarrow H^+ + T^-$$

where HT/T^- are the non-bicarbonate buffers, the only ones that can intervene in pH defense in these acid-base disorders.

As can be seen in the buffer reaction scheme, for each HCO_3^- produced, a T^- buffer base is consumed, so that buffer base, i.e. the sum HCO_3^- + T^-, remains unchanged, and therefore BE = 0. Instead, in metabolic acidosis (for example), the buffer reaction involves both bicarbonate buffer and non-bicarbonate buffers

$$H^+ + \begin{cases} \nearrow + HCO_3^- \rightarrow CO_2 \\ \searrow + T^- \rightarrow HT \end{cases}$$

therefore the sum $[HCO_3^-] + [T^-]$, that is BE, varies, decreasing in the metabolic acidosis and increasing in the metabolic alkalosis.

Nevertheless, the validity of these diagnostic indicators is limited by the fact that they are defined, determined, and calculated in vitro, and do not take into account the in vivo distribution of bicarbonate and other buffer bases. They do not remain limited to the vascular space but spread in the wider extracellular compartment, and in certain conditions even in the intracellular compartment: therefore there is no certainty that a deficit or a base excess is a specific index of a metabolic disorder, as the theory claims.

The limitations of BE were highlighted above all by the studies of researchers at the Boston school, which we will discuss later, and thus stimulated the elaboration of a correction of BE, the standard base excess (SBE). It is calculated in a similar way to the traditional BE, but at a hemoglobin concentration of 50 g/L, approximately the average concentration of the hemoglobin extended to the extracellular space, thus simulating the extension of the calculation of buffer bases to all that compartment. The SBE is in fact also called BE_{ECF}

$$\mathbf{SBE = 0.9287 \times (HCO_3^- - 24.4 + 14.83 \times [pH - 7.4]} \quad (4)$$

So, after corrected, this indicator has certainly improved its diagnostic reliability. As we shall see later, in more recent years, further integrations with specific correction factors allow their placement among the currently most widespread diagnostic interpretation criteria.

The Boston school: the physiological limits of in vivo adaptation

Researchers at the Boston school (W. Schwartz, A. Relman, R.W. Winters, K. Engel, R.B. Dell) who highlighted the inadequacy of BE, developed diagnostic criteria, this time not more in vitro but in vivo. Using the blood gas parameters pH, PCO_2, HCO_3^- in statistically valid samples of patients affected by simple acid-base disorders, that is certainly not complicated by mixed forms, both respiratory and metabolic, they compared the parameter that measures the magnitude of the disorder (PCO_2 in respiratory disorders, HCO_3^- in those of metabolic type) with the parameter that measures the response of defense and adaptation (HCO_3^- in respiratory disorders, PCO_2 in metabolic disorders).

The results of these studies made it possible to ascertain that in simple acid-base disorders of both respiratory and metabolic type: 1) the adaptation response is reproducible and predictable with 95% confidence interval; 2) in the absence of corrective therapeutic interventions, the adaptation response, while limiting the alteration of the blood pH, is not able to restore normal values, except for the chronic forms of respiratory alkalosis.

The adaptation limits thus determined, called physiological adaptation limits "in vivo" have been calculated with a 95% probability for each of the simple acid-base disorders of both respiratory and metabolic type (**Table 3.1**) and constitute over fifty years the most useful and reliable diagnostic evaluation criteria in clinical practice, as will be amply demonstrated in the following chapters. In addition to blood gas parameters, the physiological adaptation limits were also calculated for BE (Table 3.1).

Alongside these advances in the interpretation of the blood gas profile, since the 1970s, thanks above all to M. Emmett, R.G. Narins, D.W. Seldin, G. Giebisch, M.L. Halperin, M.B. Goldstein, the importance of plasma electrolytic profile, and frequently also the urinary, has become increasingly evident in the diagnostic interpretation of acid-base disorders.

Figure 3.1 lists the diagnostic indications that can provide a change in the ratio between sodium and plasma chloride. The normal ratio is on average 1.4:1.0 (Na^+ 140 mEq/L, Cl^- 100 mEq/L). As is known, the main alterations of these electrolytes are due to pathologies of water-electrolyte homeostasis, alterations that however retain the normal Na^+/Cl^- ratio.

Therefore, alterations of these electrolytes with alteration of their relationship are an indication of another pathology.

Alterations of plasmatic chloride alone, with preservation of sodium in normal values, are an indication of an acid-base disorder: for example, a decrease in plasma chloride without a decrease in sodium suggests a metabolic alkalosis.

If there is also an alteration of the plasma sodium, however disproportionate compared to the normal Na^+/Cl^- ratio, there is an indication of the coexistence of a water-electrolyte disorder and an acid-base disorder: for example, a hypernatremia with a decrease in

TABLE 3.1 Expected adaptations in simple acid-base disorders.

Disorder	PCO_2 or SBE response	PCO_2 or HCO_3^- response
Acute respiratory acidosis	SBE = 0 ± 2 mmol/L	HCO_3^- increases by 0.1 mEq/L for each 1 mmHg increase in PCO_2
Chronic respiratory acidosis	SBE + 0.4 x (PCO_2 – 40)	HCO_3^- increases by 0.35 mEq/L for each 1 mmHg increase in PCO_2
Acute respiratory alkalosis	SBE = 0 ± 2 mmol/L	HCO_3^- decreases by 0.2 mEq/L for each 1 mmHg decrease in PCO_2
Chronic respiratory alkalosis	SBE = – 0.4 x (PCO_2 – 40)	HCO_3^- decreases by 0.4 mEq/L for each 1 mmHg decrease in PCO_2
Metabolic acidosis	Δ PCO_2 = SBE	PCO_2 decreases by 1.2 mmHg for each 1 mEq/L decrease in HCO_3^-
Metabolic alkalosis	Δ PCO_2 = + 0.6 SBE	PCO_2 increases by 0.7 mmHg for each 1 mEq/L increase in HCO_3^-

SBE: standard base excess.

SODIUM/CHLORIDE RATIO IN ACID-BASE DIAGNOSIS

Proportionate variations (Na^+) e (Cl^-) (1.4:1.0)
Disorders of water-electrolyte balance

Variations of (Cl^-), but not (Na^+)
Acid-base disorder
(Cl^-) ↓ respiratory acidosis or metabolic alkalosis
(Cl^-) ↑ respiratory alkalosis or hyperchloremic metabolic acidosis

Disproportionate variations of (Na^+) and (Cl^-)
Disorders of water balance + acid-base disorders
(Na^+) ↑ (Cl^-) n ↓ dehydration + resp. ac. or met. alk.
(Na^+) ↓ (Cl^-) n ↑ hyperhydratation + resp. alk. or hyperchloremic met. ac.
(Na^+) ↑ (Cl^-) ↓↓ hyperhydratation + resp. ac. or met. alk.
(Na^+) ↑ (Cl^-) ↑↑ dehydration + resp. alk. or hyperchloremic met. ac.

Figure 3.1 Variations in the Na^+/Cl^- ratio.
By the term hyperhydratation and dehydration, in this context, it is meant that the total body water is increased or decreased respectively with reference to the total body sodium.

plasma chloride is an indication of a water deficit state associated with primary or secondary metabolic alkalosis. Since chloride follows sodium in its concentration variations, in cases where it is not clear how much chloride value depends on the variations of sodium or chloride itself, it is useful to calculate the sodium/chloride ratio which, as written above, is 1.4.

Variations of ± 0.15 of the value of this ratio point towards an acid-base disorder; in the sense of primary or secondary metabolic alkalosis, when the value of the ratio increases and in the sense of the hyperchloremic metabolic acidosis when it is reduced. Naturally these directions have an indicative value, useful for a first evaluation which must be followed by a confirmatory analysis.

The electrolyte profile is however an useful aid in acid-base diagnosis, which is frequently the diagnostic resolution rather than the blood gas profile, and is almost always indispensable in the evaluation of therapeutic treatment.

Stewart: SID, SIG, dependent and independent variables

What Stewart proposed in the 1980s, although hailed as a "Copernican revolution", is not a new theory, but rather an interpretation of the acid-base biochemistry that strictly respects the physico-chemical principles. According to this interpretation, the acid-base balance depends only on three independent variables: 1) the difference between strong ions, strong ion difference (SID); 2) total nonvolatile weak acids (Atot), mainly inorganic phosphate and albumin, considered as such and not as a function of their possible buffer function; 3) PCO_2, the only familiar member whose alterations can cause respiratory acid-base disorders.

Since we alredy discussed this last independent variable both in its physiological and pathophysiological aspects, we instead turn our attention to the other two, emphasizing that only on these depends the acid-base balance, including blood pH and bicarbonate, secondary and dependent entities (above all these statements suggested the title of "Copernican revolution").

With the difference between strong ions, the physiological biochemistry of body fluids electrolyte composition, particularly the plasma one, takes on fundamental importance in the acid-base balance.

The strong ions are those completely dissociated in body fluids, in analogy with the strong acids as we have described in Chapter 2: among the main cations sodium, potassium, calcium, magnesium; among the main anions chloride.

In aqueous solution pH remains neutral if anions and cations are in equivalent concentration (**Figure 3.2**); if anions concentration is greater than cations concentration, the excess of the negative charges is neutralized by water that dissociates H^+ up to cover the difference: the result is an acid solution; if on the other hand it is the cations that exceed, like in plasma, water dissociates OH^-, making the solution alkaline, just as it is in blood plasma.

Therefore a solution is acid or alkaline, not because H^+ have been added or removed, but because alterations

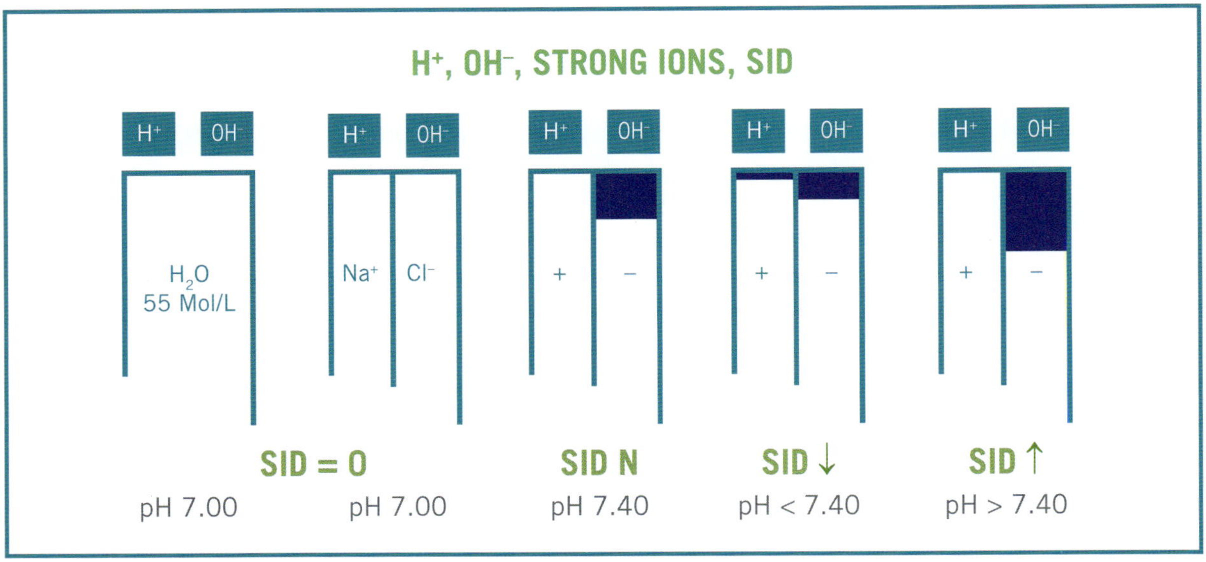

Figure 3.2 Difference between strong ions, SID.

of the positive or negative charges have caused a SID variation.

In normal plasma the difference between strong cations and strong anions is about 40 mEq/L, with cationic excess: in the most simplified form this difference, called apparent SID, is calculated by the formula

$$SID_{app} = [Na^+] + [K^+] - [Cl^-] \quad (5)$$

As shown in **Figure 3.3**, the space corresponding to the anionic difference is occupied by the plasmatic components that we already know and that we have seen performing, at least according to the traditional interpretation, an important function in acid-base homeostasis: bicarbonate, proteins (in particular albumin), inorganic phosphates: in other words bicarbonate and non-bicarbonate buffers, as we described in the Chapter on physiological biochemistry.

The SID is therefore identified with these buffers, and is also identified with the buffer bases or base excess of Siggaard-Andersen.

Stewart himself, in order to avoid possible uncertainties of an index calculated indirectly as the apparent SID, proposes the direct determination of SID by the analytical measurement of bicarbonate, of albumin, and of phosphates, in an additional index that he calls SID effective.

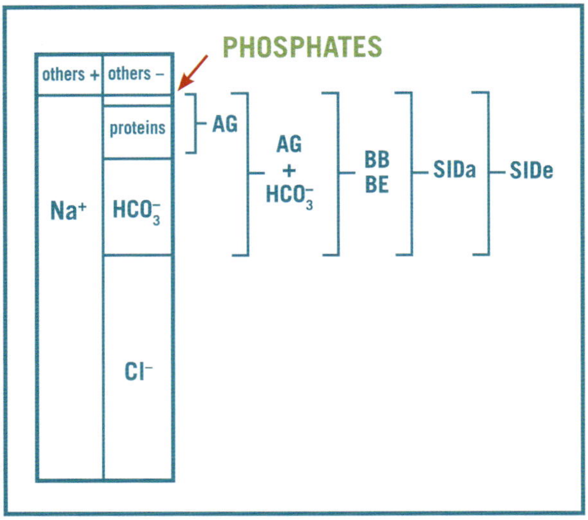

Figure 3.3 Plasmatic electrolyte composition.

According to this interpretation, therefore, in the acid-base physiology the three independent variables now described take on a role of primary importance, while traditional factors such as the buffer defense it-

self and also the physiological adaptations, although admitted, fall back to a very secondary role.
The kidney role remains important, but its intervention mechanism in the acid-base homeostasis is not so much urine acidification by means of titratable acidity and ammoniagenesis, but rather the regulation of electrolytes elimination in order to maintain SID plasmatic composition: that is, urinary SID is regulated so as to preserve or correct plasma SID. In this regulation, chloride takes on a role of primary importance, and its elimination is associated with ammonium, a cation to be eliminated, instead sparing carefully sodium or potassium, cations with physiological importance.
In conclusion, therefore, as can be seen in Figure 3.3, SID is nothing more than the sum of the bicarbonate and non-bicarbonate buffer bases, that is the buffer bases or base excess.
In accordance with the principle of electroneutrality, necessarily SID alterations result in BB or BE alterations.
It is therefore clear how, after a careful analysis, we essentially reach identical conclusions both with the traditional interpretation based on the Henderson equation, and with Stewart's interpretation based on SID, Atot, PCO_2, as most clinical studies in literature demonstrate.

The anion gap

This parameter is limited to the diagnosis of metabolic acidosis, but it is however of not secondary importance, because it allows to distinguish the two main groups of this acid-base disorder.
The anion gap (AG) includes, in fact, in the anion column of the plasma electrolyte composition, the anions of the organic and inorganic acids produced by the metabolism (Figure 3.3), which are not usually measured, and whose increase indicates that the cause of the acidosis is due to the increase of one or more of these metabolic acids.
Based on plasma electrolyte composition, it is calculated subtracting main cations from anions.
In the simplest and most commonly spread form in clinical practice

$$\mathbf{AG = [Na^+] - ([Cl^-] + [HCO_3^-])} \quad (6)$$

with normal values between 12 ± 4 mEq/L, which increase to 16 ± 4 mEq/L if potassium is also included among the cations. The AG can also be defined as the difference between unmeasured anions (UA) and unmeasured cations (UC) (Figure 3.3).
Since all the inorganic and organic acids produced by cellular metabolism have pK much lower than the physiological pH, they behave like strong acids dissociating completely, therefore the released H^+ accumulated in the blood, combine with the extra- and intracellular bicarbonate and non-bicarbonate buffers, while the corresponding anion remains in the plasma where it replaces the buffer bases consumed in pH defense reactions, adding itself to the unmeasured anions that form the anion gap, increasing its plasma concentration.
The AG clinical utility also extends to mixed disorders diagnosis, an aspect of particular interest in critically ill patients, where complex acid-base disorders are more the rule than the exception, as will be amply illustrated in the following chapters. Starting from the assumption that the anion increase – and therefore of the AG – must be stoichiometrically equivalent to the H^+ consumed in the buffer reaction, and therefore to the decrease of HCO_3^-, the buffer most immediately involved in the defense reaction, there must be stoichiometric equivalence between the increase of the AG (ΔAG) and the decrease of the HCO_3^- (ΔHCO_3^-), that is the ratio Δ/Δ (as it is symbolized) must be around 1:1. If the decrease in HCO_3^- is disproportionate (≥ 6 mEq/L) compared to the increase in AG, it means that there is another cause of HCO_3^- decrease, therefore another non AG metabolic acidosis that is added to AG acidosis. If, on the other hand, the decrease in HCO_3^- is lower (≤ 6mEq/L) than expected from the increase in AG, the presence of a metabolic alkalosis in addition to AG acidosis can be suspected.
In reality the ratio Δ/Δ 1:1 is simplistic, because it does not take into account the participation of other non-bi-

carbonate buffers, the different space of distribution of hydrogen ions and of the conjugated base, and the duration of acidosis. Studies report variable values for the different metabolic acids, with limits ranging from 0.8:1 to 1.8:1.

Diagnostic criteria, revision and correction of diagnostic indices

The evolution of the diagnostic criteria of metabolic acidosis has promoted an important revision and correction of traditional diagnostic indices.
First of all the anion gap calculation, where a correction has been inserted that takes into account any variations in plasma albumin:

$$AG_{corr} = AG_{obs} + 0.25 \times ([Albumin]_{nor} - [Albumin]_{obs}) \quad (7)$$

Regarding Atot, based on equilibrium constants, concentration, and buffer capacity, the equivalent values in mmol/L were calculated for each component both for the total concentration and for the part dissociated as anion:

[Albumin]: total 15 mmol/L, [Albumin⁻] 12 mmol/L

[Globulin]: total 4.52 mmol/L, [Globulin⁻] 3.65 mmol/L

[Phosphates]: total 1.00 mmol/L, [Phosphates⁻] 0.85 mmol/L

From which

$$[A_{tot}] = 15 + 4.5 + 1 \text{ mmol/L} = 20.5 \text{ mmol/L} \quad (8)$$

$$[A_{tot}]^- = 12 + 3.65 + 0.85 = 16.6 \text{ mmol/L} \quad (9)$$

These, together with the HCO_3^- anion (average concentration value of 24.5 mmol/L), form the overall average value of 41.1 mmol/L, which is the average value of both the SID, the BB and BE.
The interrelation between the water-electrolyte equilibrium and the acid-base balance, whose emphasis is also due to the interpretative Stewart's theory, has also promoted correction factors to be taken into account in the evaluation of electrolyte alterations and of BE (**Table 3.2**).
To better understand these interrelationships, consider for example a patient with initial Na^+ and Cl^- values of 140 and 100 mEq/L respectively, therefore with SID = 40 mEq/L: if enough water is added to the extracellular space to dilute at half the concentrations, the $[Na^+]$ and $[Cl^-]$ halve to 70 and 50 mEq/L respectively, and the SID also halves to 20 mEq/L, with consequent deviation of the pH in acid direction. Apart from these more exemplary than real alterations, it is clear, however, that sodium and chloride levels in particular are affected to a greater or lesser extent by the alterations in free water balance. Therefore, it is appropriate to correct the chloride concentration based on the sodium concentration:

$$[Cl^-]_{corr} = (140 / [Na^+]) \times [Cl^-] \quad (10)$$

The BE also has been integrated with correction factors: first of all the SBE, which we have discussed above, has been further corrected to take into account the instability that can derive from variations of the PCO_2 (12):

$$SBE_{corr} = (HCO_3^- - 24.4) + ([8.3 \times albumin \times 0.15] + [0.29 \times phosphate \times 0.32]) \times (pH - 7.4) \quad (11)$$

TABLE 3.2 Variables indicative of metabolic acidosis according to the traditional method, BE, Stewart.

	Anion gap	Physical-chemical	Base excess
Free water excess	—	↓ SID ↓ $[Na^+]$	$-BE_{fw}$
Hyperchloremia	↔AG ↑ $[Cl^-]$	↓ SID ↑ $[Cl^-]_{corr}$	$-BE_{Cl^-}$
Unmeasured anions	↑ AG_{corr}	↓ SID ↑ SIG	$-BE_{XA^-}$
Hyperalbuminemia	↓ AG_{corr}	↑ [Albumin]	$-BE_{Alb}$

corr = corrected; obs = observed; nor = normal; tot = total

Furthermore, also based on the pathophysiological principles that can cause a metabolic acid-base disorder – deficit or excess of free water, chloride alterations, alterations of plasma proteins, in particular albumin; accumulation of unmeasured anions – Gilfix and coll showed that BE as supplied by the laboratory is the sum of these four components:

$$\mathbf{BE_{lab} = BE_{fw} + BE_{Cl^-} + BE_{alb} + BE_{XA^-}} \quad (12)$$

where BE_{fw} is the component due to free water, BE_{Cl-} the one due to chloride, BE_{alb} is due to albumin and BE_{XA-} the one due to metabolic acids. The correction factors for each component were calculated:

$$\mathbf{BE_{fw}\ (mEq/L) = 0.3\ ([Na^+] - 140)} \quad (13)$$

$$\mathbf{BE_{Cl^-}\ (mEq/L) = 102 - [Cl^-]_{corr}} \quad (14)$$

$$\mathbf{BE_{Alb}\ (mEq/L) = 0.34\ ([Albumin\ g/L]_{nor} - [Albumin\ g/L])_{obs}} \quad (15)$$

BE_{XA-} is calculated by difference from (12) once the other three components are known.

Conclusion

Three methods are currently available (physiological approach, base excess approach and physico-chemical approach) for the diagnostic interpretation of acid-base disorders, whose theoretical and pathophysiological assumptions are equally valid.

A useful criterion of choice is the correlation of the diagnostic indicators proposed with mortality prediction. Since it has been shown that the mortality in lactic acidosis (56%) and in acidosis from organic non-lactate anions (39%) is significantly higher than in hyperchloremic acidosis (29%) and in controls (25%), the identification of unmeasured anions takes on primary diagnostic importance.

Clinical studies of comparison between the three methods are now numerous in literature, and almost all show an excellent correlation between the different interpretative criteria.

The AG method is based on an extended length of service and is familiar in clinical practice: however, its validity requires an empirical correction factor for albumin variability.

Furthermore, the simplistic assumptions for the calculation of Δ/Δ can limit its diagnostic sensitivity. Finally, it does not take into account the correction of chloride due to free water alterations.

The BE, especially its version calculated for the extracellular space, BE standard, is also very useful and is widely used in clinical practice, especially as, it has been sensitized and improved with the corrections we have described above. Stewart's method is precise and accurate, – even if the "Copernican revolution" with which it was announced is not revealed by careful examination – it has its admirers, and has had the merit of stimulating insights and important clarifications in many concepts and principles of acid-base biochemistry.

References

- Adroguè HJ, Gennari FJ, Galla JH et al. Assessing acid-base disorders. Kidney Int. 2009;76(12):1239-47.
- Albert MS, Dell RB, Winters RW. Quantitative displacement of acid-base equilibrium in metabolic acidosis. Ann Intern Med. 1967;66(2):312-22.
- Anstey CM. Comparision of three strong ion models used for quantifying the acid-base status of human plasma with special emphasis on the plasma weak acids. J Appl Physiol. 2005;98(6):2119-25.
- Asch MJ, Dell RB, Williams GS et al. Time course for development of respiratory compensation in metabolic acidosis. J Lab and Clin Med. 1969;73(4):610-5.
- Boron WF, Boulpaep EL. Medical physiology: a cellular and molecular approach. Philadelphia. Elsevier Saunders 2005.
- Chawla LS, Shih S, Davison D et al. Anion gap, anion gap corrected for albumin, base deficit and unmeasured anions in critically ill patients: implications on the assessement of metabolic acidosis and the diagnosis of hyperlactatemia. BMC Emerg Med. 2008;8:1-18.
- Constable PD. Clinical assessement of acid-base status: comparison of the Henderson-Hasselbalch and strong ion approaches. Vet Clin Pathol. 2000;29(4):115-28.
- Doberer D, Funk GC, Kirchner K et al. A critique of Stewart's approach: the chemical mechanism of dilutional acidosis. Intensive Care Med. 2009;35(12):2173-80.

- Emmett M. Anion gap interpretation: the old and the new. Nat Clin Pract Nephrol. 2006;2(1):4-5.
- Emmett M, Narins RG. Clinical use of the anion gap. Medicine (Baltimore). 1977;56(1):38-54.
- Feldman M, Soni N, Dickson B. Influence of hypoalbuminemia or hyperalbuminemia on the serum anion gap. J Lab Clin Med. 2005;146(6):317-20.
- Fidkowski C, Helstrom J. Diagnosing metabolic acidosis in the critically ill: bridging the anion gap, Stewart, and base excess methods. Can J Anaesth. 2009;56(3):247-56.
- Figge J, Jabor A, Kazda A et al. Anion gap and hypoalbuminemia. Crit Care Med. 1998;26(11):1807-10.
- Filley GF. Acid-Base and Blood Gas Regulation. Philadelphia. Lea & Febiger 1971.
- Gabow PA. Disorders associated with an altered anion gap. Kidney Int. 1985;27(2):472-83.
- Gabow PA, Kaehny WD, Fennessey PV et al. Diagnostic importance of an increased serum anion gap. N Eng J Med. 1980;303(15):854-8.
- Gattinoni L, Carlesso E, Maiocchi G et al. Dilutional acidosis: where do the protons come from? Intensive Care Med. 2009;35(12):2033-43.
- Gilfix BM, Bique M, Magder S. A physical chemical approach to the analysis of acid-base balance in the clinical setting. J Crit Care. 1993;8(4):187-97.
- Hasselbalch, KA. Die Berechnung der Wasserstoffzahl des Blutes aus der freien und gebundenen Kohlensäure desselben und die Sauerstoffbindung des Blutes als Funktion der Wasserstoffzahl. Biochem Z. 1917;78:112-44.
- Henderson LJ. The theory of neutrality regulation in the animal organism. Am J Physiol. 1908;21:427-48.
- Jones NL. Blood gases and acid-base physiology. 2nd ed. New York. Thieme Medical Publishers 1987.
- Jorgensen K, Astrup P. Standard bicarbonate, its clinical significance, and a new method for its determination. Scand J Clin Lab Invest. 1957;9(2):122-32.
- Kassirer JP, Bleich HL. Rapid estimation of plasma carbon dioxide tension from pH and total carbon dioxide content. N Engl J Med. 1965;272:1067-8.
- Kellum JA, Elbers PWG. Stewart's textbook of acid-base. 2nd ed. Amsterdam, AcidBase.org 2009.
- Kraut JA, Madias NE. Serum anion gap: its uses and limitations in clinical medicine. Clin J Am Soc Nephrol. 2007;2(1):162-74.
- Kurtz I, Kraut J, Ornekian V et al. Acid-base analysis: a critique of the Stewart and bicarbonate-centered approaches. Am J Physiol Renal Physiol. 2008;294(5):1009-31.
- Lang W, Zander R. The accuracy of calculated base excess in blood. Clin Chem Lab Med. 2002;40(4):404-10.
- Levraut J, Bounatirou T, Ichai C et al. Reliability of anion gap as an indicator of blood lactate in critically ill patients. Intensive Care Med. 1997;23(4):417-22.
- Matousek S, Handy J, Rees SE. Acid-base chemistry of plasma: consolidation of the traditional and modern approaches from a mathematical and clinical perspective. J Clin Monit Comput. 2011;25(1):57-70.
- Narins RG, Emmett M. Simple and mixed acid-base disorders: a practical approach. Medicine (Baltimore). 1980;59(3):161-87.
- Narins RG, Gardner LB. Simple acid-base disturbances. Med Clin North Am. 1981;65(2):321-46.
- Nguyen MK, Kao L, Kurtz I. Calculation of the equilibrium pH in a multiple-buffered aqueous solution based on partitioning of proton buffering: a new predictive formula. Am J Physiol Renal Physiol. 2009;296(6):1521-9.
- Oh MS, Carrol HJ. The anion gap. N Engl J Med. 1977;297(15):814-7.
- Park M, Macil A, Noritomo D et al. Effect of pCO_2(a) variation on standard base excess value in critically ill patients. J Crit Care. 2009;24:484-91.
- Peake MJ, White GH. Arterial blood gas analysis: selecting the clinically appropriate option for calculating base excess. Ann Clin Biochem. 2002;39(Pt 6):614-5.
- Rastegar A. Use of the DeltaAG/DeltaHCO_3^- ratio in the diagnosis of mixed acid-base disorders. J Am Soc Nephrol. 2007;18(9):2429-31.
- Robinson JR. Fundamentals of acid-base regulation. Oxford. Blackwell Scientific Publications 1961.
- Schlichtig R, Grogono AW, Severinghaus JW. Human $PaCO_2$ and standard base excess compensation for acid-base imbalance. Crit Care Med. 1998;26(7):1173-9.
- Schwartz WB, Relman AS. A critique of the parameters used in the evaluation of acid-base disorders. N Engl J Med. 1963;268:1382-8.
- Severinghaus JW. Siggaard-Andersen and the "Great Trans-Atlantic Acid–Base Debate". Scand J Clin Lab Invest Suppl. 1993;214:99-104.
- Severinghaus JW, Bradley AF. Electrodes for blood pO_2 and pCO_2 determination. J Appl Physiol. 1958;13:515-20.
- Siggaard-Andersen O. The van Slyke equation. Scand J Clin Lab Invest Suppl. 1977;146:15-20.
- Siggaard-Andersen O. Titratable acid or base of body fluids. Ann N Y Acad Sci. 1966;133(1):41-58.
- Siggaard-Andersen O, Engel K. A new acid-base nomogram. An improved method for the calculation of the relevant blood acid-base data. Scand J Clin Lab Invest. 1960;12:177-86.
- Siggaard-Andersen O, Engel K, Jorgensen K et al. A micro method for determination of pH carbon dioxide tension, base excess and standard bicarbonate in capillary blood. Scand J Clin Lab Invest. 1960;12:172-6.
- Siggaard-Anderson O, Fogh-Andersen N. Base excess or buffer base (strong ion difference) as measure of a non-respiratory acid-base disturbance. Acta Anaesthesiol Scand Suppl. 1995;107:123-8.
- Singer RB, Hastings AB. An improved clinical method for the estimation of disturbances of the acid-base balance of human blood. Medicine (Baltimore). 1948;27(2):223-42.
- Stewart PA. Modern quantitative acid-base chemistry. Can J Physiol Pharmacol. 1983;61(12):1444-61.
- Story DA, Morimatsu H, Bellomo R. Strong ions, weak acids and base excess: a simplified Fencl-Stewart approach to clinical acid-base disorders. Br J Anaesth. 2004;92(1):54-60.
- White A, Handler P, Smith EL et al. Principles of Biochemistry. New York. McGraw-Hill 1959.

Clinical interpretation of simple acid-base disorders

Ivo Casagranda

Introduction

Doctors and medical students consider the study of acid-base balance to be particularly difficult and complex and are convinced that its interpretation requires specific knowledge of chemistry and biochemistry. Probably this attitude is due to the fact that for years it has been considered indispensable, to correctly interpret the acid-base disorders, to study in depth Henderson-Hasselbalch equation and the way in which it was derived. Furthermore, many textbooks dealing with this topic focus mainly at the presentation of simple disorders, barely mentioning or ignoring mixed disorders that are very frequent in clinical activity.

In a case series of Song, referring to critically ill patients, the simple disorders were 20% (64% metabolic acidosis, 21% respiratory alkalosis, 14% respiratory acidosis and 1% metabolic alkalosis) and the mixed ones 80%. Among the double the two most frequent disorders were metabolic acidosis + respiratory alkalosis and respiratory acidosis + metabolic acidosis.

In a case series of the Author of about 300 patients arrived in the emergency department, where blood gas analysis was indicated, 35% were normal, 33% had a simple disorder and 32% a mixed disorder.

In this chapter a step by step method will be presented and rules will be proposed, some of which already discussed in the previous chapters, which will be the keys to opening the interpretative doors of acid-base disorders.

Consistent with the textbook and chapter title, each disorder will be introduced by a clinical case that will represent the main educational tool and will be the track covered in the discussion of the single topic. Before discussing the contents of this section it is important to have read and studied Chapters two and three.

Arterial blood gas parameters

Before discussing the interpretation of acid-base disorders, it was decided to insert a table with the measured and calculated blood gas parameters and the normal ranges referred to arterial blood (**Table 4.1**).

TABLE 4.1 Arterial blood gas parameters and normal values.

pH	7.35-7.45
$PaCO_2$	35-45 mmHg
HCO_3^-	22-26 mEq/L
PaO_2	70-100 mmHg*
SaO_2	95-98%
P50	24-28 mmHg
FO_2Hb	94-99%
FHHb	<9%
FCOHb	<3%
FMetHb	<2%
Hb	12-16 g/dL
$P(A\text{-}a)O_2$	Age/4 + 4
P/F	>300**
CaO_2	16-22 mLO_2/dL
Serum lactate	<1.6 mmol/L
Serum sodium	135-145 mEq/L
Serum potassium	3.5-5.0 mEq/L
Serum chloride	95-105 mEq/L
AG $Na^+ - (Cl^- + HCO_3^-)$	12 ± 4 mEq/L
Base excess	0 ± 2 mEq/L

* PaO_2 varies with age and position (lying/sitting).

** Berlin definition of ARDS (2012).

For completeness, values concerning oxygenation have also been included, even if there will be no specific treatment.
There are many arterial blood gas parameters currently available to the clinician, but some of these are of little use in daily practice. Only the basic parameters for the clinical activity are presented in the table.

NOTE

For the correct interpretation of some parameters it is advisable to read the following clarifications.
Actual and standard bicarbonate (HCO_3^-) – To date, blood gas analysis equipment do not directly measure blood bicarbonate concentration. This parameter is calculated using the Henderson-Hasselbalch equation starting from pH and PCO_2. The resolution of this equation provides the so-called actual bicarbonate and is the one that should be routinely evaluated and that will be used, in this text, in the discussion of clinical cases. The standard bicarbonate refers instead to the concentration of plasma bicarbonate of a blood sample in its entirety, in equilibrium with a gas mixture with $PO_2 > 100$ mmHg and $PCO_2 = 40$ mmHg at a temperature of 37 °C. The standard bicarbonate is devoid of the respiratory component, so a reduction in plasma concentration of the standard bicarbonate indicates metabolic acidosis, while an increase of the same metabolic alkalosis. It should be emphasized that measured pH and PCO_2 determine only the actual bicarbonate, whose values in arterial blood vary from 22 to 26 mEq/L.
Base excess/Base deficit – The base excess (BE) expresses the amount of strong acid that must be added to a liter of completely oxygenated blood to bring pH back to 7.40, at a temperature of 37 °C and a PCO_2 of 40 mmHg. The base deficit expresses, on the contrary, the quantity of strong bases that must be added under the same conditions to reach pH of 7.40. In the laboratory practice two other variables are also used: *actual base excess* (ABE) which is actually present in blood and *standard base excess* (SBE), whose value is expressed with hemoglobin at 5 g/dL and better expresses the BE in extracellular fluids. In practice, this diagnostic index (BE) is the sum of blood buffer bases $[HCO_3^-] + [T^-]$ (non-bicarbonate buffer bases), whose average normal value is 48 mEq/L and which is expressed in relative terms with the value of 0 mEq/L with a normal range of ± 2 mEq/L. The diagnostic interest of this index is that it would allow to distinguish a pure respiratory acid-base disorder from a mixed metabolic-respiratory disorder. In this textbook the BE is not used in the interpretation of acid-base disorders, because it is not very effective.

The role of the Kassirer-Bleich equation in the understanding of acid-base disorders

The Kassirer-Bleich equation is very useful for understanding the relationship between $[H^+]$, PCO_2 and $[HCO_3^-]$ and to understand how, as a equation term changes, there must be a variation of the other to keep hydrogen ions concentration constant. Depending on how these variations occur, we get very useful elements for correctly interpreting acid-base disorders:

$$[H^+]\ \text{nmol/L} = 24 \times \frac{PCO_2}{[HCO_3^-]}$$

This equation tells us that serum concentration of the hydrogen ions $[H^+]$ is directly proportional to blood CO_2 partial pressure (PCO_2) and inversely proportional to the concentration of serum bicarbonate $[HCO_3^-]$; furthermore, it suggests that $[H^+]$ remains constant until the $PCO_2/[HCO_3^-]$ ratio does not change.
As is known, the hydrogen ions concentration in solution is commonly expressed in pH units (pH = – log10 $[H^+]$ Eq/L).
This way of expressing $[H^+]$ is especially useful for very low concentrations, such as those present in blood or other biological liquids.

The well-known Henderson-Hasselbalch equation (pH = 6.10 + log [HCO_3^-]/0.03 PCO_2) expresses, in an inverse proportional way, the [H^+] in the blood (see Chapter 2, page 28).
pH determination starting from [H^+] is possible with the use of specific conversion tables or the calculator (**Table 4.2**).
The table shows the inverse and non-linear relationship between hydrogen ions concentration and pH (the more [H^+] increases the more the pH drops). Changes in pH from 7.40 to 7.10 are equal to the doubling of hydrogen ions.

TABLE 4.2 Conversion table of [H^+] expressed in nmol/L to pH.

[H^+] nmol/L	pH
16	7.80
20	7.70
26	7.60
32	7.50
40	7.40
50	7.30
63	7.20
80	7.10
100	7.00
125	6.90
160	6.80

Clinical case A 28-year-old diabetic woman arrives in the emergency department with a fever and dyspnea.
After clinical evaluation, blood chemistry tests are required including arterial blood gas (ABG).
The ABG report shows the following values: $PaCO_2$ 28 mmHg, HCO_3^- 14 mEq/L. The blood glucose is 479 mg/dL and the search for urinary ketone bodies is positive (++ – –).

$$[H^+]\ \text{nmol/L} = 24 \times \frac{28}{14} = 48$$

The Kassirer-Bleich equation tells us that the hydrogen ions concentration [H^+] is 48 nmol/L which corresponds to a pH of 7.32.
The patient is then sent to the internal medicine ward with a diagnosis of diabetic ketoacidosis and subjected to insulin therapy and normal saline infusion. Two hours after admission the general conditions seem to have improved, but not the dyspnea.
A new ABG is performed: $PaCO_2$ 33 mmHg, HCO_3^- 14 mEq/L. The blood glucose is 350 mg/dL.

$$[H^+]\ \text{nmol/L} = 24 \times \frac{33}{14} = 56\ (\text{pH } 7.25)$$

Six hours after admission, the patient's condition declines with worsening dyspnea. Chest X-ray shows significant parenchymal densification of most of the lung right lower lobe. Subsequently a third ABG is carried out: $PaCO_2$ 49 mmHg, HCO_3^- 18 mEq/L, blood glucose 230 mg/dL.

$$[H^+]\ \text{nmol/L} = 24 \times \frac{49}{18} = 65\ (\text{pH } 7.18)$$

What does the Kassirer-Bleich equation supported by the clinical case tell us?
In addition to highlighting the lung role in eliminating volatile acids (CO_2) and kidney in eliminating fixed acids (H^+) and regenerating and reabsorbing bicarbonate (HCO_3^-), it suggests four important rules:

1) For the maintenance of [H^+] within tolerable limits, when one of the equation elements increases or decreases, the other follows in the same direction. For example, if the bicarbonate concentration is reduced, $PaCO_2$ must decrease (*first part of the clinical case where the acid-base disorder is a metabolic acidosis*).
2) If one of the elements of the equation increases or decreases, the other follows in the same direction as much as required by the expected adaptation rule. If this does not happen, we are faced with a mixed acid-base disorder (*second part of the clinical case where the disorder is a metabolic acidosis with respiratory acidosis*).
3) If one of the elements of the equation increases or decreases and the other goes in the opposite direction, we are faced, even in this case, with a mixed acid-base disorder (*third part of the clinical case where the disorder is constituted from metabolic acidosis with respiratory acidosis more*

severe than what was found in the second part of the clinical case).

4) In the presence of a simple acid-base disorder, the lack of the adaptation mechanism, due to the occurrence of a second disorder that limits it, determines a sensitive deviation of pH value as is shown, in sequence, in the first, second and third part of the clinical case.

NOTE

If pH, obtained with the conversion table of the $[H^+]$ calculated with the Kassirer-Bleich equation or obtained with the Henderson-Hasselbalch equation is different from the one present on the report obtained from the blood gas analyzer, one should think of an error in the analytical phase, for example problems with pH electrode: this will also determine an error in the calculation of the bicarbonate concentration as it is obtained starting from pH and PCO_2 values.

NOTE

For the expected adaptation rule and its values see page 52.

NOTE

To better understand the clinical case described, it is necessary to consider as a reference value 40 mmHg for $PaCO_2$ and 24 mEq/L for $[HCO_3^-]$.

How to proceed in reading the ABG report and its interpretation

What will be described in the following lines is a method that we consider effective for the interpretation of acid-base alterations and that in addition to the simple disorders allows us to also highlight the mixed double, triple and even quadruple ones. It may not be immediately understandable, but it will become so, at least we hope so, at the end of that step-by-step path explained in the introduction.

Some concepts, already presented in the general part, will be repeated here to link them to the clinical interpretation of the acid-base disorders.

The fundamental steps for a correct interpretation of the acid-base balance are:

- Evaluate the accuracy and reliability of the test.
- Collect the medical history and make the patient's clinical examination.
- Consider by order pH, $PaCO_2$ and $[HCO_3^-]$.
- Identify the primary disorder.
- Evaluate electrolytes and other laboratory data.
- Calculate the anion gap.
- Determine if there is a mixed disorder by thinking about the expected adaptations and the Δgap.
- Calculate the Na^+/Cl^- ratio.
- In some cases measure urine pH and electrolytes and calculate the anion and osmolal gap.

NOTE

For methodological reasons we will discuss later the anion gap, the Δgap and the Na^+/Cl^- ratio.

Test accuracy and reliability

Test accuracy and reliability are fundamental in blood gas analysis process, also considering that 85% of the samples on which the blood gas analysis is performed come from critical areas.

Keeping in mind that some blood gas parameters are not measured, but calculated starting from those measured, it becomes clear how the exam reliability is a fundamental requirement.

According to the National Committee for Clinical Laboratory Standards (NCCLS C27-A), blood gas and pH analysis has greater immediacy and potential impact on patient care than any other laboratory measure and an incorrect result may be more deleterious to the patient than the lack of results.

Patient history and clinical examination

The collection of medical history and a careful clinical examination are fundamental in allowing an accurate interpretation of the acid-base disorders. It is inadvisable to interpret a blood gas report without knowing the patient's clinical conditions to which it refers.

In particular, it is important to collect the pharmacological (i.e., use of diuretics, steroids, etc.) and the toxicological history (i.e., poisoning with ethylene glycol, acetylsalicylic acid, methanol, etc.). It is also essential to know if the patient is suffering from cardiopulmonary or metabolic diseases such as diabetes mellitus. Clinical examination is obviously important to highlight a heart disease and/or a state of hypoxemia (cyanosis, disorders of consciousness), dehydration or shock.

pH, $PaCO_2$ and $[HCO_3^-]$

The meaning of these three variables and their relationships have already been defined in Chapter 2 and at the beginning of this chapter, when the Kassirer-Bleich equation was presented.

pH

pH is the key element to define blood acid-base status. For terminological clarity, the terms acidemia and alkalemia should be distinguished from those of acidosis and alkalosis.

While acidemia and alkalemia respectively mean a reduction or increase in blood pH, acidosis or alkalosis mean the underlying respiratory or metabolic disorder that leads to pH changes.

A pH greater than 7.45 means alkalemia. In this case we will certainly have an acid-base disorder attributable to metabolic and/or respiratory alkalosis.

However, an alkaline pH does not exclude the simultaneous presence of metabolic and/or respiratory acidosis (mixed disorder).

The same is true when pH is lower than 7.35 (acidemia): an acid pH does not exclude the presence of a metabolic or respiratory alkalosis (mixed disorder) (see clinical cases Chapter 5).

A normal pH (7.35-7.45) does not mean the absence of acid-base disorders: in fact, in the presence of abnormal values of $PaCO_2$ and/or $[HCO_3^-]$, indicates the existence of a counterbalancing mixed disorder (the only exception is chronic respiratory alkalosis and according to some Authors also uncomplicated chronic respiratory acidosis at normal pH).

$PaCO_2$

$PaCO_2$ increase over 45 mmHg is a marker of respiratory acidosis and is always determined by alveolar hypoventilation. An increase in $PaCO_2$ is also present during metabolic alkalosis for respiratory adaptation reasons.

$PaCO_2$ reduction below 45 mmHg is instead a marker of respiratory alkalosis and is always determined by alveolar hyperventilation. During metabolic acidosis there is a reduction in $PaCO_2$ for respiratory adaptation reasons.

$[HCO_3^-]$

$[HCO_3^-]$ increase over 26 mEq/L is a marker of metabolic alkalosis. An increase in $[HCO_3^-]$, due to metabolic and renal adaptation, is present during respiratory acidosis.

$[HCO_3^-]$ reduction below 22 mEq/L is a marker of metabolic acidosis.

During respiratory alkalosis there is a reduction of $[HCO_3^-]$ always for reasons of metabolic and renal adaptation.

Identification of primary disorder

At this point, having the patient's clinical picture clear and having a set of measurments offered by the laboratory (pH, $PaCO_2$ and HCO_3^-) in hand, the identification of the primary disorder in simple disorders should not be difficult (**Table 4.3**). In case of mixed disorders (respiratory and/or metabolic), their highlighting is more complex and should follow a path that we will see in the next chapter.

Evaluation of electrolytes

Serum electrolytes evaluation is important and their use is necessary for calculating the anion gap, but not only; just think of chloride ion role in maintaining electroneutrality and how its variation, with modification of the Na^+/Cl^- ratio, can quickly lead us to suspect some

TABLE 4.3 Simple disorders: pH, primary disorder, adaptation mechanism and expected adaptation.

Simple disorder	pH	Primary disorder (marker of the disorder)	Adaptation mechanism	Expected adaptation
Acute respiratory acidosis	↓	↑ $PaCO_2$	↑ HCO_3^-	**0.1** mEq/L increase in HCO_3^- for every 1 mmHg increase in $PaCO_2$
Chronic respiratory acidosis				**0.35** mEq/L increase in HCO_3^- for each 1 mmHg increase in $PaCO_2$
Acute respiratory alkalosis	↑	↓ $PaCO_2$	↓ HCO_3^-	**0.2** mEq/L reduction of HCO_3^- for each 1 mmHg decrease in $PaCO_2$
Chronic respiratory alkalosis	→			**0.4** mEq/L reduction of HCO_3^- for each 1 mmHg decrease in $PaCO_2$
Metabolic acidosis	↓	↓ HCO_3^-	↓ $PaCO_2$	**1.2** mmHg reduction of $PaCO_2$ for each 1 mEq/L reduction of HCO_3^-
Metabolic alkalosis	↑	↑ HCO_3^-	↑ $PaCO_2$	**0.7** mmHg increase in $PaCO_2$ for each 1 mEq/L increase in HCO_3^-

For practicality the same values can be used multiplied by 10 (for example, for acute respiratory acidosis an increase of 1 mEq/L of HCO_3^- for each increase of 10 mmHg of $PaCO_2$). It is a less precise method but some clinicians find it more immediate.

acid-base disorders (see also Chapter 3, page 41). The attention on blood potassium is fundamental, also for proceding to therapeutic decisions.

Calculation of the anion gap

Anion gap calculation is a fundamental moment in the interpretative path of the blood gas report. The blood gas analyzers which also measure the electrolytes calculate it automatically, printing it in the report.

Its evaluation is important both for the diagnosis of some types of metabolic acidosis and to highlight some mixed disorders through the calculation of Δgap.

For methodological reasons we will deal with these aspects later, when we will study the metabolic acidosis.

Expected adaptations and their clinical use

Expected adaptations were also discussed in Chapter 3, page 40.

The adaptations evaluation together with anion gap calculation is the other pillar that allows us to correctly interpret acid-base disorders (Table 4.3). The reference value for calculation of the expected adaptation for $PaCO_2$ is 40 mmHg, while for $[HCO_3^-]$ it is 24 mEq/L. Here we introduce two rules that will help as soon as we tackle the simple disorders.

First rule of expected adaptation

During acidosis or alkalosis both respiratory and metabolic, the organism tends to bring its pH back within the physiological limits, activating the adaptation mechanisms.

However, adaptation is never complete: pH does not completely normalize. This physiological limit can be calculated in the individual patient (expected adaptation) and its deviation from the theoretical value (with a tolerance of ± 2 or ± 3) is useful to highlight a mixed disorder. The only exception to the rule is chronic respiratory alkalosis, where pH often falls within normal values and, according to some Authors, even chronic uncomplicated respiratory acidosis at normal pH.

Second rule of expected adaptation

A normal pH in the presence of an alteration of both $PaCO_2$ and/or HCO_3^- values means that we are facing not a "compensated" disorder, but a mixed disorder. An exception, as already mentioned, is chronic respiratory alkalosis.

pH, electrolytes, urinary anion gap and urinary osmolal gap

The determination of urinary pH can be useful in the differential diagnosis of some acid-base disorders, while the determination of urinary electrolytes has a greater diagnostic significance: think of the differential diagnosis of metabolic alkalosis or, as we will see later, of renal tubular acidosis (RTA).

The calculation of the urinary anion gap (UAG) may be useful in differential diagnosis of some hyperchloremic metabolic acidosis (**Table 4.4**)

$$\mathbf{UAG = ([Na^+] + [K^+]) - [Cl^-]}$$

the value in normal subjects is equal to zero or has a positive value.

The accuracy of UAG values is not absolute and should be interpreted indicatively.

In metabolic acidosis, with a functioning kidney, urinary anion gap is negative. While it is positive in case of metabolic acidosis due to renal failure or in tubular acidosis type I and IV: in these cases the pH and UAG determination allows to reach the diagnosis.

In case of diabetic ketoacidosis, the UAG may be misleading in two phases, the initial one and during the treatment, or during hypovolemia with increased sodium reabsorption.

The osmolal gap of urine:

$$\mathbf{UOG = measured\ osmolality - calculated\ osmolality\ [2\ (Na^+ + K^+) + urea\ and\ glucose]}$$

may be useful in some cases (i.e., inhalation of toluene, see case report on page 79).

In normal subjects this gap is 80-100 mOsmol/Kg H_2O.

Clinical interpretation of simple acid-base disorders

After having explained in the introductory part the method that will be used in dealing with acid-base disorders, we can now discuss the diagnostic details of the simple ones.

By simple disorder we mean the presence, in a given patient, of only one disorder in the area of acidosis or alkalosis being that respiratory or metabolic. Therefore simple disorders of the acid-base balance are acute and chronic respiratory acidosis, acute and chronic respiratory alkalosis, metabolic alkalosis and metabolic acidosis.

TABLE 4.4 Clinical conditions associated with changes in the urinary anion gap.

Negative UAG ($Cl^-_u > Na^+_u + K^+_u$)	**Positive UAG** ($Cl^-_u < Na^+_u + K^+_u$)
Diarrhea	Distal tubular acidosis
Chloride salts of NH_4, arginine, choline	Chloride diarrhea from villous adenoma
Acute respiratory acidosis	Chloride-losing diarrhea
Recovery from chronic respiratory alkalosis	Intake of K^+ (vegetable fruit) and Na^+ salts (alkaline salts); toluene intoxication
Recovery from diabetic ketoacidosis	Acute respiratory alkalosis
Administration of lithium, use of cereals	Recovery from chronic respiratory acidosis
	Initial phase of diabetic ketoacidosis
In case of unexplained metabolic alkalosis	
UAG < 50	UAG > 50
Active vomiting, bicarbonate intake	Recent abuse of diuretics or laxatives

Respiratory acidosis

Definition

Respiratory acidosis or primary hypercapnia refers to a primary acid-base disorder, characterized by an increase in $PaCO_2 > 45$ mmHg, an increase in the concentration of blood $HCO_3^- > 26$ mEq/L and a reduction in pH < 7.35 (acidemia).

Secondary hypercapnia refers to the increase in $PaCO_2$ due to adaptation mechanism during metabolic alkalosis.

Respiratory acidosis can be acute or chronic.

Pathophysiology

The cause of this disorder is alveolar hypoventilation, determined either by a reduction of pulmonary pump function without alteration of the ventilation/perfusion ratio ($\dot{V}/\dot{Q}$) or by a deficiency of the same due to a $\dot{V}A/\dot{Q}$ alteration that determines an increase in the physiological dead space

$$PaCO_2 = K\,\frac{\dot{V}CO_2}{\dot{V}A} \qquad PaCO_2 = K\,\frac{\dot{V}CO_2}{\dot{V}E\,(1 - V_D/V_T)}$$

The PCO_2 equation both in its synthetic and in the more articulated form, with the highlighting of the component linked to the physiological dead space, clearly shows how the reduction of alveolar ventilation ($\dot{V}A$) increases $PaCO_2$.

The CO_2 retained in the blood hydrates to the formation of carbonic acid (H_2CO_3) which dissociates into H^+ and HCO_3^-.

The formation of carbonic acid causes blood acidification.

$$CO_2 + H_2O \rightarrow H_2CO_3 \rightarrow H^+ + HCO_3^-$$

This reaction occurs both in blood, especially in red blood cells which are rich in carbonic anhydrase (CA) able to catalyze the hydration of CO_2, and in renal tubular cells with the same mechanism. The dissociation of carbonic acid leads to the production of H^+ and HCO_3^-. H^+ is buffered by hemoglobin proteins in the case of intracellular reaction or eliminated by kidney when the reaction occurs in renal tubular cells. Bicarbonate is transferred into plasma from the red blood cells in exchange with Cl^- (an important mechanism in the acute phase of hypercapnia) or reabsorbed by the kidney (a prevalent mechanism in chronic hypercapnia) (**Figure 4.1**).

The adaptation mechanism during acute respiratory acidosis is given by the buffer system consisting of proteins, in particular hemoglobin, and phosphates with bicarbonate production coming from red blood cells (acute respiratory acidosis).

With the continuation of the disorder, renal H^+ elimination takes place followed by a greater reabsorption of bicarbonate (chronic respiratory acidosis) (**Figure 4.2**; see also Chapter 2).

Acute respiratory acidosis

Acute respiratory acidosis is caused by an acute failure of the alveolar ventilation, which is responsible for $PaCO_2$ increase (> 45 mmHg), pH reduction (< 7.35) and a modest but fundamental increase in serum bicarbonate.

Causes of acute respiratory acidosis

The causes of acute hypercapnia and therefore of acute respiratory acidosis are many and can be divided into two groups: those due to a pump deficit with or without increase of the physiological dead space (**Table 4.5**).

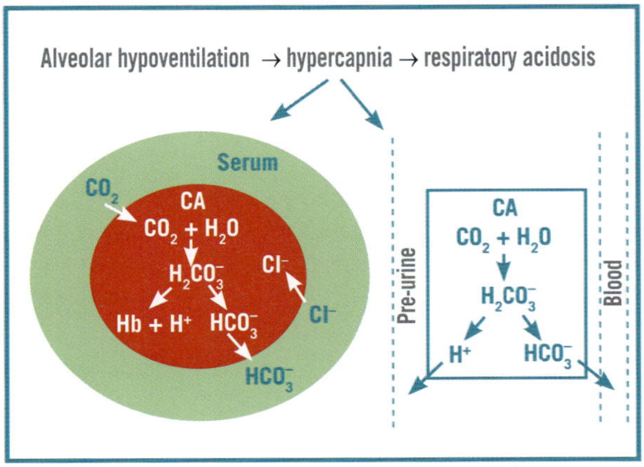

Figure 4.1 Hydration of CO_2 in the red blood cell and renal tubular cell.

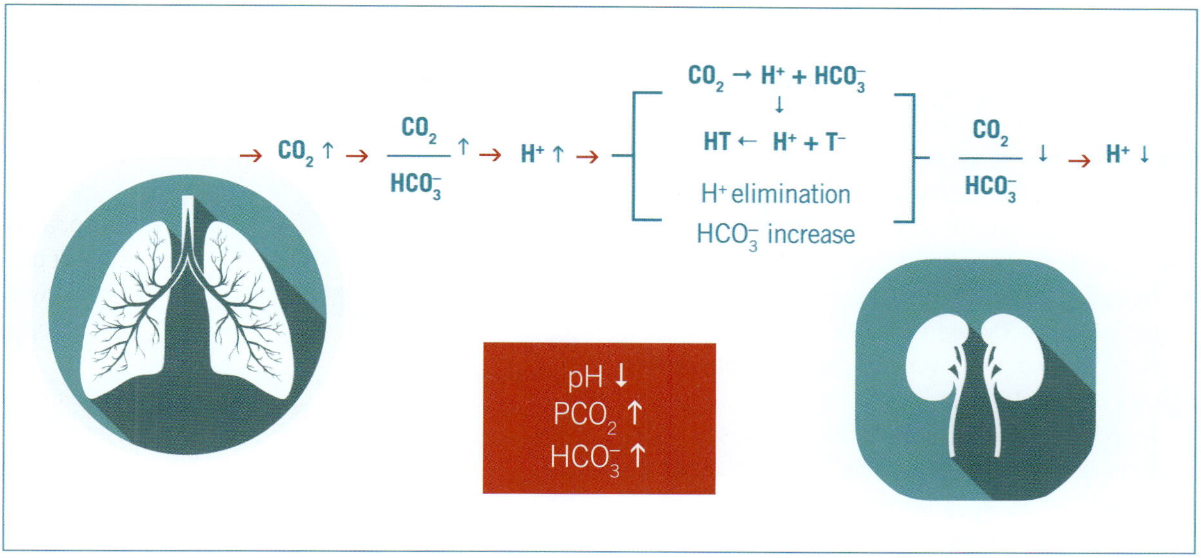

Figure 4.2 Respiratory acidosis: buffer and adaptive mechanisms.

TABLE 4.5 Causes of acute hypercapnia.

Pump deficit without increase of the physiological dead space	
Depression of the central nervous system (CNS)	Overdose of sedatives with or without alcohol Head trauma Acute cerebrovascular accidents (stroke) Acute encephalitis
Acute neuromuscular diseases	High injuries of spinal cord Guillain-Barré syndrome Status epilepticus Myasthenia gravis crisis Drugs or toxic agents (succinylcholine, organophosphorus)
Muscle dysfunction	Hyper or hypokalemia Fatigue
Diseases of the pleura	Pneumothorax Massive pleural effusion
Diseases of the parenchyma	Acute respiratory distress syndrome (ARDS) Multilobar pneumonia
Pump deficit with increase of the physiological dead space	
Acute pulmonary diseases	Acute bronchial asthma Acute exacerbation of chronic obstructive pulmonary disease (COPD)

Clinical features of acute respiratory acidosis

The medical history (anamnesis) should focus in particular on identifying the causes listed above but also on predisposing or risk factors.

The clinical manifestations of hypercapnia are often superimposed on those of hypoxemia, also determined by alveolar hypoventilation and are essentially neurological, cardiovascular and respiratory:

- Neurological signs and symptoms. They depend on the severity of hypercapnia, the speed with which it is manifested, the severity of the acidemia and the concomitant hypoxia.
  Acute respiratory acidosis causes vasodilation, increased cerebral blood flow and volume and increased intracranial pressure. The clinical manifestations are characterized by anxiety, irritability, aggressive agitation, confusion and headache secondary to vasodilation. The clinical examination can detect tremors, awkward speech, myoclonus, asterixis, pupillary constriction. Deep tendon reflexes are often brisk in mild to moderate hypercapnia but reduced when severe.
- Cardiovascular signs and symptoms. Mild to moderate hypercapnia causes vasodilation with increased cardiac output, increased heart rate while blood pressure may be normal or elevated.
  Hypercapnia can also cause a transient cardiac contractility reduction while the increase in arrhythmias (usually supraventricular) is determined by hypoxemia, electrolyte alterations and increased sympathetic tone. High-grade hypercapnia, combined with hypoxemia, causes arterial hypotension also due to myocardial contractility depression. At the clinical examination there is a warm and sweaty skin and a rapid and elastic arterial pulse.
- Respiratory signs and symptoms. Without central nervous system depression there is tachypnea and frequently even severe dyspnea.

Ongoing adaptation of acute respiratory acidosis

During acute respiratory acidosis the adaptive response occurs within a few minutes and is due, as already mentioned, to cellular buffers, in particular to hemoglobin and phosphates. This determines a modest increase in bicarbonate. The renal response also begins early but is slower (Figure 4.2).

Rule of expected adaptation

During acute respiratory acidosis for every 1 mmHg of $PaCO_2$ increase there is [HCO_3^-] increase equal to 0.1 mEq/L.

Clinical case A 63-year-old man is taken to the emergency department by the emergency medical service (EMS), for dyspnea that has risen sharply. From the history it emerges that the man, hypertensive since ten years, from four years is affected by exertional angina well controlled by β-blocker therapy (atenolol 100 mg/day).

He also takes an ACE inhibitor (enalapril 20 mg) for better blood pressure control.

Two hours before arriving at the emergency department he had constrictive retrosternal pain, following an effort judged by the patient to be of modest magnitude. When the pain stopped, a significant dyspnea appeared which is what led the patient to the emergency department.

On physical examination labial cyanosis and cold sweats can be seen.

The vital signs are: BP 190/115 mmHg, HR 74 bpm, RR 32 bpm, SpO_2 80%. At chest thoracic auscultation diffuse bronchospasm sounds with crackling rattles at the bases are heard. No leg swelling. ECG: left ventricle overload signs. Chest ultrasound shows B lines on both lung fields. Some blood tests are required, including troponin dosage and an ABG with electrolytes.

ABG: pH 7.20, $PaCO_2$ 70 mmHg, HCO_3^- 27 mEq/L, PaO_2 44 mmHg, Na^+ 140 mEq/L, Cl^- 100 mEq/L, K^+ 4.3 mEq/L, anion gap 13 mEq/L.

ABG interpretation

pH	7.20	acidemia
$PaCO_2$	70 mmHg	high (respiratory acidosis)
HCO_3^-	27 mEq/L	increased (adaptation mechanism)
Anion gap	13 mEq/L	normal
Na^+/Cl^-	1.4	normal

Expected adaptation

Calculate the $\Delta PaCO_2$: $\Delta PaCO_2$ = (actual $PaCO_2$ – reference $PaCO_2$) 70 – 40 = 30 mmHg.

Calculate the expected increase in bicarbonate compared to the reference value (24 mEq/L) in relation to the increase of $PaCO_2$, taking into account the adaptation rule for acute respiratory acidosis (or acute hypercapnia): 30 × 0.1 = 3 mEq/L (actual bicarbonate increase) + 24 (reference bicarbonate) = 27 mEq/L (expected bicarbonate).

Final interpretation: acute respiratory acidosis.

Reasoned comment

The medical history and clinical picture point towards acute left ventricular failure (acute pulmonary edema). The combination of an acid pH, a high $PaCO_2$ and bicarbonate increase lead to a primary acid-base disorder such as respiratory acidosis.

Bicarbonate is moderately elevated due to the adaptation mechanism of cellular origin (proteins and phosphates) which is established during acute respiratory acidosis. In fact, in this case, its rise is consistent with the adaptation rule for acute respiratory acidosis.

Since $PaCO_2$ is increased by 30 mmHg with respect to the reference value which is 40 mmHg, and since bicarbonate has to rise 0.1 mEq/L for each mmHg of $PaCO_2$ increase, the expected increase of bicarbonate is 3 mEq/L which added up to the reference bicarbonate value (24 mEq/L) they give 27 mEq/L. Since the concentration of actual bicarbonate (27 mEq/L) is equal to the expected one (27 mEq/L) we can speak of expected adaptation achieved. Anion gap and Na^+/Cl^- ratio normality exclude the concomitance of any type of metabolic acidosis and other disorders of metabolic origin.

The clinical interpretation is of acute respiratory acidosis as a simple acid-base disorder, in a patient with acute pulmonary edema.

Chronic respiratory acidosis

Chronic respiratory acidosis is caused by alveolar ventilation failure which can last from a few days to several months/years.

It is characterized by $PaCO_2$ increase (> 45 mmHg), marked increase in bicarbonate concentration and pH close to normal.

According to some Authors, the renal adaptation mechanism can lead in some cases to normal pH (so-called chronic stable hypercapnia).

Causes of chronic respiratory acidosis

As for acute hypercapnia, even in chronic cases the causes can be distinguished in those with pump deficits with (most common) or without increase in the physiological dead space (**Table 4.6**).

Clinical features of chronic respiratory acidosis

Chronic hypercapnia is less dramatic than the acute one and neurological symptoms are often blurred, consisting of morning headache, modest irritability, drowsiness with inversion of the sleep/wake rhythm. Only when this is severe does headache, confusion and drowsiness occur until carbonarcotic coma.

On the motor level tremors and myoclonus are frequent, while on the respiratory level the desensitization of dyspnea can make this symptom little evident.

Ongoing adaptation of chronic respiratory acidosis

During chronic respiratory acidosis adaptation is completed in 3-5 days and is due to kidney, through H^+ excretion but above all with the bicarbonate reabsorption (Figure 4.2).

Rule of expected adaptation

There is a 0.35 mEq/L increase in [HCO_3^-] during chronic respiratory acidosis for every 1 mmHg of $PaCO_2$ increase.

TABLE 4.6 Causes of chronic hypercapnia.

Pump deficit without increase of the physiological dead space	
Depression of the central nervous system (CNS)	Central sleep apnea Hypoventilation due to obesity Brain tumors Bulbar poliomyelitis Hypothyroidism
Chronic neuromuscular diseases	High injuries of spinal cord Poliomyelitis Multiple sclerosis Amyotrophic lateral sclerosis Myasthenia gravis Muscular dystrophy Diaphragmatic paralysis
Muscle dysfunction	Myopathies
Diseases of the thoracic cage, pleura and lung	Obesity Kyphoscoliosis Chronic interstitial disease (early stage)
Pump deficit with increase of the physiological dead space	
Chronic pulmonary diseases	Chronic obstructive pulmonary disease (COPD) Pulmonary emphysema Pulmonary fibrosis (advanced phase) Pulmonary vascular disease

Clinical case A 65-year-old man arrives at the emergency department for dyspnea, accompanied by his wife. Anamnesis reveals that this disorder had begun approximately six months before after significant efforts and subsequently also efforts of modest entity. Since a few days the dyspnea is present even at rest. He claims to be a heavy smoker (25 cigarettes a day), and to have worked as a builder until he retired. For about eight years he has been suffering from a cough, first only in the morning and then present throughout the day, with mucous sputum.

On physical examination, warm skin, turgid jugular veins and labial cyanosis. Vital signs: BP 145/85 mmHg, HR 104 bpm, RR 28 bpm, T 36.7 °C, SpO_2 81%, GCS 15.

Listening to the chest reveals widespread wet sounds with medium bubbles and bronchospasm sounds. At heart auscultation the tones are distant and apparently there are no added tones. Liver inferior margin is three centimeters from the costal arch.

Modest but clearly evident pretibial edemas are present. Chest X-ray allows to appreciate an increase of the vascular tree.

ABG: pH 7.34, $PaCO_2$ 67 mmHg, HCO_3^- 35 mEq/L, PaO_2 45 mmHg, Na^+ 142 mEq/L, Cl^- 93 mEq/L, K^+ 4.2 mEq/L, anion gap 13 mEq/L.

ABG interpretation

pH	7.34	acidemia
$PaCO_2$	67 mmHg	high (respiratory acidosis)
HCO_3^-	35 mEq/L	increased (adaptation mechanism)
Anion gap	13 mEq/L	normal
Na^+/Cl^-	1.52	in range but increased (secondary metabolic alkalosis, from adaptation)

Expected adaptation

Calculate the $\Delta PaCO_2$: $\Delta PaCO_2$ (actual $PaCO_2$ – reference $PaCO_2$) 67 – 40 = 27 mmHg.
Calculate the expected increase in bicarbonate compared to the reference value (24 mEq/L) in relation to the increase in $PaCO_2$ taking into account the expected adaptation rule for chronic respiratory acidosis: 27 × 0.35 = 9.45 mEq/L (increase of the actual bicarbonate) + 24 (reference bicarbonate) = 33.45 mEq/L (expected bicarbonate).

Final interpretation: chronic respiratory acidosis.

Reasoned comment

History and clinical picture point towards a chronic obstructive pulmonary disease with chronic respiratory failure and initial congestive heart failure.
The combination of an acid pH, a high $PaCO_2$ and an increase in bicarbonate, lead to a primary acid-base disorder such as respiratory acidosis. Bicarbonate is elevated due to adaptation mechanism of renal origin that is established during respiratory acidosis that lasts since 4-5 days. In our case their increase is consistent with the expected adaptation rule for chronic respiratory acidosis.
In fact, since $PaCO_2$ is rised by 27 mmHg with respect to the reference value which is 40 mmHg, and since bicarbonate increases by 0.35 mEq/L for each mmHg of $PaCO_2$ increase, the expected augmentation is 9.45 mEq/L which added up to the reference value (24 mEq/L) it gives 33.45 mEq/L. Since the concentration of actual bicarbonate (35 mEq/L) is almost equal to the expected one (33.45 mEq/L ± 2) we can speak of expected adaptation achieved.
Anion gap nornality and the absence of hyperchloremia exclude the concomitance of any type of metabolic acidosis.
Hypochloremia and Na^+/Cl^- = 1.52 ratio are compatible with metabolic alkalosis secondary to chronic hypercapnia.
Therefore, the clinical interpretation is of chronic respiratory acidosis as a simple acid-base disorder in a patient with chronic obstructive pulmonary disease (COPD).

Respiratory alkalosis

Definition

By respiratory alkalosis or primary hypocapnia, we mean a primary acid-base disorder characterized by a decrease in $PaCO_2$ < 35 mmHg, a reduction in the concentration of HCO_3^- < 22 mEq/L and a pH > 7.45 (alkalemia).
Secondary hypocapnia refers to the reduction of $PaCO_2$ secondary to the adaptation mechanism during metabolic acidosis.
Respiratory alkalosis may be acute or chronic.

Pathophysiology

The cause of this disorder is alveolar hyperventilation which causes hypocapnia and therefore respiratory alkalosis.

$$PaCO_2 = K \frac{\dot{V}CO_2}{\dot{V}A}$$

The PaCO2 equation clearly shows how the increase in alveolar ventilation ($\dot{V}A$) reduces $PaCO_2$.
The reaction that follows blood alkalinization is in some aspects specular and inverse with respect to respiratory acidosis:

$$CO_2 + H_2O \leftarrow H_2CO_3 \leftarrow H^+ + HCO_3^-$$

The resulting response to limiting pH excursions in the alkaline sense is plasma acidification.
Acute alkalinization is followed by H^+ release from hemoglobin and extracellular buffers such as H_2PO_4, resulting in bicarbonate consumption. This mechanism of the acute phase (acute respiratory alkalosis) starts after a few minutes and lasts a few hours.
A second response reaches the steady state after 48-72 hours: the renal response. This is characterized by a reduction in H^+ secretion at the proximal and distal tubule (reduction of the activity of the Na^+/K^+ exchangers) which causes an increased elimination of $NaHCO_3^-$.
The decreased $PaCO_2$ causes a reduction in the regeneration and reabsorption of renal bicarbonate (**Figure 4.3**). $NaHCO_3^-$ loss causes a transient loss of extracellular fluids.

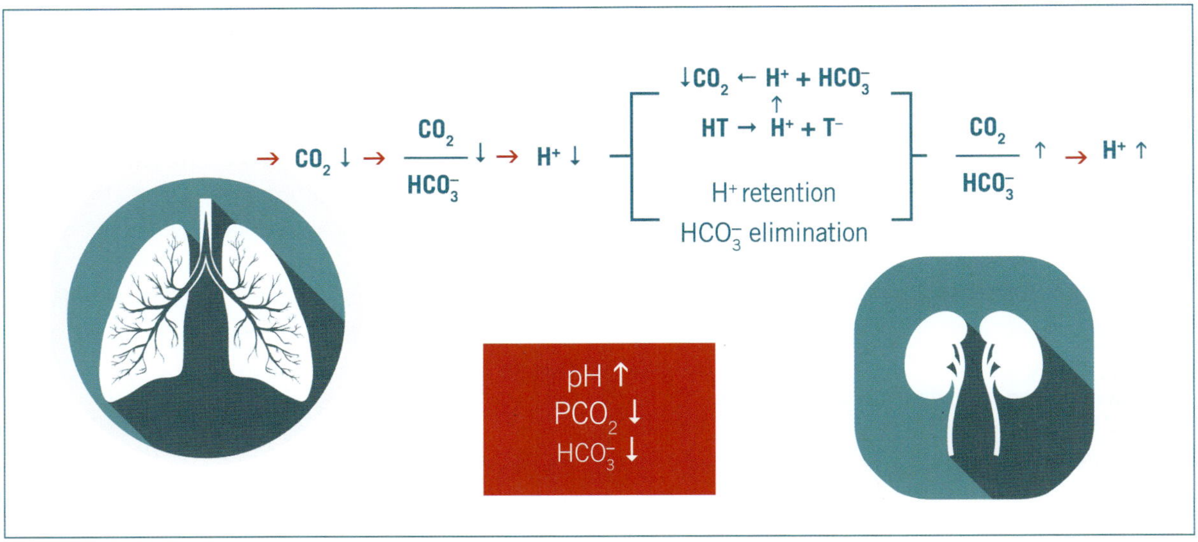

Figure 4.3 Respiratory alkalosis: buffer and adaptive mechanisms.

During the acute and chronic phase hyperchloremia may be present, aiming to maintain the electroneutrality, due to bicarbonate concentration reduction. In the acute phase the increase in chloride is due to a shift from the red blood cells, while in the chronic phase to the contraction of the ECF.

In acute respiratory alkalosis, there is often a modest increase in plasma potassium concentration due to α-adrenergic hyperactivity, while in the chronic phase transient hypokalemia (72-96 hours) appears due to urinary potassium loss and intracellular shift.

Calcium ion also undergoes changes, particularly in the acute phase, due to pH increase which causes a reduction of about 0.4 mmol/L per pH unit. Instead only small variations are observed for magnesium.

Causes of respiratory alkalosis

The causes of respiratory alkalosis are multiple and can lead to acute respiratory alkalosis at the beginning and, if persistent, to chronic respiratory alkalosis. These causes can be divided into three groups (**Table 4.7**).

In the first group, the reason for hyperventilation is due to hypoxemia of pulmonary origin (intrapulmonary shunt): reduced PaO_2 stimulates the respiratory drive and on the arterial blood gas level we can see hypocapnia with hypoxemia and increased alveolar-arterial difference $P(A-a)O_2$.

In the second group, the reason for hyperventilation is due to pulmonary diseases that cause hypoxemia without intrapulmonary shunts, with normal $P(A-a)O_2$.

In the third group, the cause is due to tissue hypoxia or conditions that stimulate breath center independently of PaO_2.

In these cases the classical arterial blood gas framework is characterized by hypocapnia and often by high PaO_2 with reduced or normal $P(A-a)O_2$.

Clinical features of respiratory alkalosis

History, even in this disorder, should be oriented to search for the causes that produced the respiratory alkalosis.

The clinical manifestations are present almost exclusively in acute forms whereas in chronic ones the pH often normalizes.

Symptoms are related to both alkalemia which is a reason for the reduction of ionized calcium, and to hypocapnia which causes vasoconstriction at the level of the central nervous system and coronary circulation (**Table 4.8**).

TABLE 4.7 Causes of pulmonary hyperventilation.

Causes of hyperventilation with intrapulmonary shunt hypoxemia with increased $P(A-a)O_2$
Pneumonia
Pulmonary embolism
Atelectasis
Pulmonary contusion
Early cardiogenic acute pulmonary edema
Acute respiratory distress syndrome
Pulmonary causes without intrapulmonary shunt with normal $P(A-a)O_2$
Bronchial asthma
Interstitial pulmonary fibrosis (initial phase)
High airway obstruction
Pneumothorax
Hemothorax
Causes of hyperventilation from tissue hypoxia or CNS stimulation with hypocapnia and normal $P(A-a)O_2$
Reduced FiO_2
Anemia
Drugs or hormones
Salicylates
Progesterone
Xanthines
Catecholamines
Nicotine
Anxiety
Sepsis
Hyperthyroidism
Heart failure
Pain
Temperature
Pregnancy (progesterone)
Liver cirrhosis

Neurological symptoms and signs

They are the most frequent. Those related to the central nervous system are characterized by dizziness, a sense of instability, anxiety, euphoria, forgetfulness, hallucinations up to convulsive crises.

Peripheral disorders are due to hypocalcemia nerve excitability and are characterized by perioral paresthesia, fingers paresthesia up to carpopedal spasm and tetany.

Cardiovascular symptoms and signs

Mostly they consist of tachycardia and the appearance of ventricular and supraventricular arrhythmias. A characteristic and fairly frequent symptom is chest pain which can be secondary to cardiac or non-cardiac causes.

Cardiac causes are due to myocardial ischemia secondary to coronary vasoconstriction, increased affinity of oxygen to hemoglobin and increased myocardial oxygen consumption caused by increased contractility and peripheral resistance.

Furthermore, hypocapnia can favor a coronary thrombotic event due to platelets increase and their aggregation. Reversible alterations of the S-T tract can be seen on the ECG.

Patients who experience chest pain may have an undamaged coronary circulation or be suffering from coronary artery disease.

Chest pain due to non-cardiac causes is often caused by esophageal spasms.

In addition to symptoms hereby described there may be other disorders characterized by nausea, vomiting and alterations of the gastrointestinal motility and also bronchospasm in asthmatic subjects.

Acute respiratory alkalosis

Acute respiratory alkalosis is caused by an acute increase in pulmonary ventilation which is responsible for $PaCO_2$ reduction (< 35 mmHg), followed by pH increase (> 7.45) and a reduction in serum bicarbonate (< 22 mEq/L).

Ongoing adaptation of acute respiratory alkalosis

During acute respiratory alkalosis the adaptive response occurs within a few minutes and is due to the H^+ released by the buffer system consisting of hemoglobin, followed by a modest reduction in bicarbonate (see pathophysiology).

Rule of expected adaptation

During acute respiratory alkalosis for every 1 mmHg of $PaCO_2$ reduction there is a decrease in serum HCO_3^- concentration equal to 0.2 mEq/L.

TABLE 4.8 Clinical manifestations of acute respiratory alkalosis.

Type of manifestation	Signs and symptoms
Neurological	**Central** Dizziness Sense of instability Anxiety Euphoria Forgetfulness Hallucinations Seizure crisis **Peripheral** Perioral paresthesia, fingers paresthesia Carpopedal spasm Tetany
Cardiovascular	Tachycardia Arrhythmias Chest pain of coronary origin or from esophageal spasm ECG: reversible alterations of the ST-T segment
Lower airways	Bronchospasm
Hematologic	Increased white blood cells and platelets

Clinical case A 52-year-old woman, rather weak, is accompanied to the emergency department after developing a fever for about two days.

The woman suffers from multiple sclerosis with neurological bladder. In her history there have been frequent episodes of urinary tract infection from gram-negative bacteria. She reports dysuria, hematuria and some episodes of vomiting.

On objective examination, skin and mucous membranes are moderately dehydrated and in addition to the reported neurological picture, there are no important pathological findings in the physical examination of chest and abdomen.

The vital signs show: BP 100/70 mmHg, HR 110 bpm, RR 32 bpm, T 39.5 °C, SpO_2 98%.

Blood is collected for tests and a urine sample for culture.

ABG: pH 7.55, $PaCO_2$ 23 mmHg, HCO_3^- 20 mEq/L, PaO_2 102 mmHg, Na^+ 143 mEq/L, Cl^- 105 mEq/L, K^+ 3.2 mEq/L, anion gap 18 mEq/L.

ABG interpretation

pH	7.55	alkalemia
$PaCO_2$	23 mmHg	reduced (respiratory alkalosis)
HCO_3^-	20 mEq/L	reduced (adaptation mechanism)
Anion gap	18 mEq/L	increased (from alkalemia)
Na^+/Cl^-	1.36	normal

Expected adaptation

Calculate the $\Delta PaCO_2$: (reference $PaCO_2$ – actual $PaCO_2$) 40 – 23 = 17 mmHg.

Calculate the expected bicarbonate reduction with respect to the reference value (24) in relation to $PaCO_2$ reduction taking into account the rule of adaptation for acute respiratory alkalosis: (reference bicarbonate) 24 – (bicarbonate reduction) 3.4 mEq/L (17 × 0.2) = 20.6 mEq/L (expected bicarbonate).

Final interpretation: acute respiratory alkalosis.

Reasoned comment

History and clinical picture guide for an acute infection of the urinary tract.

The combination of an alkaline pH, a reduced $PaCO_2$ accompanied by a [HCO_3^-] reduction, orientates towards a primary acid-base disorder such as respiratory alkalosis.

Bicarbonate has moderately decreased due to the mechanism of adaptation of cellular origin. In this case their decrease is consistent with the adaptation rule for acute respiratory alkalosis.

In fact, since $PaCO_2$ is reduced by 17 mmHg with respect to the reference value which is 40 mmHg, and since bicarbonate should drop by 0.2 mEq/L for every mmHg reduction of $PaCO_2$, the expected bicarbonate reduction is 3.4 mEq/L which subtracted from reference value (24 mEq/L) it gives 20.6 mEq/L. Since the concentration of the actual bicarbonate (20 mEq/L) is almost equal to the expected (20.6 mEq/L ± 2) we can speak of an expected adaptation achieved.

The moderately high anion gap does not reveal a concomitant metabolic acidosis but is due to an increase in the negative charges of plasma proteins (amphoteric), linked to the alkaline environment in which they are found.

Moreover, during alkalemia there is an increased lactic acid production due to a rise in the pH-dependent activity of the enzyme 6-phosphofructokinase.

After three days the urine culture results positive for *Escherichia coli* (gram-negative). It is known that gram-negative bacteria produce an endotoxin that acts directly on the breathing center (medulla oblongata) causing hyperventilation.

Therefore the clinical interpretation is of acute respiratory alkalosis as a simple acid-base disorder, in the course of gram-negative sepsis.

Chronic respiratory alkalosis

Chronic respiratory alkalosis is due to an increase in alveolar ventilation lasting several days and is characterized by a $PaCO_2$ reduction (< 35 mmHg) and a marked bicarbonate reduction (< 22 mEq/L) with a pH that is often normal.

Causes of chronic respiratory alkalosis

The causes of chronic respiratory alkalosis, as already mentioned, are the same as those of acute respiratory alkalosis, what changes is their duration over time.

Ongoing adaptation of chronic respiratory alkalosis

In the course of chronic respiratory alkalosis adaptation is completed in 3-5 days and is due to kidney that intervenes through the H^+ retention and the reduction of the bicarbonate reabsorption (see pathophysiology).

Rule of expected adaptation

During chronic respiratory alkalosis, for every 1 mmHg of $PaCO_2$ reduction there is a decrease in the HCO_3^- concentration equal to 0.4 mEq/L. This is the only simple acid-base disorder in which the adaptation mechanism leads to pH normalization.

Clinical case A 38-year-old woman arrives in the emergency department accompanied by her husband because she has been suffering dyspnea for five days, which suddenly began after trans-oceanic airplane flight.

The woman has always been well, she has never used drugs, except progestogens for contraceptive purposes since about six years. At the physical examination, nothing relevant except varicose veins affecting the saphenous vein bilaterally. Regular chest and abdomen examination.

The vital signs show: BP 110/70 mmHg, HR 105 bpm, RR 33 bpm, T 36.5 °C, SpO_2 96%, GCS 15. Chest X-ray is negative. Some blood tests are required including ABG.

ABG: pH 7.43, $PaCO_2$ 30 mmHg, HCO_3^- 20 mEq/L, PaO_2 88 mmHg, Na^+ 138 mEq/L, Cl^- 107 mEq/L, K^+ 3.2 mEq/L, anion gap 11 mEq/L.

Evaluating of the clinical picture and ABG, the D-dimer dosage and a venous compressive ultrasound (CUS) of the lower limbs were performed and subsequently to their positivity, a chest CT scan was requested.

ABG interpretation

pH	7.43	normal
$PaCO_2$	30 mmHg	reduced (respiratory alkalosis)
HCO_3^-	20 mEq/L	reduced (adaptation mechanism)
Anion gap	11 mEq/L	normal
Na^+/Cl^-	1.28	normal

Expected adaptation

Calculate the $\Delta PaCO_2$: $\Delta PaCO_2$ (reference $PaCO_2$ – actual $PaCO_2$) 40 – 30 = 10 mmHg.
Calculate the expected reduction of bicarbonate compared to the reference value (24 mEq/L) in relation to the reduction of $PaCO_2$, taking into account the expected adaptation rule in the course of chronic respiratory alkalosis: $10 \times 0.4 = 4$ mEq/L; (reference bicarbonate) 24 – (bicarbonate reduction) 4 = 20 mEq/L (expected bicarbonate).

Final interpretation: chronic respiratory alkalosis.

Reasoned comment

History and clinical picture guide to pulmonary embolism. The combination of a normal pH, reduced $PaCO_2$ and bicarbonate can guide to a primary acid-base disorder such as chronic respiratory alkalosis.
Bicarbonate is reduced due to the adaptation mechanism of renal origin. In this case their decrease is consistent with the adaptation rule for chronic respiratory alkalosis.
In fact, since $PaCO_2$ is reduced by 10 mmHg with respect to the reference value which is 40 mmHg, and since bicarbonate should drop by 0.4 mEq/L for every mmHg of $PaCO_2$ reduction, the expected reduction is $10 \times 0.4 = 4$ mEq/L which subtracted from the reference value (24 mEq/L) it gives 20 mEq/L.
Since the concentration of actual bicarbonate (20 mEq/L) is equal to the expected one (20 mEq/L) we can speak of expected adaptation achieved.
In this case the adaptation mechanism led to the pH normalization.
Meanwhile, after CUS positivity, the venous compression of the lower limbs, the D-dimer dosage appears to be 7 ng/mL. CT scan performed after an hour from the arrival highlights the presence of a thrombus in the main branch of the right pulmonary artery.
Therefore, the clinical interpretation is of chronic respiratory alkalosis as a simple acid-base disorder, in a patient with pulmonary embolism.

NOTE

Although the text does not deal with disorders concerning oxygenation and its diagnostics, the majority have noticed that the value of PaO_2 is too low compared to the $PaCO_2$ of 30 mmHg. In fact, if we calculate P(A - a) O_2 this will be equal to 24 mmHg, which means the presence of intrapulmonary shunts, the cause of hypoxemia and therefore of hyperventilation.

Metabolic alkalosis

Definition

Metabolic alkalosis is a primary acid-base disorder characterized by a rise in serum bicarbonate concentration > 26 mEq/L, an increase in pH > 7.45 and in $PaCO_2$ > 45 mmHg, related to the adaptation mechanisms.

Classification

Although there are some more recent pathophysiological classifications, such as that based on the centrality of ion transport stimulation in collecting ducts, it is still very popular and more suited to this textbook purposes, the one which is based on the dependence or not of metabolic alkalosis from chloride ion depletion.
According to this classification, there are metabolic alkaloses due to chloride ion depletion, also called chloride-responsive and others, largely related to K^+ depletion, named chloride-resistant.

The term chloride-responsive means that the metabolic alkalosis merged into this group are not corrected by administration of K^+ or by the volume expansion with fluids without chloride ion, but only by Cl^- administration. On the contrary those chloride-resistant are not corrected by Cl^- administration.

Pathophysiology

From a pathophysiological point of view there are two questions to be answered: how is the metabolic alkalosis generated and how it is maintained.

Generation of metabolic alkalosis

Metabolic alkalosis generation is essentially due to the loss of chloride ion (Cl^- depletion alkalosis) or potassium ion (K^+ depletion alkalosis).

There are also some cases, the pathogenesis of which is not attributable to the mechanisms mentioned above.

Chloride-depletion or chloride-responsive alkalosis

It is the most common form of metabolic alkalosis. The loss of Cl^- can occur through the stomach (vomiting, nasogastric tube), the colon (villous adenoma or congenital forms of altered ion transport), the kidney (thiazide or loop diuretics) or the skin (cystic fibrosis). In the case of chloride ion loss from the stomach a HCO_3^-, reabsorption follows, produced during the formation of HCl, unbalanced by the concomitant Cl^- reabsorption, because it is eliminated by the stomach.

In the case of thiazide or loop diuretics there is a Cl^- loss together with the loss of Na^+ and K^+. To counterbalance the Cl^- loss the kidney reabsorbs HCO_3^- at the proximal tubule.

This mechanism is accelerated by fluid reabsorption, secondary to the contraction of extracellular volume (ECF) by loss of Na^+ and water and is promoted by the renin-aldosterone mechanism with increased H^+ secretion and HCO_3^- reabsorption in the collecting ducts.

In the case of the villous rectum adenoma, this can secrete Na^+, K^+ or Cl^-, depending on the cellular type. If the chloride secretion prevails, the acid-base disorder that follows is metabolic alkalosis.

Potassium depletion or chloride-resistant alkalosis

It is a type of metabolic alkalosis caused by a reduction in total body potassium that can only be corrected by potassium administration.

It is almost always accompanied by hypochloremia, but in this case the administration of chloride does not correct the acid-base alteration, on the contrary it worsens it.

Potassium loss can occur by renal or intestinal route.

In the first case the loss is due to an excess of mineralocorticoids (for example, primary hyperaldosteronism) or genetic alterations that determine an altered transport of electrolytes at the tubule level with loss of chloride ion.

Intestinal causes may depend on continuous K+ loss from laxative abuse or a potassium-free diet.

The generation of the metabolic alkalosis due to renal causes is probably due to to an increased ammoniagenesis with elimination of NH_4^+ and followed by the production of HCO_3^- and subsequent reabsorption.

In non-renal causes the generation of metabolic alkalosis is due to a shift of H^+ within non-renal cells which causes an increase in HCO_3^-, while the shift in renal tubular cells increases HCO_3^- reabsorption by causing intracellular acidosis.

Maintenance of metabolic alkalosis

The key to understanding the maintenance of metabolic alkalosis lies in the kidney, where there is an increased bicarbonate reabsorption in the proximal tubule, which is not secreted in the distal tubule as it should.

The kidney loses the ability to efficiently eliminate bicarbonate and paradoxically reabsorbs it due to the causes shown in Table 4.4 (**Figure 4.4**).

Metabolic alkalosis and pH defense

In metabolic alkalosis the pH defense affects both classes of buffers, which react by yielding hydrogen ions from their protonated forms.

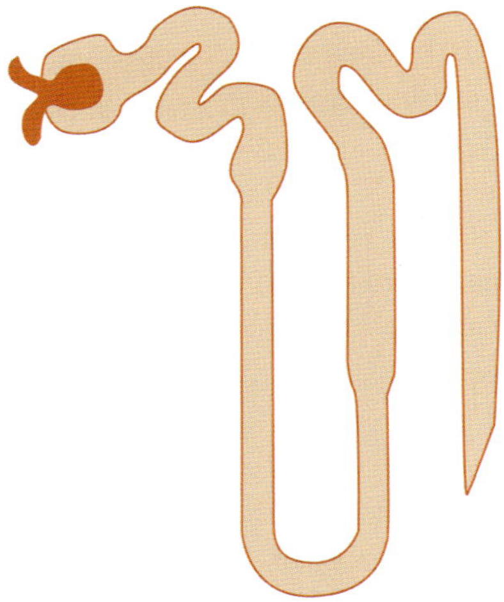

Figure 4.4 Factors that contribute to the generation and maintenance of metabolic alkalosis.
ECF: extracellular fluid; ICF: intracellular fluid; GFR: glomerular filtration rate.

Respiratory adaptation acts by reducing ventilation followed by blood PCO_2 increase, a mechanism limited by tissue oxygenation needs.

The kidney instead intervenes with a maladaptive response because PCO_2 enhances H^+ excretion followed by an increase in the plasma concentration of HCO_3^-, thus nullifying, after a few days, the adaptive respiratory effect (**Figure 4.5**).

Causes of metabolic alkalosis

The causes will be divided into chloride-responsive and chloride-resistant. This subdivision seems to be more useful, also for therapeutic management (**Table 4.9**).

Clinical features of metabolic alkalosis

The clinical manifestations (**Table 4.10**), present above all in the course of severe metabolic alkalosis, are due both to the disorders caused by the alkalemia as such and to the problems related to the lack of Cl^-, K^+, Mg^{++} ions and to the Ca^{++} variations.

Neuromuscular excitability on the neurological level is less present than in respiratory alkalosis, also in part due to the reduced concentration of Ca^{++}. Mental confusion from cerebral hypoperfusion may also be present. In the cardiovascular field there is arteriolar constriction with reduced coronary flow and reduced angina threshold.

Supraventricular and ventricular arrhythmias are frequent, mainly due to concomitant hypokalemia and hypomagnesemia.

The effect on alveolar ventilation is important, with a reduction that leads to hypercapnia (adaptation mechanism) and hypoxemia. Mucous membranes and the skin are often dehydrated in the chloride-sensitive form. The electrocardiogram shows alterations related to hypokalemia and hypomagnesemia: Q-Tc interval prolongation, U-wave appearance, ST-segment depression.

Laboratory tests

Laboratory tests are particularly important during metabolic alkalosis and show a reduction in serum concentration of chloride, potassium, ionized calcium, magnesium. The Na^+/Cl^- ratio is often ≥ 1.55.

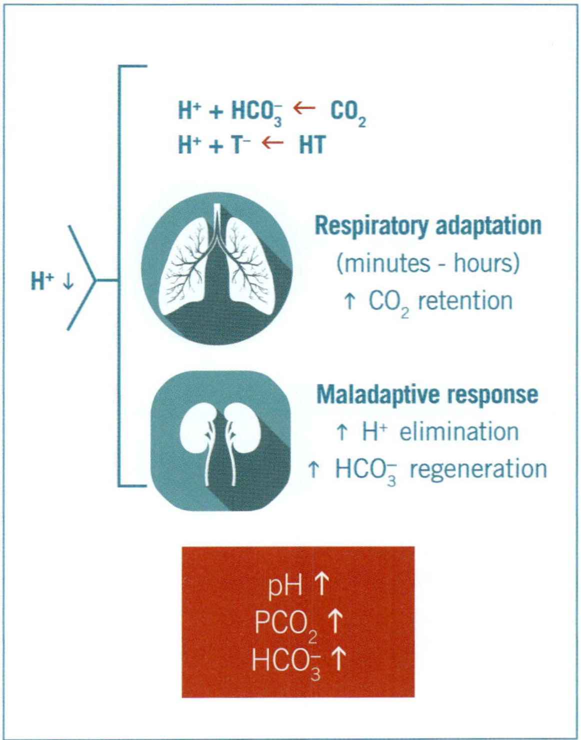

Figure 4.5 Buffer mechanisms, respiratory adaptation and maladaptive response of the kidney.

The dosage of chloride and urinary potassium is useful to differentiate between chloride-responsive and chloride non-responsive forms.

Chloride-responsive forms are characterized by low urinary chloride (< 15 mEq/L). Care should be taken that in the forms caused by thiazide or loop diuretics, chloride concentration in the urine is reduced after discontinuation of the diuretic while it is elevated during intake.

Chloride non-responsive forms (with or without hypertension) are characterized by a urinary chloride > 20 mEq/L.

In some special conditions the cause of metabolic alkalosis may remain undetermined. In these cases the determination of pH and urinary anion gap (UAG) may be useful.

A pH ≥ 7 or UAG < 50 testifies for active vomiting or bicarbonate intake, while a pH ≤ 6 or UAG > 50 points towards an abuse of laxatives or recent use of diuretics.

TABLE 4.9 Causes of metabolic alkalosis.

Chloride-responsive alkalosis
Gastric fluid loss (vomiting, nasogastric tube)
Diuretics (thiazides and loop diuretics)
Loss of intestinal secretions (villous adenoma)
Cystic fibrosis
Post-hypercapnic
Chloride-resistant alkalosis
With arterial hypertension
Primary and secondary hyperaldosteronism
Cushing syndrome
Intake of glucocorticoids and mineralocorticoids
Genetic deficiency of 11β-HSD2 or its inhibition by licorice, carbenoxolone, chewing tobacco
Deficiency of 11β and 17β-hydroxylase which leads to an excess of deoxycorticosterone.
Renovascular hypertension
Without arterial hypertension
Bartter syndrome
Liddle syndrome
Gitelman syndrome
Pendred syndrome
Severe potassium depletion by laxatives or K^+ free diet
Hypomagnesemia
Miscellaneous
Administration of alkali
Milk-alkali syndrome
Feeding after prolonged fasting
Hypercalcemia
IV administration of penicillin
Massive blood transfusion

Adaptation during metabolic alkalosis

Alveolar hypoventilation with increased $PaCO_2$ is the adaptation mechanism that allows to maintain the pH values.

This mechanism, however, is limited by PaO_2 reduction, that below a certain threshold determines a resumption of the respiratory rate.

An increase in $PaCO_2$ above 55 mmHg is uncommon, even if values > 60 mmHg are reported during severe metabolic alkalosis.

TABLE 4.10 Clinical manifestations of metabolic alkalosis.

Type of manifestation	Signs and symptoms
Neurological	Neuromuscular excitability up to tetany Alteration of mental state Apathy Confusion
Cardiovascular	Angina Arrhythmias ECG: alterations due to hypokalemia and hypomagnesemia
Respiratory	Hypoventilation

Rule of expected adaptation

During metabolic alkalosis for every 1 mEq/L increase in [HCO_3^-], there is a $PaCO_2$ increase of 0.7 mmHg (with the limit due to hypoxemia).

Clinical case A 78-year-old man arrives in the emergency department due to confusion and severe dehydration.

According to the history he results affected by congestive heart failure which is now difficult to treat due to continuous relapse, even shortly after being discharged from hospital.

At the end of his last stay in hospital, ten days earlier, he was advised for home therapy with enalapril, furosemide and metolazone.

In recent days he has had several vomiting episodes of unclear cause.

The physical examination shows dehydrated mucous membranes and skin, absence of leg swelling and pleural effusion that he used to have during previous hospitalizations. He answers questions confusingly.

The vital signs are: BP 90/70 mmHg, HR 108 bpm, RR 14 bpm, T 36.5 °C, SpO_2 94%, GCS 13. ECG: sinus rhythm, lengthened QTc and presence of U waves.

Performed blood tests show renal failure with creatinine 2.5 mg/dL and blood urea 110 mg/dL.

ABG: pH 7.52, $PaCO_2$ 48 mmHg, HCO_3^- 38 mEq/L, PaO_2 75 mmHg, Na^+ 148 mEq/L, Cl^- 92 mEq/L, K^+ 2.2 mEq/L, anion gap 18 mEq/L.

ABG interpretation

pH	7.52	alkalemia
$PaCO_2$	48 mmHg	high (adaptation mechanism)
HCO_3^-	38 mEq/L	increased (metabolic alkalosis)
Anion gap	18 mEq/L	increased (due to alkalemia)
Na^+/Cl^-	1.60	increased (metabolic alkalosis)

Expected adaptation

Calculate the ΔHCO_3^- (actual HCO_3^- – reference HCO_3^-) 38 – 24 = 14 mEq/L.

Calculate the expected increase in $PaCO_2$ with respect to the reference value (40 mmHg) in relation to the increase in bicarbonate, taking into account the expected adaptation rule: 0.7 × 14 = 9.8 mmHg + (reference $PaCO_2$) 40 mmHg = 49.8 mmHg (expected $PaCO_2$).

Final interpretation: metabolic alkalosis.

Reasoned comment

History and clinical picture point to a state of dehydration/hypovolemia due to diuretics intake (furosemide and metolazone) and to vomiting.

The combination of a frankly alkaline pH, increased bicarbonate and $PaCO_2$ point toward a primary acid-base disorder such as metabolic alkalosis.

$PaCO_2$ is increased by the respiratory adaptation mechanism, consistent with the adaptation rule for metabolic alkalosis. In fact, since bicarbonate concentration is

increased by 14 mEq/L with respect to the reference value of 24 mEq/L, and since $PaCO_2$ increases by 0.7 mmHg for every mEq/L rise in bicarbonate, the expected increase in $PaCO_2$ is 9.8 which added to the reference value (40 mmHg) gives 49.8 mmHg.
Since the actual $PaCO_2$ (48 mmHg) is close to the expected one (49.8 mmHg ± 2) we can speak of expected adaptation achieved.
The moderately high anion gap does not stand for a concomitant metabolic acidosis, but is due to the rise in the negative charges of the plasma proteins (amphoteric), linked to the alkaline environment in which they are found.
Also in course of alkalemia there is a production of lactic acid caused by to an increase of the activity of phosphofructokinase, a pH-dependent enzyme.
Therefore, the clinical interpretation is of metabolic alkalosis as a simple acid-base disorder, in a dehydrated/hypovolemic patient due to diuretic intake and vomiting.

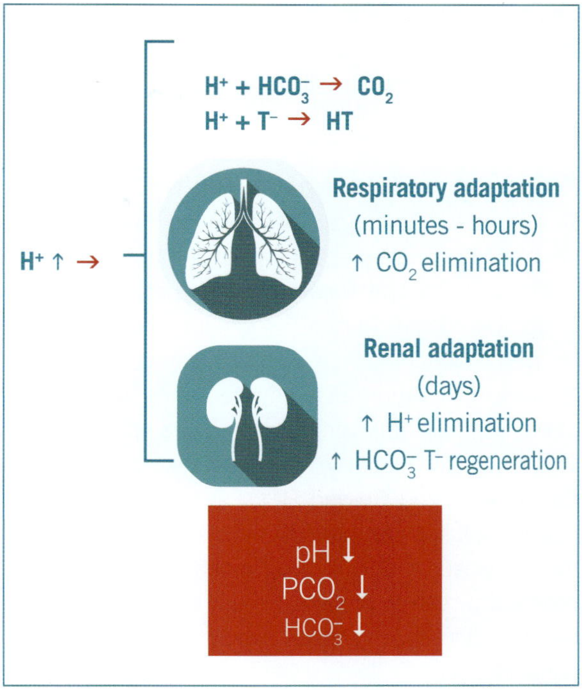

Figure 4.6 Metabolic acidosis and pH defense mechanisms.

Metabolic acidosis

Definition
Metabolic acidosis is a primary acid-base disorder characterized by a decrease in serum HCO_3^- concentration < 22 mEq/L followed by lowering of pH < 7.35 and the reduction of $PaCO_2$ < 35 mmHg due to the adaptation mechanism.

Pathophysiology
In metabolic acidosis, bicarbonate concentration is reduced either by consumption (buffer function) or by its loss from the intestinal tract (i.e., diarrhea) or kidney (i.e. renal tubular acidosis).
Both the bicarbonate buffer and the non-bicarbonate buffers contribute to pH defense (**Figure 4.6**) with consumption of the HCO_3^- and T^- bases.
In addition to this immediate defense, both physiological adaptation functions are involved.
Within a few minutes the respiratory one is activated, caused by the reduction of pH which activates the peripheral chemoreceptors of aorta, carotids and the central ones located on brainstem ventral face, determining an increase in the frequency and depth of the ventilation with consequent $PaCO_2$ reduction.
Kidney intervention takes place more slowly, increasing H^+ elimination, especially in the form of ammonium and with the simultaneous recovery and restoration of the bases consumed in buffer defense.

Diagnosis of metabolic acidosis
For the diagnosis of metabolic acidosis and its causes (from bicarbonate consumption or loss) the calculation of the anion gap is extremely useful.
In fact, two other methods have also been proposed which are the calculation of the base excess (BE) and the strong ion difference (SID), which have been mentioned in Chapter 3.
Our choice, however, was to use anion gap calculation for several reasons, particularly because it is a method that works well and is quite well understandable.

Therefore, before addressing the two types of metabolic acidosis, we will try to understand the significance of the anion gap, its clinical utility and what its limits are.

Anion gap and its clinical utility

To understand anion gap meaning and its utility in the clinic, it is necessary to briefly mention the principle of electroneutrality that states: in body fluids the number of positive charges (cations) is equal to that of negative charges (anions).

This principle is represented by the James Gamble ionogram (Gamblegram) highlighted in **Figure 4.7**.

The laboratory routinely measures the Na^+, K^+, Mg^{++}, Ca^{++} cations and Cl^- and HCO_3^- anions but not phosphates, sulfates and proteins as anions. Since most of the unmeasured anions, in a normal subject, are represented by serum proteins (mainly albumin), it follows that the difference between cations and anions is not equal to zero.

This difference, due to unmeasured anions, is called anion gap (AG) (**Figure 4.8**).

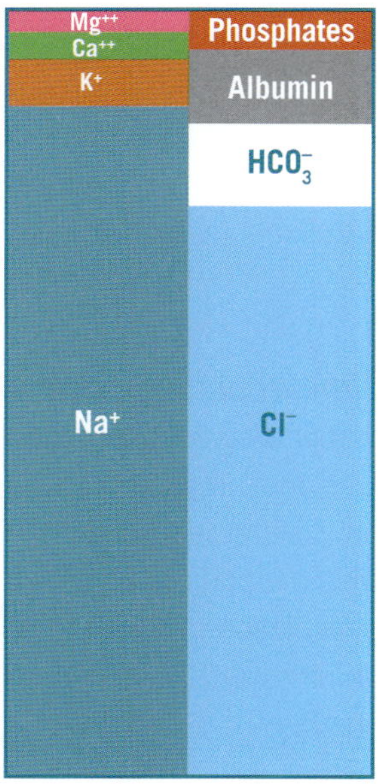

Figure 4.7 Gamble ionogram.

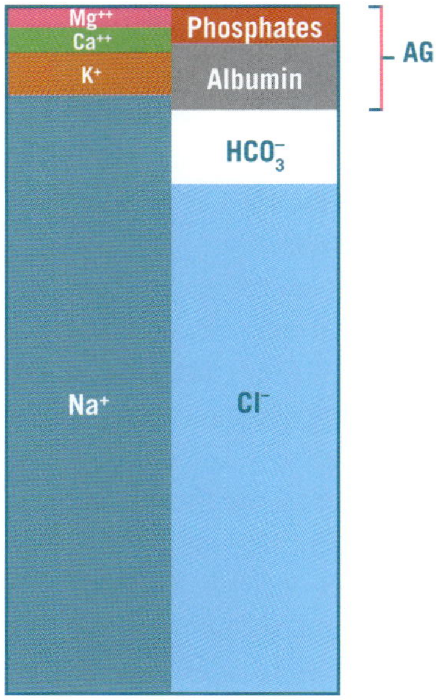

Figure 4.8 Gamble ionogram and the anions whose unmeasured charges constitute the anion gap.

If we use for the calculation $(Na^+ + K^+) - (Cl^- + HCO_3^-)$ which are the quantitatively relevant ions, the difference is equal to 16 mEq/L (± 4). Since most Authors exclude K^+ from the calculation, because it is quantitatively not very significant, in this case the anion gap value is 12 mEq/L (± 4) (**Figure 4.9**).

$$\text{anion gap} \quad (Na^+ + K^+) - (Cl^- + HCO_3^-) = 16\ \text{mEq/L} \pm 4$$

$$\text{anion gap} \quad Na^+ - (Cl^- + HCO_3^-) = 12\ \text{mEq/L} \pm 4$$

While the cation compartment, dominated by sodium, is quite stable and the possible variations in the potassium concentration do not create particular problems in terms of electroneutrality, the anion compartment, as we will see later, is instead very variable in its main components (Cl^- and HCO_3^-).

Anion gap calculation has been proposed as an useful diagnostic tool in three situations:

- Diagnosis of metabolic acidosis type and its causes.

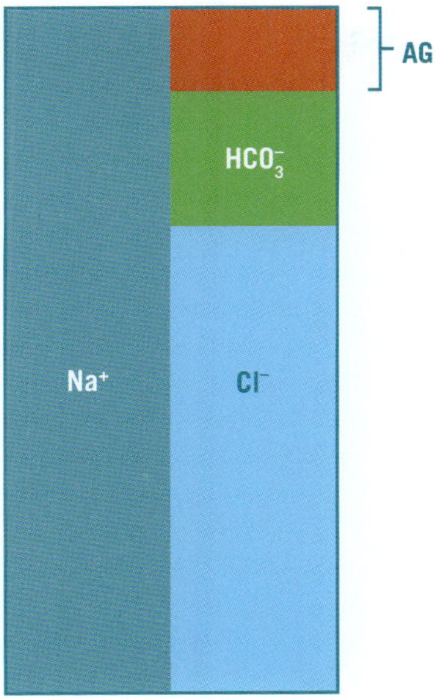

Figure 4.9 Main cations and anions and depiction of the anion gap (red rectangle).

- Diagnosis of mixed disorders: Δgap and ΔAG/ ΔHCO$_3$.
- Diagnosis of particular clinical situations in presence of reduced or increased anion gap (outside AG metabolic acidosis).

Diagnosis of metabolic acidosis type and its causes

As already expressed in the definition, metabolic acidosis is a primary acid-base disorder characterized by a bicarbonate reduction due to consumption (by buffer function) or loss followed by a pH and $PaCO_2$ decrease.

Metabolic acidosis due to bicarbonate consumption

In the course of accumulation of endogenous acids (i.e., lactic acid), failure to eliminate H^+ (renal failure) or introduction of exogenous acids or toxic substances, whose metabolites are acids (i.e., ethylene, glycol) a bicarbonate consumption occurs.

These, like all acids, consist of a hydrogen ion (H^+) and an anion (A^-); for example for lactic acid: H^+ + lactate$^-$.

In plasma the produced H^+ consume bicarbonate according to this reaction:

$$HCO_3^- + H^+ \rightarrow H_2CO_3 \rightarrow H_2O + CO_2$$

followed by a reduction, in the anion compartment, of the negative charges related to the consumed bicarbonate (HCO_3^-). These consumed negative charges are replaced, in an equivalent manner, by the negative charges of the anion (A^-) to which H^+ were related, thus restoring electrical neutrality.

Since these anions are not routinely measurable (unmesured anions), the anion gap is increased without changes in chloride concentration. So the acidosis that occurs with this pathophysiological mechanism is called metabolic acidosis with elevated anion gap (AG metabolic acidosis).

From what has been written above it is possible to derive an important rule: during AG metabolic acidosis, serum bicarbonate concentration is reduced (approximately) by as many mEq/L as those due to the increase in the anion gap, starting from the reference value of 12 mEq/L (**Figure 4.10 B**).

Metabolic acidosis due to bicarbonate loss

Bicarbonate loss occurs mainly through the intestinal (diarrhea) or renal (renal tubular acidosis) route and causes a net reduction of negative charges in the anion compartment. This loss, due to electroneutrality reasons, is replaced by the negative charge of chloride anion (Cl^-) which thus increases its serum concentration. In this case there is no change in anion gap (**Figure 4.10 C**).

The metabolic acidosis that occurs with this pathophysiological mechanism is called metabolic acidosis with normal anion gap, hyperchloremic (hyperchloremic metabolic acidosis).

Diagnosis of mixed disorders: Δgap *and* ΔAG/ΔHCO$_3^-$

The second area where anion gap calculation can be useful is while searching for a mixed metabolic disorder. This can be highlighted by calculating the Δgap, which is obtained by calculating the difference between the ΔAG value (actual anion gap – 12 mEq/L as refer-

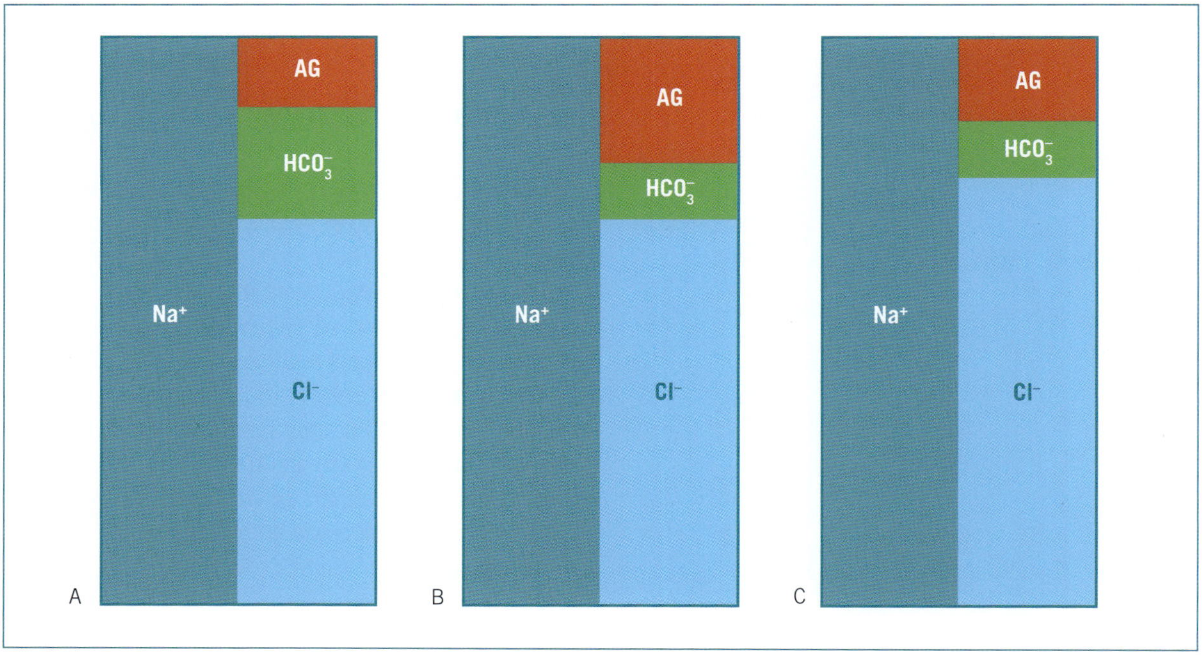

Figure 4.10 A-C It shows the different behavior of anions depending on whether it is AG acidosis (B) or hyperchloremic acidosis (C) and compared to the normal condition (A).

ence value) and the ΔHCO_3^- value (24 mEq/L bicarbonate reference value – actual bicarbonate value): $\Delta gap = (\Delta AG - \Delta HCO_3^-)$.

The normal value is 0 ± 6 mEq/L. This calculation is based, as already mentioned above, on the assumption that for every mEq of acid added to body fluids there is an increase of (approximately) a similar equivalent of anion gap (unmeasured anions), followed by an almost equivalent bicarbonate reduction: protons (H^+) that make up the acid will consume bicarbonate, conjugated bases of acid (A^-) will take part of the "compartment" of the anion gap, as they cannot be routinely dosed (Figure 4.10 B).

This means that when serum $[HCO_3^-]$ is reduced less than expected by the increase in AG ($\Delta AG > \Delta HCO_3^-$), there is a bicarbonate excess (metabolic alkalosis); so in addition and associated to AG metabolic acidosis there is a metabolic alkalosis (**Figure 4.11 A**).

Instead, when HCO_3^- is reduced more than expected by the increase in AG ($\Delta AG < \Delta HCO_3^-$), it means that there is also a bicarbonate loss (hyperchloremic metabolic acidosis) and therefore, in this case, two types of

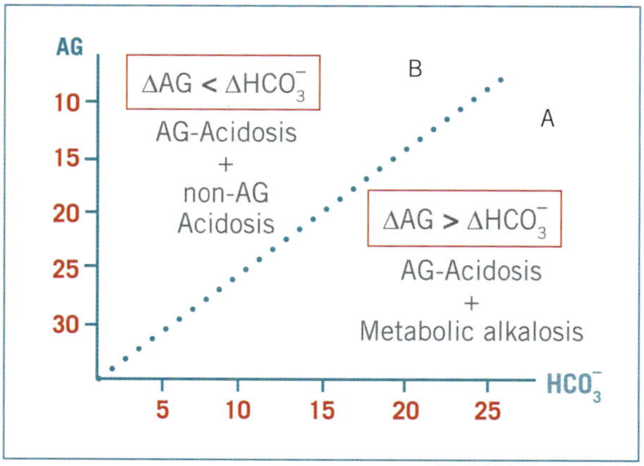

Figure 4.11 A, B Diagram of the Δgap for highlighting the double metabolic disorder.

metabolic acidosis are present: the high anion gap and the hyperchloremic one (**Figure 4.11 B**).

More simply: when the Δgap is significantly positive (> 6 mEq/L) metabolic alkalosis is very likely, on the contrary if the Δgap is significantly negative (< 6 mEq/L) hyperchloremic acidosis is also present. This rule should be applied with caution in the case of lactic acidosis where the $\Delta AG/\Delta HCO_3^-$ ratio is not 1 but 1.6 because the protons (H^+) are dispersed in a larger volume of distribution and are also buffered in the intracellular area.

The same rule must be applied, with the same caution, in the course of particularly serious metabolic acidosis. Another very practical tool is the use of the $\Delta AG/\Delta HCO_3^-$ ratio as shown in **Figure 4.12**, **Table 4.11**.

Clinical use limits of the anion gap calculation

In assessing anion gap the clinician's attitude should be cautious, considering that it is a very specific tool (high positive predictive value) but not very sensitive (low negative predictive value).

This means that in the presence of an anion gap (in its simplified formula without K^+) $\geq$ 19 mEq/L, the diagnosis of AG metabolic acidosis is almost certain (we will see how this is important in the interpretative study of mixed disorders), while in the case of metabolic acidosis with normal AG without hyperchloremia, an increase in unmeasured anions cannot be excluded.

Some Authors have underlined anion gap scarce sensitivity in detecting, for example, clinically significant increases in lactate.

Diagnosis of particular clinical situations in the presence of reduced or increased anion gap (outside AG metabolic acidosis)

The anion gap may also increase without metabolic acidosis.

This may be due to the laboratory test itself or to the presence of the so-called conflict factors.

On the other hand, AG can also be much lower than reference values when the unmeasured anions are in turn reduced, as happens during hypoalbuminemia (low blood albumin). In this case it is possible to correct the error with the Figge's formula, that allows us to bring back the anion gap within the useful values for its clinical use:

Corrected AG = actual AG + 2.5 × ([normal albumin] – [actual albumin])

For each 1 g/dL reduction in serum albumin concentration (with a reference value of 4.5 g/dL) AG decreases by 2.5 mEq/L.

Furthermore, the anion gap can be reduced when there is a significant increase in cations (potassium, magnesium, calcium) or in case of lithium intoxication. But the most significant condition is found in presence of paraproteins (IgG and IgM) which have excess positive charges and therefore behave like cations.

In conclusion, the presence of AG < 8 mEq/L should make us suspect the existence of some disorders, such as those just discussed (**Table 4.12**).

NOTE

Some Authors consider helpful, in metabolic acidosis, the use of the Cl^-/Na^+ ratio (not to be confused with Na^+/Cl^-) as an alternative to the anion gap, where values < 0.75 would suggest a metabolic acidosis with excess of unmeasured ions, while if > 0.79 there would be a metabolic acidosis due to bicarbonate loss.

In the discussion of clinical cases we will not use this tool.

TABLE 4.11 Decision values of $\Delta AG/\Delta HCO_3^-$ ratio.

< 0.4	Hyperchloremic MA
0.4-0.8	Hyperchloremic MA + MA with high AG
> 0.8-2	MA with high AG
> 2	MA with high AG + metabolic alkalosis

MA = metabolic acidosis

TABLE 4.12 Variations in anion gap and conflict factors.

Conflict factors reducing the anion gap	
Interference or laboratory error	Presence of bromide in the blood or error in the determination of Cl^-
Hyperviscosity	It underestimates sodium concentration (automatic analyzer)
Hypoalbuminemia	It is the most frequent cause. It can be corrected with Figge's formula
Monoclonal and polyclonal gammopathies	In particular IgG because they have a prevalent positive charge and IgM due to the size (macromolecules with positive charge)
Hyperkaliemia, hypermagnesemia and hypercalcemia	Ralely they can reduce anion gap
Lithium and bromide	If taken at high doses (toxicological doses)
High levels of lipids or proteins in the blood	Because it determines pseudohyponatremia (artifact inexistent with the blood gas analyzers)
Hypernatremia	Underestimation of sodium value (not with blood gas analyzers)
Hyponatremia	In patients with SIADH
Polymyxin B	High doses and preparations with chloride
Conflict factors causing a negative anion gap	
Laboratory error	Most common cause
Bromide intoxication	Second most common cause
Conflict factors increasing the anion gap	
Laboratory error	
Carbenicillin and albumin	If administered in large quantities
Alkalemia	Increase in protein negative charges, in particular albumin and increase in lactic acid due to increased phosphofructokinase activity
Increased anionic paraproteins	Increased negative charges
Severe hyperphosphatemia	Increased negative charges

Causes of metabolic acidosis

Metabolic acidosis causes are divided into two groups: those causing bicarbonate consumption and are responsible for the AG metabolic acidosis and those causing loss or lack of regeneration/reabsorption of bicarbonate to which the hyperchloremic metabolic acidosis can be attributed.

Metabolic acidosis with high anion gap

AG metabolic acidosis is substantially due to three causes: the excessive production of organic acids (organic acidosis) such as lactic acid or ketoacids, a reduced acids elimination such as in acute and chronic renal failure (mineral acidosis) and finally the introduction of toxic substances or drugs that cause a state of acidosis directly, through their own metabolites or through the production of lactic acid, ketoacid or others (**Table 4.13**, **Figure 4.12**)

Hyperchloremic metabolic acidosis

The main causes of hyperchloremic metabolic acidosis are due to intestinal bicarbonate loss, direct renal

TABLE 4.13 Causes of AG metabolic acidosis.

Endogenous organic acidosis (organic acidosis)	Inorganic acidosis (mineral acidosis)	Acidosis caused by drugs and toxic substances (main)
Lactic acidosis (L and D) Diabetic ketoacidosis Alcoholic ketoacidosis Ketoacidosis due to starvation	Acute and chronic renal failure (phosphates and sulphates, hyppurate and urate)	Ethylene glycol Methanol Ethanol $CaCl_2$ Acetylsalicylic acid Cyanide salts Carbon monoxide Theophylline Acetaminophen Salbutamol Tricyclic antidepressants Metformin SGLT2-inhibitors

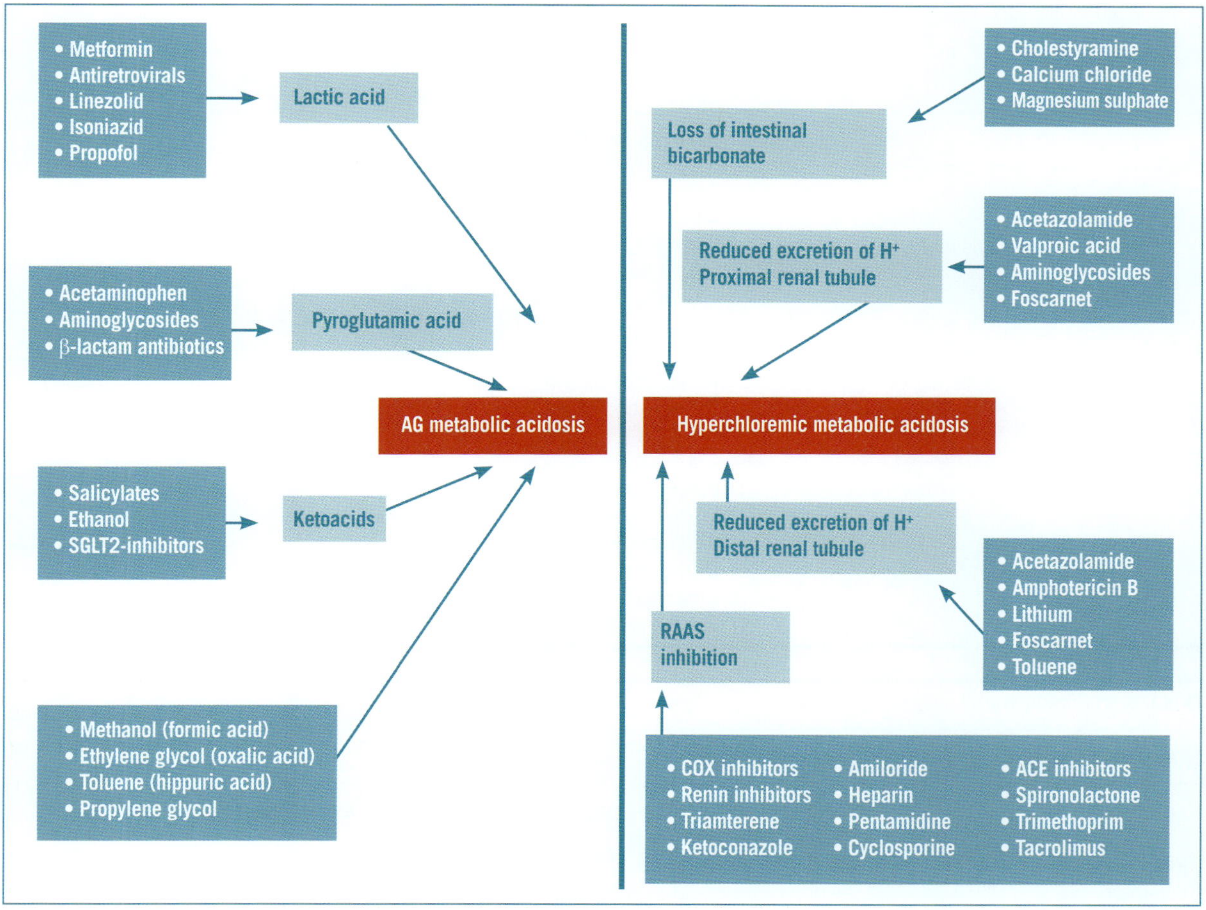

Figure 4.12 Drugs and toxic substances that can determine AG metabolic acidosis or hyperchloremic metabolic acidosis and their mechanism of action. RAAS: renin-angiotensin-aldosterone system.

loss of bicarbonate due to lack of tubular reabsorption or indirect loss due to H^+ retention or reduced NH^+_4 production (**Table 4.14 and Fig. 4.12**).

Clinical features of metabolic acidosis

History

The history must be very careful and oriented to the search for the above mentioned causes. In particular, in the course of hyperchloremic metabolic acidosis, a positive history of diarrhea is important since this is its most frequent cause, as well as attention to the search for renal tubular acidosis.

In case of AG metabolic acidosis, besides considering the most common causes such as lactic acidosis, renal failure and ketoacidosis during type I diabetes mellitus, it is also necessary to look for ketoacidosis from starvation and alcohol use.

The metabolic acidosis that develops during intestinal ischemia/infarction should also be considered.

If these causes are excluded it is important to look for those of toxicological origin (with or without lactates).

TABLE 4.14 Causes of hyperchloremic metabolic acidosis.

Intestinal causes	**Renal causes from bicarbonate loss**
Diarrhea Ureterosigmoidostomy Adrenal insufficiency Pancreatic fistula Intestinal fistula	Proximal renal tubular acidosis (RTA) Carbonic anhydrase inhibitors Fanconi syndrome
	Renal causes due to reduced excretion of H^+
	Distal tubular renal acidosis (RTA type 1) – familiar Distal tubular renal acidosis (RTA type 4) – from interstitial tubule disease – from NSAIDs Addison's disease From potassium-sparing diuretics From initial uremia By ingestion of HCl, NH_4Cl^-, arginine HCl
	Other causes
	Recovery from prolonged hypocapnia During the treatment of diabetic ketoacidosis Inhalation of toluene in healthy kidney Other (see Figure 4.12)

TABLE 4.15 Clinical manifestations of metabolic acidosis.

Type of manifestation	**Signs and symptoms**
Neurological	Headache, reduced level of consciousness, reduced muscle tone and tendon reflexes, muscle tremors
Cardiovascular	Warm skin, reduced blood pressure, arrhythmias
Respiratory	Dyspnea, Kussmaul's breathing
Gastroenterological	Nausea and vomiting, abdominal pain

TABLE 4.16 Renal tubular acidosis and determination of UAG.

Type of RTA	Type II (proximal)	Type I classic	Type I from retro-diffusion	Type IV acidosis	From CDK
Defect	Reduced proximal reabsorption of HCO_3^-	Reduced distal acidification	Hydrogen ions retro-diffusion	Aldosterone deficit or resistance	Inability to produce or secrete NH_4^+
UAG	Positive or negative	Positive	Positive	Positive	Positive

Signs and symptoms

Signs and symptoms often depend on the etiology of the metabolic disorder. Frequent symptoms are hyperventilation, Kussmaul's breathing, nausea, vomiting accompanied by abdominal pain. There may be disorders of the central nervous system, characterized by alteration of the state of consciousness up to coma or seizures (**Table 4.15**).

Acidemia causes cardiac contractility depression and peripheral vasodilation which is counterbalanced by hyperactivity of the sympathetic system and by catecholamines increase. It also reduces the effectiveness of vasopressor drugs. It should be emphasized that severe acidemia is arrhythmogenic.

Laboratory tests

ABG remains the fundamental test. There is often potassium increase due to cell shift (H^+ in exchange of K^+). Chloremia can be normal or increased depending on whether it is an AG metabolic acidosis or a hyperchloremic metabolic acidosis. Frequent detection of increased in creatinine and blood urea.

In the suspected toxic alcohol poisoning the osmolal gap is measured (measured osmolality - calculated osmolality (nv < 10 mOsm/Kg H_2O). If tubular acidosis is suspected as first screening, the determination of the urinary anion gap is useful (**Table 4.16**) (see also page 53).

Respiratory adaptation

Alveolar hyperventilation with $PaCO_2$ reduction is the adaptation mechanism that allows to maintain pH values, within acceptable limits reaching its maximum after 12-24 hours.

Rule of expected adaptation

During metabolic acidosis, $PaCO_2$ is reduced by 1.2 mmHg for every 1 mEq/L of reduction in HCO_3^-.

Clinical case A 24-year-old woman arrives in the emergency department accompanied by her parents after the appearance of fever and mental confusion.

The history shows that the girl has always been well. Only in the last three days she began to suffer from asthenia and low-grade temperature and for two days now, polyuria and polydipsia.

On physical examination the patient presents hot, dehydrated skin as well as xerostomia. The abdomen palpation shows widespread tenderness, while chest auscultation is negative, except for tachycardia when listening to heart sounds. Vital signs are: BP 95/70 mmHg, HR 115 bpm, RR 34 bpm, T 38.2 °C, SpO_2 97%, GCS 14. Some blood tests (blood glucose 396 mg/dL), urine test (ketone ++++) are required.

ABG: pH 6.98, $PaCO_2$ 13 mmHg, HCO_3^- 3.0 mEq/L, PaO_2 96 mmHg, Na^+ 140 mEq/L, Cl^- 103 mEq/L, K^+ 5.0 mEq/L, anion gap 34 mEq/L.

ABG interpretation

pH	6.98	acidemia
$PaCO_2$	13 mmHg	reduced (adaptation mechanism)
HCO_3^-	3.0 mEq/L	decreased (metabolic acidosis)
Anion gap	34 mEq/L	increased
Na^+/Cl^-	1.35	normal

Calculate the ΔAG: (actual AG – reference AG) 34 – 12 = 22 mEq/L.
Calculate the ΔHCO_3^--: (reference HCO_3^- – actual HCO_3^-) 24 – 3 = 21 mEq/L.
Calculate the bicarbonate gap: ($\Delta AG - \Delta HCO_3^-$) 22 – 21 = 1 or $\Delta AG/\Delta HCO_3^-$ (22 : 21 = 1) which confirms the previous data of the presence of an AG metabolic acidosis alone.
Na+/Cl– = 1.35 (normal).

Expected adaptation

Calculate the expected reduction of $PaCO_2$ with respect to the reference value (40 mmHg) in relation to the reduction of bicarbonate, keeping in mind the adaptation rule: 1.2 × 21 = 25.2 mmHg; (reference $PaCO_2$) 40 – 25.2 (reduction of $PaCO_2$) = 14.8 mmHg (expected $PaCO_2$).

Final interpretation: metabolic acidosis with high anion gap.

Reasoned comment

Medical history, clinical picture and laboratory tests point to diabetic ketoacidosis.
The combination of a frankly acidic pH, the decrease in bicarbonate and $PaCO_2$ and the considerable increase in anion gap guide towards a primary acid-base disorder such as AG metabolic acidosis.
The anion gap has risen by 22 mEq/L (ΔAG) and the bicarbonate has fallen by 21 mEq/L (ΔHCO_3^-) so Δgap = + 1 (or $\Delta AG/\Delta HCO_3^- = 1$), which excludes the presence of another acid-base disorder of the metabolic type (also confirmed by the normal Na^+/Cl^- ratio). $PaCO_2$ is reduced due to the respiratory adaptation mechanism. In this case its decrease is consistent with the expected adaptation rule for metabolic acidosis. In fact, since bicarbonate is 3.0 mEq/L with respect to the reference value of 24 mEq/L, it means that it has fallen fallen by 21 mEq/L.
Since $PaCO_2$ decreases by 1.2 mmHg for every mEq/L decrease in bicarbonate, the expected $PaCO_2$ decrease will be 1.2 × 21 = 25.2 mmHg which, subtracted from the reference value (40 mmHg) gives 14.8 mmHg.
Being the actual $PaCO_2$ (13 mmHg) we can speak of expected adaptation achieved (14.8 mmHg ± 2).

Therefore, the clinical interpretation is of AG metabolic acidosis in a patient with ketoacidosis at onset of type I diabetes mellitus.

Clinical case 2 A 71-year-old woman is taken to the emergency department because she has had diarrhea for about six days.
According to the history she has been prescrived therapy with antibiotics for 15 days, due to a pneumonia interesting the right lower lobe.
At pneumonia resolution she began to have several diarrheal discharges a day, without the common generic antidiarrheal therapies having any benefit. On physical examination the patient presents moderately dehydrated skin and mucous membranes, she is suffering and anxious.
The clinical examination of the abdomen does not detect anything pathological outside of a diffuse tenderness, however modest, and also chest examination does not show alterations worthy of note except increased heart rate.
Vital signs: BP 100/70 mmHg, HR 103 bpm, RR 32 bpm, T 37.4 °C, SpO_2 97%, GCS 15.
At the end of the clinical examination some blood tests are required, including ABG.
Stool sample culture is also requested and the *Clostridium difficile* toxin is found to be positive.
ABG: pH 7.29, $PaCO_2$ 28 mmHg, HCO_3^- 14 mEq/L, PaO_2 96 mmHg, Na^+ 141 mEq/L, Cl^- 115 mEq/L, K^+ 3.0 mEq/L, anion gap 12 mEq/L.

ABG interpretation

pH	7.29	acidemia
$PaCO_2$	28 mmHg	reduced (adaptation mechanism)
HCO_3^-	14 mEq/L	decreased (metabolic acidosis)
Anion gap	12 mEq/L	normal
Na^+/Cl^-	1.22	reduced

Calculate the ΔHCO_3^-: (reference HCO_3^- – actual HCO_3^-) 24 – 14 = 10 mEq/L.

Calculate the Δgap of bicarbonate: since the anion gap is normal, it is not calculated.
Na^+/Cl^- = 1.22 (decreased) confirms hyperchloremia.

Expected adaptation

Calculate the expected $PaCO_2$ reduction with respect to the reference value (40 mmHg) in relation to bicarbonate reduction, taking into account the expected adaptation rule 1.2 × 10 = 12 mmHg; (reference $PaCO_2$) 40 – 12 (reduction of $PaCO_2$) = 28 mmHg (expected $PaCO_2$).

Final interpretation: hyperchloremic metabolic acidosis.

Reasoned comment

The history, clinical picture and laboratory tests point to *Clostridium difficile* diarrhea.

The combination of a frankly acidic pH, the decrease in bicarbonate and $PaCO_2$ indicate a primary acid-base disorder such as metabolic acidosis. Hyperchloremia, the value of the Na^+/Cl^- ratio = 1.22 and the normal anion gap define it as a hyperchloremic metabolic acidosis.

$PaCO_2$ is reduced due to the respiratory adaptation mechanism. In this case its decrease is consistent with the expected adaptation rule for metabolic acidosis. In fact, since bicarbonate is 14 mEq/L with respect to the reference value which is 24 mEq/L and since $PaCO_2$ decreases by 1.2 mmHg for every mEq/L of bicarbonate reduction, the expected $PaCO_2$ decrease is 1.2 × 10 = 12 mmHg which subtracted from the reference value (40 mmHg) gives 28 mmHg. Since the actual $PaCO_2$ (28 mmHg) is equal to the expected value (28 mmHg) we can speak of expected adaptation achieved.

The value of the anion gap is normal while chloride concentration has increased significantly for reasons of electroneutrality due to the loss of negative charges from the loss of bicarbonate with diarrhea.

Therefore, the clinical interpretation is of hyperchloremic metabolic acidosis as a simple acid-base disorder, in a patient with Clostridium difficile *diarrhea.*

Clinical case 3 A 22-year-old man is taken by a EMS vehicle to the local emergency department.

Parents report seeing their son euphoric, with an ataxic gait, "as if he had been drinking". He had just come from the cellar of a friend who lives in the same building.

Before the ambulance arrived, he had a short duration seizure.

In the emergency department he is confused, asthenic, with reduced muscle strength of upper and lower limbs. The vital signs: BP 105/75 mmHg, HR 100 bpm, RR 28 bpm, SpO2 97%, GCS 13. ECG: Regular sinus rhythm, Q-Tc interval prolongation with present U wave.

ABG: pH 7.30, PCO_2 25 mmHg, HCO_3^-, 12 mEq/L, PaO_2 100 mmHg, Na^+ 141mEq/L, Cl^- 116 mEq/L, K^+ 2.4 mEq/L, anion gap 13 mEq/L.

ABG interpretation

pH	7.30	acidemia
$PaCO_2$	25 mmHg	reduced (adaptation mechanism)
HCO_3^-	12 mEq/L	reduced (metabolic acidosis)
Anion gap	13 mEq/L	normal
Chloride	116 mEq/L	increased
Na^+/Cl^-	1.21	reduced

Expected adaptation

Calculate the expected reduction of $PaCO_2$ with respect to the reference value (40 mmHg) in relation to the reduction of bicarbonate, taking into account the adaptation rule 1.2 × 12 = 14.4 mmHg; (reference $PaCO_2$) 40 – 14.4 (reduction of $PaCO_2$) = 25.6 mmHg (expected $PaCO_2$).

Final interpretation: hyperchloremic metabolic acidosis.

At this point, after correctly interpreting the arterial blood gas, the cause of the hyperchloremic metabolic acidosis remains to be established. The young man has no diarrhea and has never had kidney problems.

After a few hours the father arrives with some small cans containing glue, found in the cellar, and which raised the first suspicions. The pH, the dosage of sodium, chloride, potassium, glucose and urea is required on the urine collected in the observation unit, where the young man was hospitalized.

pH	5.9
Na^+	20 mEq/L
K^+	22 mEq/L
Cl^-	4
Glucose	0 mg/dL
Urea	9 mg/dL

UAG calculation: $(Na^+ + K^+ - Cl^-) = (20 + 22 - 4) = 38$ mEq/L. UOG calculation: measured osmolality (218 mOsm/Kg H_2O) – calculated osmolality [2 (20 + 22) + 0 + 9 = 93 mOsm/Kg H_2O] = 218 - 93 = 125 mOsm/Kg H_2O.

Reasoned comment

ABG interpretation is quite simple. It is a hyperchloremic metabolic acidosis with a respiratory adaptation consistent with bicarbonate reduction (expected $PaCO_2$ 25.6 mmHg and actual $PaCO_2$ 25 mmHg).

The problem is to understand the cause of this metabolic acidosis mostly is found during diarrhea and renal tubular acidosis.

At this point, the determination of UAG which is very positive and of UOG, which is also positive, is useful.

Considering the clinical picture, characterized by evident neurological disorders, and the laboratory one with hypokalemia, hyperchloremic metabolic acidosis, UAG and UOG decidedly positive, the orientation was for acute poisoning due to toluene aspiration.

In fact the containers brought by the father contained glue. Further investigations confirmed the diagnosis.

Therefore, the clinical interpretation is of hyperchloremic metabolic acidosis with positive UAG and UOG from voluntary toluene intake.

References

Relating to clinical interpretation

- Adrogué HJ, Gennari FJ, Galla JH et al. Assessing acid-base disorders. Kidney Int. 2009; 76(12):1239-47.
- Adrogué HJ, Wilson H, Boyd AE et al. Plasma acid-base patterns in diabetic ketoacidosis. N Engl J Med. 1982;307(26):1603-10.
- Arieff AI, Defronzo RA. Fluid, electrolyte, and acid-base disorders. New York, Churchill Livingstone 1995.
- Batlle DC, Hizon M, Cohen E et al. The use of the urinary anion gap in the diagnosis of hyperchloremic metabolic acidosis. N Engl J Med. 1988;318(10):594-9.
- Berend K. Diagnostic Use of base excess in acid-base disorders. N Engl J Med. 2018;378(15):1419-28.
- Berend K, de Vries AP, Gans RO. Physiological approach to assessment of acid-base disturbances. N Engl J Med. 2014;371(15):1434-45.
- Burnett RW, Noonan DC. Calculation and correction factors used in determination of blood pH and blood gases. Clin Chem. 1974;20(12):1499-506.
- Burtis CA, Burns DE. Tietz fundamentals of clinical chemistry and molecular diagnosis. 7th edition. Elsevier 2014.
- Emmet M. Diagnosis of simple and mixed disorders. In: Dubose T Jr, Hamm L (eds). Acid-base and electrolyte disorders: a companion to Brenner & Rector's The Kidney. Philadelphia, Saunders 2002.
- Emmett M, Seldin DW. Evaluation of acid-base disorders from plasma composition. In: Seldin W, Giebisch G (eds). The regulation of acid-base balance. New York. Raven Press 1989.
- Gennari FJ, Adrogué HJ, Galla JH et al.. Acid-base disorders and their treatment. Boca Raton, Taylor &Francis Group 2005.
- Ghosh AK. Diagnosing acid-base disorders. J Assoc Physicians India. 2006;54:720-4.
- Gluck SL. Acid-base. Lancet. 1998;352(9126):474-9.
- Kamel KS, Halperin ML. Fluid, electrolyte and acid-base physiology. A problem-based approach. 5th edition. Elsevier 2016.
- Kassirer JP, Bleich HL. Rapid estimation of plasma carbon dioxide tension from pH and total carbon dioxide content. N Engl J Med. 1965;272:1067-8.
- Kraut JA, Madias NE. Approach to patients with acid-base disorders. Respir Care. 2001;46(4):392-403.
- Martin L. All you really need to know to interpret arterial blood gases. Philadelphia. Lippincott Williams & Wilkins 1999.
- Narins RG, Emmett M. Simple and mixed acid-base disorders: a practical approach. Medicine (Baltimore). 1980;59 (3):161-87.
- Narins RG, Jones ER, Stom MC et al. Diagnostic strategies in disorders of fluid, electrolyte and acid-base homeostasis. Am J Med. 1982;72(3):496-520.
- Oh M, Carroll HJ. Value and determinants of urine anion gap. Nephron. 2002;90(3):252-5.
- Palmer BF. Approach to fluid and electrolyte disorders and acid-base problems. Prim Care 2008;35(2):195-213.

- Palmer BF, Clegg DJ. The Use of Selected Urine Chemistries in the Diagnosis of Kidney Disorders. Clin J Am Soc Nephrol. 2019;14(2):306-16.
- Raphael KL, Gilligan S, Ix JH. Urine Anion Gap to Predict Urine Ammonium and Related Outcomes in Kidney Disease. Clin J Am Soc Nephrol. 2018;13(2):205-12.
- Raphael KL, Ix JH. Correlation of Urine Ammonium and Urine Osmolal Gap in Kidney Transplant Recipients. Clin J Am Soc Nephrol. 2018;13(4):638-40.
- Rose BD, Post TW. Clinical physiology of acid-base and electrolyte disorders. New York. McGraw-Hill 2001.
- Song ZF, Gu WH, Li HJ et al. The incidence and types of acid-base imbalance for critically ill patients in emergency. Hong Kong J Emerg Med. 2012;19:13-17.

Respiratory acidosis

- Adrogué HJ, Madias NE. Secondary responses to altered acid-base status: the rules of engagement. J Am Soc Nephrol. 2010;21(6):920-3.
- Brackett NC Jr, Wingo CF, Muren O et al. Acid-base response to chronic hypercapnia in man. N Engl J Med. 1969; 280(3):124-30.
- Epstein SK, Singh N. Respiratory acidosis. Respir Care. 2001;46(4):366-83.
- Gennari FJ, Goldstein MB, Schwartz WB. The nature of the renal adaptation to chronic hypocapnia. J Clin Invest. 1972;51(7):1722-30.
- González SB, Menga G, Raimondi GA et al. Secondary Response to Chronic Respiratory Acidosis in Humans: A Prospective Study. Kidney Int Rep. 2018;3(5):1163-70.
- Kassirer JP, Madias NE. Respiratory acid-base disorders. Hosp Pract. 1980;15(12):57-9.
- Krachman S, Criner GJ. Hypoventilation syndromes. Clin Chest Med. 1988;19(1):139-55.
- Madias NE, Cohen JJ. Respiratory acidosis. In: Cohen JJ, Kassirer JP (eds.). Acid-Base, Boston, Little Brown 1982.
- Madias NE, Wolf CJ, Cohen JJ. Regulation of acid-base equilibrium in chronic hypercapnia. Kidney Int. 1985;27(3): 538-43.
- Martinu T, Menzies D, Dial S. Re-evaluation of acid-base prediction rules in patients with chronic respiratory acidosis. Can Respir J. 2003;10(6):311-5.
- Norman LJ. Acidemie sans acidose respiratoire. Can Respir J. 2003;10:301-3.
- Polak A, Haynie GD et al. Effects of chronic hypercapnia on electrolyte and acid-base equilibrium. I. Adaptation. J Clin Invest. 1961;40:1223-37.
- Schwartz WB, Brackett NC Jr, Cohen JJ. The response of extracellular hydrogen ion concentration to graded degrees of chronic hypercapnia: The physiologic limits of the defense of pH. J Clin Invest. 1965;44:291-301.
- Van Ypersele de Striho, Brasseur L, De Coninck JD. The "carbon dioxide response curve" for chronic hypercapnia in man. N Engl Med. 1966;275(3):275:117-22.
- Weinberger SE, Schwartzstein RM, Weiss JW. Hypercapnia. N Engl J Med. 1989;321(18):1223-31.

Respiratory alkalosis

- Arbus GS, Herbert LA, Levesque PR et al. Characterization and clinical application of the "significance band" for acute respiratory alkalosis. N Engl Med 1969;280(3):117-23.
- Eldridge F, Salzer J. Effect of respiratory alkalosis on blood lactate and pyruvate in humans. J Appl Physiol. 1967;22 (3):461-8.
- Foster GT, Vaziri ND, Sassoon CS. Respiratory alkalosis. Resp Care. 2001;46(4):384-91.
- Gennari FJ, Goldstein MB, Schwartz WB. The nature of the renal adaptation to chronic hypocapnia. J Clin Invest. 1972;51(7):1722-30.
- Krapf R, Caduff P, Wadgi P et al. Plasma potassium response to acute respiratory alkalosis. Kidney Int. 1995;47(1):217-24.
- Kreisberg RA. Lactate homeostasis and lactic acidosis. Ann Intern Med. 1980;92:227-37.
- Laffey JG, Kavanagh BP. Hypocapnia. N Engl J Med. 2002; 347(1):43-53.
- Maddock RJ. The lactic acid response to alkalosis in panic disorder: an integrative review. J Neuropsychiatry Clin Neurosci. 200;13(1):22-34.
- Yoon S, Zuccarello M, Rapoport RM. pCO(2) and pH regulation of cerebral blood flow. Front Physiol. 2012;3:365.

Metabolic alkalosis

- Anderson LE, Henrich WL. Alkalemia-associated morbidity and mortality in medical and surgical patients. South Med J. 1987;80(6):729-33.
- Galla JH. Metabolic alkalosis. J Am Soc Nephrol. 2000;11(2): 369-75.
- Galla JH, Gifford JD, Luke RG et al. Adaptations to chloride-depletion alkalosis. Am J Physiol. 1991;261(4 Pt 2): R771-81.
- Gennari FJ. Pathophysiology of metabolic alkalosis: a new classification based on the centrality of stimulated collecting duct ion transport. Am J Kidney Dis. 2011;58(4):626-36.
- Hamm LL, Nakhoul N, Hering-Smith KS. Acid-base homeostasis. Clin J Am Soc Nephrol. 2015;10(12):2232-42.
- Hodgkin JE, Soeprono FF, Chan DM. Incidence of metabolic alkalemia in hospitalized patients. Crit Care Med. 1980;8(12):725-8.
- Javaheri S, Kazemi H. Metabolic alkalosis and hypoventilation in humans. Am Rev Respir Dis. 1987;136(4):1011-6.
- Javaheri S, Shore NS, Rose BD et al. Compensatory hypoventilation in metabolic alkalosis. Chest. 1982;81(3):296-301.
- Khanna A, Kurtzman NA. Metabolic alkalosis. Resp Care. 2001;46(4):354-65.
- Laski ME, Sabatini S. Metabolic alkalosis, bedside and bench. Semin Nephrol. 2006;26(6):404-21.
- Luke RG, Galla JH. It is chloride depletion alkalosis, not contraction alkalosis. J Am Soc Nephrol. 2012;23(2):204-7.
- Madias NE, Adrogué HH, Cohen JJ. Maladaptive renal response to secondary hypercapnia in chronic metabolic alkalosis. Am J Physiol. 1980;238(4):F283-9.
- Norris SH, Kurtzman NA. Does chloride play an independent role in the pathogenesis of metabolic alkalosis? Semin Nephrol. 1988;8(2):101-8.

- Pela I, Bigozzi M, Bianchi B. Profound hypokalemia and hypochloremic metabolic alkalosis during thiazide therapy in a child with Pendred syndrome. Clin Nephrol. 2008;69(6):450-3.
- Ring T. Potassium and metabolic alkalosis. Am J Kidney Dis. 2012;59(2):315.
- Seldin DW, Rector FC Jr. The generation and maintenance of metabolic alkalosis. Kidney Int. 1972;1:306-21.

Metabolic acidosis

- Berkman M, Ufberg J, Nathanson LA et al. Anion gap as a screening tool for elevated lactate in patients with an increased risk of developing sepsis in the Emergency Department. J Emerg Med 2009;36(4):391-94.
- Brenner BE. Clinical significance of the elevated anion gap. Am J Med. 1985;79(3):289-96.
- Bushinsky DA, Coe FL, Katzenberg C et al. Arterial PCO_2 in chronic metabolic acidosis. Kidney Int. 1982; 22(3):311-4.
- Camara-Lemarroy CR, Rodríguez-Gutiérrez R, Monreal-Robles R et al. Acute toluene intoxication-clinical presentation, management and prognosis: a prospective observational study. BMC Emerg Med. 2015;15:19.
- Carlisle EJ, Donnelly SM, Vasuvattakul S et al. Glue-sniffing and distal renal tubular acidosis: sticking to the facts. J Am Soc Nephrol. 1991;1(8):1019-27.
- Chawla LS, Shih S, Davison D et al. Anion gap, anion gap corrected for albumin, base deficit and unmeasured anions in critically ill patients: implications on the assessment of metabolic acidosis and the diagnosis of hyperlactatemia. BMC Emerg Med. 2008;8:18.
- Emmett M. Anion gap interpretation: the old and the new. Clin Pract Nephrol. 2006;2(1):4-5.
- Emmett M, Narins RG. Clinical use of the anion gap. Medicine (Baltimore). 1977;56(1):38-54.
- Feldman M, Soni N, Dickson B. Influence of hypoalbuminemia or hyperalbuminemia on the serum anion gap. J Lab Clin Med. 2005;146(6):317-20.
- Figge J, Jabor A, Kazda A et al. Anion gap and hypoalbuminemia. Crit Care Med. 1998;26(11):1807-10.
- Gabow P. Disorders associated with an altered anion gap. Kidney Int. 1985;27(2):472-83.
- Gabow PA, Kaehny WD, Fennessey PV et al. Diagnostic importance of an increase serum anion gap. N Engl J Med. 1980;303:854-58.
- Goldstein RJ, Lichtenstein NS, Souder D. The myth of the low anion gap. JAMA 1980;243(17):1737-8.
- Hatherill M, Waggie Z, Purves L et al. Correction of the anion gap for albumin in order to detect occult tissue anions in shock. Arch Dis Child. 2002;87(6):526-9.
- Iberti TJ, Leibowitz AB, Papadakos PJ et al. Low sensitivity of the anion gap as a screen to detect hyperlactatemia in critically ill patients. Crit Care Med. 1990;18(3):275-77.
- Ishihara K, Szerlip HM. Anion gap acidosis. Semin Nephrol. 1998;18(1):83-97.
- Jurado RL, del Rio C, Nassar G et al. Low anion gap. South Med J. 1998;91(7):624-9.
- Keshgegian AA. Anion gap and immunoglobulin concentration. Am J Clin Pathol 1980;74(3):282-4.
- Kokko JP, Tannen RL (eds.). Metabolic acid-base disorders. In: Fluids and electrolytes. Philadelphia, WB Saunders 1990.
- Kraut JA, Madias NE. Lactic acidosis. N Engl J Med. 2015; 372(11):1078-9.
- Kreisberg RA, Wood BC. Drug and chemical-induced metabolic acidosis. Clin Endocrinol Metab. 1983;12(2):391-411.
- Levraut J, Bounatirou T, Ichai C et al. Reliability of anion gap as an indicator of blood lactate in critically ill patients. Intensive Care Med. 1997;23(4):417-22.
- Lynd LD, Richardson KJ, Purssell RA et al. An evaluation of the osmole gap as a screening test for toxic alcohol poisoning. BMC Emerg Med. 2008;8:5.
- Kraut JA, Madias NE. Serum anion gap: its uses and limitations in clinical medicine. Clin J Am Soc Nephrol. 2007; 2(1):162-74.
- Marino PL. Primary metabolic disorders in acid-base interpretation. In: The ICU Book. Philadelphia. Lippincott Williams & Wilkins 1998.
- Moss AH, Gabow PA, Kaehny WD et al. Fanconi's syndrome and distal renal tubular acidosis after glue sniffing. Ann. Intern Med. 1980;92(1):69-70.
- Murray T, Long W, Narins RG. Multiple myeloma and the anion gap. N Engl J Med. 1975;292(11):574-5.
- Oh MS, Carroll HJ. The anion gap. N. Engl J Med. 1977;297 (15):814.7.
- Oster JR, Perez GO, Materson BJ. Use of anion gap in clinical medicine. South Med J. 1988;81(2):229-37.
- Perez GO, Oster JR. Acid-base disorders. Part II. Use of AG/ HCO_3^- in evaluating mixed acid-base disorders: a patient management problem. South Med J. 1986;79:882-6.
- Pierce NF, Fedson DS, Brigham KL et al. The ventilatory response to acute base deficit in humans. Time course during development and correction of metabolic acidosis. Ann Intern Med. 1970;72(5):633-40.
- Reilly RF, Anderson RJ. Interpreting the anion gap. Crit Care Med. 1998;26(11):1771-2.
- Roberts WL, Johnson RD. The serum anion gap. Has the reference interval really fallen? Arch Pathol Lab Med. 1997;121(6):568-72.
- Rastegar A. Use of the DeltaAG/Delta HCO_3^- ratio in the diagnosis of mixed acid-base disorders. J Am Soc Nephrol 2007;18(9):2429-31.
- Rosival V. Reliability of the anion gap. Crit Care Med. 2000; 28(5):1693.
- Salem MM, Mujais SK. Gaps in the anion gap. Arch Intern Med. 1992;152(8):1625-9.
- Swenson ER. Metabolic acidosis. Respir Care. 2001;46(4): 342-53.
- Whittington JE, La'ulu SL, Hunsaker JJ et al. The osmolal gap: what has changed? Clin Chem. 2010;56(8):1353-5.
- Wrenn K. The delta (delta) gap: an approach to mixed acid-base disorders. Ann Emerg Med. 1990;19(11):1310-3.

Clinical interpretation of mixed acid-base disorders

Ivo Casagranda

Definition

A mixed disorder is a clinical condition characterized by the simultaneous presence of two or more alterations of the acid-base balance.

Many disorders may be concomitant in a single patient, except for the simultaneous presence of respiratory alkalosis superimposed on respiratory acidosis; an exception is the patient with chronic lung disease and CO_2 retention, subjected to mechanical ventilation in such a way as to cause a sharp reduction in $PaCO_2$ and therefore to determine an acute respiratory alkalosis on a pre-existing condition of chronic respiratory acidosis.

Classification of mixed disorders

Double respiratory disorders

- Acute respiratory acidosis superimposed on chronic respiratory acidosis.
- Acute respiratory acidosis superimposed on chronic respiratory alkalosis.
- Acute respiratory alkalosis superimposed on chronic respiratory alkalosis.
- Acute respiratory alkalosis superimposed on chronic respiratory acidosis (from mechanical ventilation).

Double metabolic disorders

- AG metabolic acidosis or hyperchloremic metabolic acidosis and metabolic alkalosis.
- AG metabolic acidosis and hyperchloremic metabolic acidosis.

Double respiratory and metabolic disorders

- Respiratory acidosis (acute or chronic) with
  – metabolic acidosis (AG or hyperchloremic)
  or with
  – metabolic alkalosis.
- Respiratory alkalosis (acute or chronic) with
  – metabolic acidosis (AG or hyperchloremic)
  or with
  – metabolic alkalosis.

Triple respiratory and metabolic disorders

- Metabolic alkalosis with chronic respiratory acidosis and overlap of acute respiratory acidosis.
- Respiratory alkalosis with metabolic alkalosis and metabolic acidosis (AG or hyperchloremic).
- Respiratory acidosis with metabolic alkalosis and metabolic acidosis (AG or hyperchloremic).

Quadruple respiratory and metabolic disorders

- Metabolic acidosis (AG or hyperchloremic) and metabolic alkalosis with chronic respiratory acidosis and overlapping of acute respiratory acidosis (more frequent disorder among quadruple disorders).

NOTE

The disorders consisting of a double alkalosis or double acidosis are defined additives with a very alkaline pH in the first case and a very acid in the second. Those in which there is the simultaneous presence of alkalosis and acidosis whether respiratory and/or metabolic are defined counterbalancing disorders and disclose with pH often normal.

When to suspect the presence of a mixed acid-base disorder

At this point it seems appropriate to review some principles already discussed in Chapter 4 that can help us understand when we are dealing with a mixed disorder. It also seemed appropriate to propose these interpretative elements as rules.

First rule (mother rule) or the Kassirer-Bleich equation disregarded

As already explained in Chapter 4, this equation tells us that to keep the serum hydrogen ion concentration $[H^+]$ constant and within the physiological limits, the ratio between the two terms of the equation ($PaCO_2/HCO_3^-$) must remain constant. It follows, and this is the rule, that when one of the two terms goes in one direction (increases or decreases), the other should go in the same direction (increase or decrease); for example, if $PaCO_2$ increases or decreases $[HCO_3^-]$ must also increase or decrease and vice versa.

If, on the contrary, one of the two terms proceeds in the opposite direction, it means that we are dealing with a mixed disorder.

Second rule or failure to comply with adaptation

When one of the two terms that should adapt to the changes of the other, varies in excess or in defect with respect to the rules of adaptation we have seen for each disorder, it means that we are dealing with a mixed disorder. This rule can be considered a corollary of the mother rule.

Third rule or pH false compensation

A normal pH range (7.35, 7.45), in the presence of values of $PaCO_2$ and/or $[HCO_3^-]$ out of range, is indicative of a mixed disorder (counterbalancing disorders). The exception is chronic respiratory alkalosis which often brings the pH back to normal.

Fourth rule or the Δgap ($\Delta AG - \Delta HCO_3^-$) or the $\Delta AG/\Delta HCO_3^-$ ratio

When the rule is not respected that (approximately) for each mEq/L increase in anion gap there is a reduction of an analogous bicarbonate equivalent, we are dealing with a mixed disorder.

The difference between anion gap increase and $[HCO_3^-]$ reduction is called Δgap and the normal values are 0 ± 6 mEq/L.

The Δgap can be normal (0 ± 6 mEq/L), positive (> +6 mEq/L), negative (< –6 mEq/L).

If the Δgap is positive, in the sense that bicarbonate is not reduced by how much it should with respect to the increase in the anion gap ($\Delta AG > \Delta HCO_3^-$), it means that metabolic alkalosis coexists next to AG metabolic acidosis. If it is negative, in the sense that bicarbonate is reduced too much compared to the expected value ($\Delta AG < \Delta HCO_3^-$), it means that a hyperchloremic metabolic acidosis accompanies an AG metabolic acidosis. For the $\Delta AG/\Delta HCO_3^-$ ratio see Chapter 4, page 72, Figure 4.11.

Fifth rule or the Na^+/Cl^- ratio

The evaluation of the Na^+/Cl^- ratio, whose normal value is 1.40, can be useful to highlight the presence of metabolic alkalosis or hyperchloremic acidosis in the presence of AG metabolic acidosis.

This evaluation can support the calculation of the Δgap as it confirms it.

In practice, if the ratio value is ≥ 1.55 the presence of metabolic alkalosis is probable. If there is a value ≤ 1.25 the presence of hyperchloremic metabolic acidosis is probable.

Furthermore, the evaluation of this relationship is very useful during hyponatremia in case it is not possible to understand if the hypochloremia is due only to hyponatremia or there is also a concomitant metabolic alkalosis.

Flow chart for the identification of mixed acid-base disorders

On the basis of these interpretative keys and those previously seen, when we discussed the simple disorders, we suggested to adopt in the clinical practice the following path to identify, with reasonable certainty, the mixed disorders:

Evaluate pH (normal, acid, alkaline), $PaCO_2$ and $[HCO_3^-]$

- If pH is normal, in the presence of values of $PaCO_2$ and/or $[HCO_3^-]$ out of range, think of a mixed disorder (acidosis + alkalosis).
- If pH is acid there is certainly an acidosis (metabolic and/or respiratory) but this does not exclude the concomitance of another disorder (i.e., double acidosis and alkalosis).
- If pH is alkaline there is certainly an alkalosis (metabolic and/or respiratory) but this does not exclude the concomitance of another disorder (i.e., double alkalosis and acidosis).

Evaluate electrolytes (Na^+ and Cl^-) and check if there is hyperchloremia or hypochloremia, calculating the Na^+/Cl^- ratio

Calculate anion gap • $Na^+ - (Cl^- + HCO_3^-)$ • despite any pH

→ **Normal anion gap**

↓

On the basis of the hypothetical disorder, check the expected adaptation (according to the rules set out in the chapter on simple disorders)

↓

Assumption of respiratory alkalosis
If $[HCO_3^-]$ is greater than expected with $Na^+/Cl^- \geq 1.55$:
concomitant metabolic alkalosis
If $[HCO_3^-]$ is lower than expected and there is hyperchloremia ($Na^+/Cl^- \leq 1.25$):
concomitant hyperchloremic metabolic acidosis

Assumption of respiratory acidosis
If $[HCO_3^-]$ is greater than expected with $Na^+/Cl^- \geq 1.55$:
concomitant metabolic alkalosis
If $[HCO_3^-]$ is lower than expected and there is hyperchloremia ($Na^+/Cl^- \leq 1.25$):
concomitant hyperchloremic metabolic acidosis

Assumption of metabolic alkalosis → Evaluate $PaCO_2$

→ **High anion gap (significant ≥ 19 mEq/L)**
AG metabolic acidosis

↓

Calculate the Δgap (v.n. 0 ± 6 mEq/L) or the $\Delta AG/\Delta HCO_3^-$ ratio (see pages 72 and 73)

→ **Normal** → Evaluate $PaCO_2$

↓

Δgap > +6 and $Na^+/Cl^- \geq 1.55$
concomitant metabolic alkalosis
Δgap < –6 and $Na^+/Cl^- \leq 1.25$
concomitant hyperchloremic metabolic acidosis

↓

Evaluate $PaCO_2$ for the calculation of the expected adaptation (± 2/± 3 mmHg)

$PaCO_2$ > to expected *concomitant respiratory acidosis*
$PaCO_2$ < to expected *concomitant respiratory alkalosis*

TABLE 5.1 (comparative) Mixed alkalosis: respiratory and metabolic.

	Normal	Respiratory alkalosis acute	Respiratory alkalosis chronic	Metabolic alkalosis	Mixed alkalosis mild	Mixed alkalosis severe
pH	7.40	7.51	7.43	7.54	7.51	7.63
$PaCO_2$ (mmHg)	40	27	30	56	40	29
HCO_3^- (mEq/L)	24	21	20	47	31	30
Na^+ (mEq/L)	139	138	138	135	135	136
K^+ (mEq/L)	4.0	3.4	3.2	2.8	3.0	2.8
Cl^- (mEq/L)	103	104	104	72	89	90
Anion gap (mEq/l)	16	13	14	16	15	16
Na^+/Cl^-	1.34	1.32	1.32	1.87	1.51	1.51

Double mixed acid-base disorders

Respiratory alkalosis and metabolic alkalosis (additive disorders)

Definition

It is a mixed acid-base disorder characterized by $PaCO_2$ reduction and a concomitant [HCO_3^-] increase.

In this case alkalemia is usually severe, because neither of the two disorders can be partially corrected by their own adaptation mechanism.

Table 5.1 shows, indicatively, what happens when two additive disorders such as metabolic alkalosis and respiratory alkalosis in their mild and severe forms occur. A normal ABG and two simple disorders has been used as a reference. When these two disorders are found simultaneously in the same patient, they produce the mentioned mixed disorder.

NOTE

This table and those that will follow in this section are inspired by those present in Narins RG, Emmett M. Simple and mixed acid-base disorders: a practical approach. Medicine (Baltimore). 1980; 59 (3): 161-87, and subsequently modified by us.

Causes

- *Critical patients:* respiratory alkalosis from sepsis, hypoxemia, pain, liver failure, central neurological lesions, massive blood transfusion, hypotension, drugs; metabolic alkalosis from nasogastric suction, vomiting, use of diuretics or steroids, excessive infusion of Ringer's lactate solution, administration of antacids.
- *Pregnancy*: respiratory alkalosis due to the increase in the circulating rate of progesterone; metabolic alkalosis from vomiting.
- *Mechanical ventilation*: this is the case in which a patient suffering from chronic respiratory acidosis with high serum bicarbonate is placed in mechanical ventilation: if the $PaCO_2$ falls too fast, while the bicarbonate concentration remains high, a double alkalosis is determined.

Clinical case A 76-year-old man, having a indwelling bladder catheter for simple prostatic hypertrophy, reaches in the emergency department because he has had a high fever for four days. In the last two days he has had frequent episodes of bilious vomiting.

The history highlights congestive heart failure and for this reason he is being treated, among other things, with loop diuretics, which he continued to take until the day he arrived at the hospital.

The patient is confused and dehydrated. The vital signs:

BP 95/70 mmHg, HR 110 bpm, RR 32 bpm, T 38.5 °C, SpO_2 97% on room air, GCS 13. Some blood tests are required.

ABG: pH 7.65, $PaCO_2$ 30 mmHg, HCO_3^- 32 mEq/L, PaO_2 96 mmHg, Na^+ 137 mEq/L, Cl^- 88 mEq/L, K^+ 2.7 mEq/L, anion gap 17 mEq/L, Na^+/Cl^- 1.55.

A urine culture is being requested.

ABG interpretation

pH	7.65	alkalemia
$PaCO_2$	30 mmHg	reduced (respiratory alkalosis)
HCO_3^-	32 mEq/L	increased (metabolic alkalosis)
Anion gap	17 mEq/L	slightly (increased due to alkaline pH)
Chloride	88 mEq/L	reduced (for electroneutrality reasons: increase in bicarbonate anions)
Na^+/Cl^-	1.55	increased (due to metabolic alkalosis)

Expected adaptation for metabolic alkalosis

It is useless to calculate, because $PaCO_2$ that should increase is even decreased thus disregarding both the Kassirer-Bleich equation and the expected adaptation rule. Conversely, if we start with respiratory alkalosis.

Final interpretation: metabolic alkalosis and respiratory alkalosis.

Reasoned comment

The clearly alkaline pH, $PaCO_2$ reduction and bicarbonate increase (rule of the disregarded Kassirer-Bleich equation) give evidence of a mixed acid-base disorder and in particular of respiratory alkalosis with metabolic alkalosis. Anion gap is slightly increased due to alkaline pH. The increased Na^+/Cl^- ratio confirms the presence of metabolic alkalosis. This double disorder is explained by the clinical picture: the metabolic alkalosis is due to diuretics use and vomiting, while the respiratory one is caused by the gram⁻ sepsis (urine culture was positive for *E. Coli*).

Therefore the diagnosis is of metabolic alkalosis and respiratory alkalosis in patients with gram⁻ sepsis, vomiting and diuretics intake.

Metabolic acidosis and respiratory alkalosis (counterbalancing disorders)

Definition

It is a mixed acid-base disorder characterized by metabolic acidosis (decrease in bicarbonates) accompanied by $PaCO_2$ reduction beyond the expected adaptation limit.

Table 5.2 shows indicatively what happens when two counterbalancing disorders occur, metabolic acidosis with high anion gap (AG) and respiratory alkalosis (mild and severe).

A normal ABG and two simple disorders has been used as a reference. When these two disorders are found simultaneously in the same patient, they produce the mentioned mixed disorder.

Causes

- *Intoxication with acetylsalicylic acid*: toxic levels of acetylsalicylic acid cause $PaCO_2$ reduction, due to a respiratory rate increase by direct stimulation of the breath center and also due to the decoupling of oxidative phosphorylation (respiratory alkalosis); the high concentration of acetylsalicylic acid causes the production of organic acids such as keto acids and lactic acid to which it is added, to a lesser extent, the same acetylsalicylic acid (AG metabolic acidosis). In children, compared to adults, during the intoxication, the metabolic acidosis intervenes first and then the respiratory alkalosis.
- *Hepatic failure*: during advanced liver disease there is a production of biogenic amines, ammonium and an increase in progesterone levels due to reduced hepatic catabolism which determines a stimulation of the breath center. Furthermore, under these conditions, there is hypoxemia caused by ventilation-perfusion alterations. All this causes respiratory alkalosis. Metabolic acidosis is due to the onset of renal tubular acidosis and furthermore lactic acid production can be increased in patients with ad-

TABLE 5.2 (comparative) Metabolic acidosis and respiratory alkalosis.

	Normal	Respiratory alkalosis acute	chronic	AG Metabolic acidosis	Metabolic acidosis and respiratory alkalosis mild	severe
pH	7.40	7.51	7.43	7.02	7.43	7.59
$PaCO_2$ (mmHg)	40	27	30	16	23	15
HCO_3^- (mEq/L)	24	21	20	4	15	14
Na^+ (mEq/L)	139	138	138	140	140	140
K^+ (mEq/L)	4.0	3.4	3.2	3.7	4.0	3.5
Cl^- (mEq/L)	103	104	104	105	106	105
Anion gap (mEq/L)	12	13	14	31	19	21
Na^+/Cl^-	1.34	1.32	1.32	1.33	1.32	1.33

vanced liver disease, reduced uptake and lactic acid metabolism by the liver.

- *Critical patients*: in these patients there can often coexist causes that cause respiratory alkalosis and metabolic acidosis such as, for example, in septic shock, in diabetic ketoacidosis with sepsis and in pneumonia with renal failure.

Clinical case An 18-year-old woman is brought to the emergency department by the EMS team, alerted by parents who found their daughter lying on the bed, sleepy.

On physical examination she has tachypnea and is easily irritabled. When stimulated, she refers to see very intense lights.

The vital signs: BP 95/70 mmHg, HR 100 bpm, RR 32 bpm, T 37.8 °C, SpO_2 97% on room air, GCS 13. Some blood tests are required.

ABG: pH 7.39, $PaCO_2$ 24 mmHg, HCO_3^- 14 mEq/L, PaO_2 102 mmHg, Na^+ 140 mEq/L, Cl^- 105 mEq/L, K^+ 4.0 mEq/L, anion gap 21 mEq/L.

After an hour the brother arrives with numerous empty blister packs, found in the bathroom, which contained acetylsalicylic acid tablets. As a consequence plasma dosage of salicylates is required, which results 80 mg/dL.

ABG interpretation

pH	7.39	normal
$PaCO_2$	24 mmHg	reduced (respiratory alkalosis)
HCO_3^-	14 mEq/L	reduced (metabolic acidosis)
Anion gap	21 mEq/L	increased
ΔAG	9 mEq/L	
ΔHCO_3^-	10 mEq/L	
Δgap	−1	normal
Chloride	105 mEq/L	normal
Na^+/Cl^-	1.33	normal

Expected adaptation for metabolic acidosis

Calculate the expected $PaCO_2$ reduction with respect to reference value (40 mmHg) in relation to bicarbonate reduction, taking into account the adaptation rule for metabolic acidosis 1.2 × 10 (bicarbonate reduction) = 12 – 40 (reference $PaCO_2$) = 28 mmHg (expected $PaCO_2$). The actual $PaCO_2$ (24 mmHg) is lower than expected (28 mmHg) and therefore there is a failure to comply with the adaptation rule, highlighting the presence of respiratory alkalosis.

Final interpretation: AG metabolic acidosis and respiratory alkalosis.

Reasoned comment

Normal pH, the reduction of $PaCO_2$ and bicarbonate (the rule of false pH compensation) point towards a mixed disorder. The high anion gap is due to metabolic acidosis. The Δgap is equal to −1 and the ratio Na^+/Cl^- = 1.33 and therefore there is no other metabolic disorder added to AG metabolic acidosis.

$PaCO_2$ is reduced as it happens during metabolic acidosis but in this case its decrease is not consistent with the adaptation rule for metabolic acidosis.

In fact, since the actual bicarbonate are 14 mEq/L and compared to reference value (24 mEq/L) they have dropped by 10 mEq/L, the $PaCO_2$ should fall by 12 mmHg (1.2 × 10 = 12 mmHg) compared to the reference of 40 mmHg, thus reaching the expected value of 28 mmHg.

Being the actual $PaCO_2$ (24 mmHg) different from the expected one (28 mmHg), it means that there is an extra stimulus that determines a ventilation frequency greater than that required by the physiological mechanism of adaptation to metabolic acidosis: this causes a further $PaCO_2$ reduction which leads to respiratory alkalosis which is added to AG metabolic acidosis.

Therefore the diagnosis is of metabolic acidosis with high anion gap with respiratory alkalosis due to intoxication by acetylsalicylic acid.

AG metabolic acidosis and respiratory acidosis (additive disorders)

Definition

It is a mixed acid-base disorder characterized by metabolic acidosis (bicarbonate reduction) accompanied by $PaCO_2$ reduction lower than that provided by the expected adaptation rule or by a real increase in it. In this case acidemia is usually severe, because neither of the two disorders can be partially corrected by their own adaptation mechanisms.

Table 5.3 shows indicatively what happens when two additive disorders occur: AG metabolic acidosis and respiratory acidosis in the mild and severe form.

A normal ABG and two simple disorders has been used as a reference. When these two disorders are found simultaneously in the same patient, they produce the mentioned mixed disorder.

Causes

- *Chronic obstructive pulmonary disease (COPD) with hypoxemia and hypercapnia*: patients with chronic hypercapnic bronchopneumopathy (respiratory acidosis) may experience episodes of exacerbation of the disease with a significant drop in PaO_2 followed by tissue hypoxia and production of lactic acid (AG metabolic acidosis). In addition to this, other conditions such as anemia, reduced cardiac output and reduced tissue perfusion due to arterial hypotension and left shift of hemoglobin's dissociation curve can contribute to tissue hypoxia.
- *Cardio-respiratory arrest*: it is the clinical emergency in which circulation absence (cardiac failure) and pulmonary insufficiency (pump and lung failure) are maximally expressed. A severe acidemia follows due to the addition of two acidifying pro-

TABLE 5.3 (comparative) Mixed acidosis: AG metabolic and respiratory.

	Normal	Respiratory acidosis		AG metabolic acidosis	Respiratory acidosis and metabolic acidosis	
		acute	chronic		mild	severe
pH	7.40	7.22	7.34	7.02	7.24	7.17
$PaCO_2$ (mmHg)	40	69	67	16	38	48
HCO_3^- (mEq/L)	24	27	35	4	16	17
Na^+ (mEq/L)	139	140	137	140	140	140
K^+ (mEq/L)	4.0	4.1	4.2	3.7	4.2	4.8
Cl^- (mEq/L)	103	102	90	105	104	102
Anion gap (mEq/L)	12	11	12	31	20	21
Na^+/Cl^-	1.34	1.37	1.52	1.33	1.34	1.37

cesses such as carbon dioxide retention and lactic acid production.

- *Acute pulmonary edema*: various acid-base disorders may occur during acute pulmonary edema. At the beginning fluids accumulation at alveolar level leads to hypoxia due to the intrapulmonary shunt, causing an increase in respiratory rate followed by respiratory alkalosis.
  As clinical conditions worsen, also due to the addition of airways obstructive component, ventilation is reduced, resulting in respiratory acidosis and severe hypoxemia.
  Furthermore, left ventricular failure causes a reduction in cardiac output and tissue perfusion that adds to hypoxemia and it is responsible for an increased production of lactic acid and therefore of AG metabolic acidosis.
- *Poisoning*: most poisonings produce mixed disorders such as metabolic acidosis and respiratory acidosis. Metabolic acidosis can be due to the toxic products direct action (i.e., hydrochloric acid), to acid metabolites derived by original chemical compound (i.e., ethylene glycol) or to interference with the cellular metabolism that causes lactic acid production and/or ketone bodies (i.e., metformin and acetylsalicylic acid) or to interference with oxygen transport and cellular respiratory chain followed by tissue hypoxia with lactic acid production (i.e., carbon monoxide and cyanide).
  Often there is respiratory acidosis from breath centers depression, from direct or indirect pulmonary toxicity, for example from aspiration of gastric contents following vomiting, frequent during intoxication.

Clinical case An 82-year-old man is transported to the emergency department by a EMS vehicle, due to severe dyspnea arose about an hour earlier. He is well known by local emergency department doctors for previous accesses for acute cardiogenic pulmonary edema.

For many years he has been suffering from arterial hypertension and chronic atrial fibrillation; four years earlier he had had an anterior myocardial infarction complicated by acute pulmonary edema.

On examination, he presents dyspnea, algid diaphoresis, skin cyanosis and turgid jugular veins. Chest auscultation detects rattles at medium bubbles and bronchospasm sounds.

The vital signs: BP 85/70 mmHg, HR 120 bpm, RR 36 bpm, T 36.2 °C, SpO_2 85% on room air.

ABG: pH 7.15, $PaCO_2$ 50 mmHg, HCO_3^- 17 mEq/L, PaO_2 50 mmHg, Na^+ 142 mEq/L, Cl^- 105 mEq/L, K^+ 4.0 mEq/L, anion gap 20 mEq/L.

ABG interpretation

pH	7.15	acidemia
$PaCO_2$	50 mmHg	elevated (respiratory acidosis)
HCO_3^-	17 mEq/L	reduced (metabolic acidosis)
Anion gap	20 mEq/L	increased
ΔAG	8 mEq/L	
ΔHCO_3^-	7 mEq/L	
Δgap	+1	normal
Chloride	105 mEq/L	normal
Na^+/Cl^-	1.35	normal

Expected adaptation for metabolic acidosis

It is useless to calculate because $PaCO_2$ that should decrease is even increased thus disregarding both the Kassirer-Bleich equation and the expected adaptation rule.

Final interpretation: AG metabolic acidosis and respiratory acidosis.

Reasoned comment

The acid pH with $PaCO_2$ increase and the reduction of the bicarbonate concentration (rule of the disregarded Kassirer-Bleich equation) point towards a mixed disorder. The high anion gap is due to metabolic acidosis.

The Δgap is normal, as is the Na^+/Cl^- ratio and therefore there is no other metabolic disorder added to metabolic acidosis.

TABLE 5.4 (comparative) Respiratory acidosis and metabolic alkalosis.

	Normal	Respiratory acidosis acute	chronic	Metabolic alkalosis	Respiratory acidosis and metabolic alkalosis
pH	7.40	7.22	7.34	7.54	7.41
$PaCO_2$ (mmHg)	40	69	67	56	68
HCO_3^- (mEq/L)	24	27	35	47	42
Na^+ (mEq/L)	139	140	137	135	140
K^+ (mEq/L)	4.0	4.1	4.2	2.8	4.0
Cl^- (mEq/L)	103	102	90	72	88
anion gap (mEq/L)	12	11	12	16	10
Na^+/Cl^-	1.34	1.37	1.52	1.87	1.59

Since actual $PaCO_2$ is even higher than the reference value in the presence of bicarbonate reduction it means that we are facing a clinical picture of respiratory acidosis that accompanies an AG metabolic acidosis.

Therefore the diagnosis is of AG metabolic acidosis with respiratory acidosis in acute pulmonary edema and cardiogenic shock.

NOTE

The presence of an elevated Na^+/Cl^- ratio in chronic respiratory acidosis (as simple disorder) indicates the presence of secondary metabolic alkalosis (from adaptation).

Respiratory acidosis and metabolic alkalosis (counterbalancing disorders)

Definition

It is a quite frequent mixed acid-base disorder in clinical practice and is characterized by respiratory acidosis (increase in $PaCO_2$) accompanied by bicarbonate increase in that exceeds the expected adaptation limit. This type of mixed disorder is often characterized by normal pH.

Table 5.4 shows indicatively what happens when two counterbalancing disorders such as respiratory acidosis and metabolic alkalosis occur.

A normal ABG and two simple disorders has been used as a reference. When these two disorders are found simultaneously in the same patient, they produce the descrised mixed disorder.

Causes

- *Patients with COPD and congestive failure*: they often present hypercapnia (respiratory acidosis) and are frequently treated with thiazide or loop diuretics and with steroids that cause metabolic alkalosis.

Clinical case A 74-year-old man arrives in the emergency department for dyspnea.

Anamnesis reveals a heavy smoke history, although suspended about 5 years ago. For a long time he has been affected from chronic obstructive pulmonary disease with numerous exacerbations, above all in the winter period. For about three years he has been on prescrived loop diuretics for congestive heart failure.

Added to diuretics, as home therapy, he uses theophylline and inhaled steroids.

In the last month he experienced worsening dyspnea

and leg edema appeared. A modest labial cyanosis, external turgid jugular veins and malleolar soft tissue swelling, bilaterally, were noticed at the physical examination.

Chest auscultation detects coarse, diffuse wet sounds and bronchospasm. Heart tones are rhythmic but muffled.

Abdomen palpation highlights the inferior margin of the liver four centimeters from the right costal arch.

The vital signs: BP 170/105 mmHg, HR 105 bpm, RR 34 bpm, T 37.4 °C, SpO_2 87% on room air.

After the clinical examination, a chest X-ray and some blood tests are required, including ABG.

ABG: pH 7.40, $PaCO_2$ 67 mmHg, HCO_3^- 40 mEq/L, PaO_2 54 mmHg, Na^+ 140 mEq/L, Cl^- 88 mEq/L, K^+ 4.0 mEq/L, anion gap 12 mEq/L.

ABG interpretation

pH	7.40	normal
$PaCO_2$	67 mmHg	elevated (respiratory acidosis)
HCO_3^-	40 mEq/L	increased (metabolic alkalosis)
Anion gap	12 mEq/L	normal
Chloride	88 mEq/L	reduced (for reasons of electroneutrality due to $[HCO_3^-]$ increase)
Na^+/Cl^-	1.59	increased (due to metabolic alkalosis)

Expected adaptation for respiratory acidosis

Calculate the expected bicarbonate increase compared to reference value (24 mEq/L) in relation to $PaCO_2$ increase (67 mmHg) with respect to reference value (40 mmHg), taking into account the adaptation rule for chronic respiratory acidosis: $27 \times 0.35 = 9.45$ mEq/L (increase in bicarbonate) + 24 (reference bicarbonate) = 33.45 mEq/L (expected bicarbonate).

The actual bicarbonate concentration (40 mEq/L) is clearly higher than the expected one (failure to comply with the expected adaptation rule) due to the presence of metabolic alkalosis.

Final interpretation: chronic respiratory acidosis and metabolic alkalosis.

Reasoned comment

History and clinical picture point towards an exacerbation of chronic obstructive pulmonary disease and congestive heart failure.

The combination of a normal pH, a high $PaCO_2$ with an important increase in bicarbonate concentration lead to a mixed acid-base disorder (rule of false pH compensation).

Bicarbonate concentration is very high not only due to the adaptation mechanism of renal origin. In fact, in this case, the increase is not consistent with the adaptation rule for chronic respiratory acidosis. Since $PaCO_2$ is increased by 27 mmHg with respect to reference value which is 40 mmHg, and since bicarbonate needs to rise by 0.35 mEq/L for every mmHg of $PaCO_2$ increase, the expected increase in bicarbonate concentration is 9.45 mEq/L which added up to the reference value (24 mEq/L) it gives 33.45 mEq/L. Since the concentration of actual bicarbonate (40 mEq/L) is much higher than the expected one (33.45 mEq/L) the disorder is characterized by metabolic alkalosis with respiratory acidosis.

The Na^+/Cl^- ratio of 1.59 confirms the presence of metabolic alkalosis.

Therefore diagnosis is of chronic respiratory acidosis and metabolic alkalosis, in a patient suffering from hypercapnic and hypoxemic chronic obstructive pulmonary disease with congestive heart failure on diuretic therapy.

Metabolic acidosis and metabolic alkalosis (counterbalancing disorders)

Definition

It is a mixed acid-base disorder characterized by metabolic acidosis (reduction of bicarbonate) and metabolic alkalosis (increase of bicarbonate). The simultane-

TABLE 5.5 (comparative) Metabolic alkalosis with AG or hyperchloremic metabolic acidosis.

	Normal	Metabolic alkalosis	AG metabolic acidosis	Hyperchloremic metabolic acidosis	Metabolic alkalosis with	
					AG acidosis	Hyperch. acidosis
pH	7.40	7.54	7.02	7.29	7.43	7.40
$PaCO_2$ (mmHg)	40	56	16	28	39	40
HCO_3^- (mEq/L)	24	47	4	14	25	25
Na^+ (mEq/L)	139	135	140	141	140	140
K^+ (mEq/L)	4.0	2.8	3.7	4.0	3.5	3.5
Cl^- (mEq/L)	103	72	105	115	90	105
Anion gap (mEq/L)	12	16	31	12	25	10
Na^+/Cl^-	1.34	1.87	1.33	1.22	1.55	1.33

ous presence of the two disorders can show a normal, increased or decreased pH and [HCO_3^-]: this depends on the relative severity of both disorders. The disorder is easily identifiable when facing metabolic alkalosis and AG metabolic acidosis, while in case of metabolic alkalosis and prevailing hyperchloremic metabolic acidosis, the only element that directs is hyperchloremia and urinary chloride dosage.

In the event that these last two disorders are very balanced between them, the serum and urinary electrolytic framework may not be decisive.

In this case, only the clinical picture can help suspect this mixed disorder.

So we will present, in succession, two clarifying clinical cases, one with the first mixed acid-base disorder and the other with the second.

Table 5.5 shows indicatively what happens when two counterbalancing disorders such as metabolic acidosis (AG or hyperchloremic) and metabolic alkalosis occur. A normal ABG and two simple disorders has been used as a reference. When these two disorders are found simultaneously in the same patient, they produce the descrised mixed disorder.

Causes of metabolic alkalosis and AG metabolic acidosis

- *Loss of gastric fluid, use of diuretics and accumulation of organic and inorganic acids*: this condition can occur during vomiting or use for a certain time of the nasogastric tube (metabolic alkalosis) in patients with diabetic ketoacidosis or with severe renal failure not subjected to dialysis treatment (AG metabolic acidosis).

  In addition, in critical patients both abundant vomiting and use of diuretics (metabolic alkalosis) can lead to hypovolemia with tissue hypoperfusion and therefore an increase in lactic acid production (AG metabolic acidosis).

Causes of metabolic alkalosis and hyperchloremic metabolic acidosis

- *Diarrhea and vomiting*: patients who simultaneously experience vomiting and diarrhea (i.e. during gastroenteritis) lose hydrochloric acid and water from the stomach followed by metabolic alkalosis and eliminate bicarbonate with diarrhea (hyperchloremic metabolic acidosis).

Clinical case 1 An 18-year-old man with type I diabetes mellitus arrives to the emergency department for biliary vomiting that has lasted for about 48 hours. Anamnesis reveals that since about 5 days, in the midst of a flu epidemic, he is suffering from high fever, cough and polyuria.

For unclear reasons, the general practitioner was not consulted. The insulin dosage was not changed from the usual one.

On physical examination the patient is oriented, dehydrated and the skin is warm.

Chest auscultation shows crackling rattles in small bubbles, bilaterally. On palpation, abdomen is painful, particularly in epigastrium.

The vital signs: BP 95/60 mmHg, HR 110 bpm, RR 26 bpm, T 39.4 °C, SpO_2 97% on room air.

After the clinical examination, a chest X-ray and some blood tests are required, including ABG.

ABG: pH 7.40, $PaCO_2$ 40 mmHg, HCO_3^- 25 mEq/L, PO_2 98 mmHg, Na^+ 140 mEq/L, Cl^- 88 mEq/L, K^+ 3.2 mEq/L, anion gap 27 mEq/L. La ricerca dei corpi chetonici nelle urine è positiva (++++).

ABG interpretation

pH	7.40	normal
$PaCO_2$	40 mmHg	normal
HCO_3^-	25 mEq/L	normal
Anion gap	27 mEq/L	increased
ΔAG	15 mEq/L	
ΔHCO_3^-	1 mEq/L	
Δgap	+14 mEq/L	increased
Chloride	88 mEq/L	reduced (for electroneutrality reason due to $[HCO_3^-]$)
Na^+/Cl^-	1.59	increased (due to metabolic alkalosis)

Expected adaptation for metabolic acidosis

It is not significant to calculate the expected adaptation limit because $[HCO_3^-]$ and $PaCO_2$ are both normal.

Final interpretation: AG metabolic acidosis and metabolic alkalosis.

Reasoned comment

Clinical picture and laboratory tests point towards a diabetic ketoacidosis secondary to an infectious process in a known diabetic patient, not adequately treated and complicated by vomiting.

Normal pH, $PaCO_2$ values and bicarbonate in the reference range would suggest an absolute normality. The only discordant evidence is chloride reduction and Na^+/Cl^- ratio = 1.59 which guide towards the presence of metabolic alkalosis.

Anion gap is the fundamental measurement that allows us to diagnose metabolic acidosis.

The ΔAG is high (+15) and this does not correspond to an equivalent reduction of bicarbonate, which is actually in range. The increased Δgap (+14 mEq/L) is due to metabolic alkalosis.

Since bicarbonate concentration is normal as well as $PaCO_2$, it makes no sense to look for $PaCO_2$ expected adaptation, as we do while facing a bicarbonate reduction during metabolic acidosis.

Therefore the diagnosis is of metabolic alkalosis and high anion gap metabolic acidosis in a patient with diabetic ketoacidosis complicated by vomiting and dehydration.

NOTE

This clinical case suggests that we should never interpret an ABG without the evaluation of sodium and chloride electrolytes. Furthermore even in the presence of metabolic acidosis the value of BE is zero underlining the limits of this parameter in acid-base disorders interpretation.

Clinical case 2 A 20-year-old man is brought to the emergency department around noon for vomiting and diarrhea.

The man has always been healthy. Going deeper into the history it is possible to understand that the gastroenteric symptoms arose after about six hours from homemade ice cream ingestion, purchased from a street seller.

Moderate xerostomia upon examination. Abdomen palpation shows only a slight diffuse tenderness. Negative chest examination. The vital signs: BP 110/70 mmHg, HR 100 bpm, RR 22 bpm, T 37.5 °C, SpO_2 97% on room air, GCS 15.

ABG: pH 7.40, $PaCO_2$ 40 mmHg, HCO_3^- 25 mEq/L, PO_2 96 mmHg, Na^+ 140 mEq/L, Cl^- 105 mEq/L, K^+ 3.6 mEq/L, anion gap 10 mEq/L.

ABG interpretation

pH	7.40	normal
$PaCO_2$	40 mmHg	normal
HCO_3^-	25 mEq/L	normal
Anion gap	10 mEq/L	normal
Chloride	105 mEq/L	normal
Na^+/Cl^-	1.33	normal

Final interpretation: normal blood gas analysis.

Reasoned comment

Hystory and clinical picture point towards an alimentary gastroenteritis from staphylococcal toxin. The importance of symptoms (incoercible vomiting and profuse diarrhea) suggest a simultaneous loss of HCl and fluids (vomiting) and bicarbonate with water (diarrhea).

ABG normality values should not be misleading because we are probably facing a case of vomiting metabolic alkalosis and a metabolic acidosis with normal anion gap from diarrhea, perfectly counterbalancing. In cases like this, only the history and the clinical picture can orient us correctly.

Mixed metabolic acidosis (additive disorders)

It is a mixed acid-base disorder characterized by a very acid pH due to the simultaneous presence of AG metabolic acidosis and hyperchloremic metabolic acidosis, with a different pathogenesis.

Table 5.6 shows indicatively what happens when two additive disorders such as AG metabolic acidosis and hyperchloramic metabolic acidosis occur.

A normal ABG and two simple disorders has been used as a reference. When these two disorders are found simultaneously in the same patient, they produce the descrived mixed disorder.

Causes

- *Severe diarrhea*: during diarrhea there is a bicarbonate loss (hyperchloremic metabolic acidosis) with volume loss followed by tissue hypoperfusion with lactic acid production (AG metabolic acidosis).
- *Diabetes mellitus*: during diabetes mellitus there may be ketoacidosis, which causes AG metabolic acidosis. At the same time there may be hyperchloremic metabolic acidosis, during the recovery phase of diabetic ketoacidosis due ketone salts loss and dilution by infusion of important quantities of normal saline and potassium chloride.
- *Interstitial nephropathy*: in the initial phase of interstitial nephropathy there is a diminished excretion of acids from insufficient glomerular filtration leading

TABLE 5.6 (comparative) Mixed metabolic acidosis (AG and hyperchloremic).

	Normal	AG metabolic acidosis	Hyperchloremic metabolic acidosis	Mixed acidosis
pH	7.40	7.02	7.29	7.17
$PaCO_2$ (mmHg)	40	16	28	18
HCO_3^- (mEqL)	24	4	14	6
Na^+ (mEq/L)	139	140	141	142
K^+ (mEq/L)	4.0	3.7	4.0	4.0
Cl^- (mEq/L)	103	105	115	117
Anion gap (mEq/L)	12	31	12	19
Na^+/Cl^-	1.34	1.33	1.22	1.21

to AG metabolic acidosis and a reduced production and excretion of ammonium which causes hyperchloremic metabolic acidosis.

Clinical case A 21-year-old woman is accompanied to the emergency department by her parents for fever and altered sensorium.

For about five days she has had polyuria associated to intense thirst and her parents also report that for two days she has also suffered from many diarrheal episodes in 24 hours.

On physical examination, the woman appears confused (GCS 13) with hot and dry skin.

Chest examination is normal, while the abdomen, however soft, is widely painful.

The vital signs: BP 90/70 mmHg, HR 100 bpm, RR 32 bpm, T 38.4 °C, SpO_2 97% in room air.

A finger glycemic stick is performed which shows hyperglicemia of 420 mg/dL. Positive urinary ketone bodies (++++).

ABG: pH 7.11, $PaCO_2$ 16 mmHg, HCO_3^- 5 mEq/L, PO_2 96 mmHg, Na^+ 142 mEq/L, Cl^- 117 mEq/L, K^+ 4.0 mEq/L, anion gap 20 mEq/L.

ABG interpretation

pH	7.11	acidemia
$PaCO_2$	16 mmHg	reduced
HCO_3^-	5 mEq/L	reduced
Anion gap	20 mEq/L	increased (metabolic acidosis with high anion gap)
ΔAG	8 mEq/L	
ΔHCO_3^-	19 mEq/L	
Δgap	−11 mEq/L	reduced
Chloride	117 mEq/L	increased (for electroneutrality reasons due to bicarbonate reduction)
Na^+/Cl^-	1.21	reduced

Expected adaptation for metabolic acidosis

Calculate the expected $PaCO_2$ reduction with respect to reference value (40 mmHg) in relation to bicarbonate reduction, taking into account the rule of adaptation during metabolic acidosis: 1.2 × 19 (bicarbonate reduction) = 22.8 – 40 (reference $PaCO_2$) = 17.2 mmHg (expected $PaCO_2$).

Final interpretation: AG metabolic acidosis and hyperchloremic metabolic acidosis.

Reasoned comment

Clinical picture and laboratory tests point towards diabetic ketoacidosis at the onset of type I diabetes mellitus, complicated by diarrhea.

The acid pH, the reduction of bicarbonate and $PaCO_2$ suggest metabolic acidosis, confirmed by high anion gap (20 mEq/L).

However, there is a marked difference between the ΔAG = 8 mEq/L and the ΔHCO_3^- = 19 mEq/L.

This means that $[HCO_3^-]$ has dropped far more than expected. In fact, with a ΔAG of 8 mEq/L the expected bicarbonate concentration is about 16 mEq/L and not 5 mEq/L which is the actual one.

In other words there was a bicarbonate loss (diarrhea) other than that consumed by the buffer mechanism.

The confirmation is in chloride increase and in Na^+/Cl^- ratio reduction, for electroneutrality reasons.

$PaCO_2$ decrease is consistent with the adaptation rule during metabolic acidosis. In fact bicarbonates are 5.0 mEq/L and compared to reference value (24 mEq/L) they have decreased by 19 mEq/L.

Since $PaCO_2$ decreases by 1.2 mmHg for every mEq/L of bicarbonate reduction, the expected reduction of $PaCO_2$ is 1.2 × 19 = 22.8 mmHg which, subtracted from the reference value (40 mmHg) gives 17.2 mmHg.

Since the current $PaCO_2$ (16 mmHg) is almost equal to the expected one (17.2 mmHg ± 2) we can speak of expected adaptation achieved.

Therefore the diagnosis is of mixed metabolic acidosis (AG and hyperchloremic) in a patient with diabetic ketoacidosis at the onset of type I diabetes mellitus, complicated by acute diarrhea.

Double mixed acid-base disorders, characterized by the superposition of an acute disorder to a chronic disorder

Acute respiratory acidosis on chronic respiratory acidosis

It is a frequent mixed acid-base disorder. In most cases the cause is the exacerbation of hypoxemic and hypercapnic chronic obstructive pulmonary disease.

Clinical case A 62-year-old man, suffering from chronic hypoxemic and hypercapnic COPD, arrives to the emergency department due to the appearance of fever, cough with mucopurulent sputum and worsening dyspnea.

On objective examination labial cyanosis, crackles and coarse rattles spread over the entire chest, tachycardia on heart tones auscultation. The vital signs: BP 160/80 mmHg, HR 104 bpm, RR 27 bpm, T 38 °C, SpO_2 88% on room air. Chest X-ray does not show infectious foci.

ABG: pH 7.24, $PaCO_2$ 76 mmHg, HCO_3^- 32 mEq/L, PaO_2 55 mmHg, Na^+ 140 mEq/L, Cl^- 93, K^+ 4.1, anion gap 15 mEq/L.

ABG interpretation

pH	7.24	acidemia
$PaCO_2$	76 mmHg	increased (respiratory acidosis)
HCO_3^-	32 mEq/L	increased (adaptation mechanism)
Anion gap	15	normal
Chloride	93 mEq/L	reduced (for electroneutrality reasons)
Na^+/Cl^-	1.50	in range elevation (due to secondary adaptation metabolic alkalosis)

Expected adaptation for respiratory acidosis

Calculate $\Delta PaCO_2$ (actual PCO_2 76 – 40 reference PCO_2) = 36 mmHg. If it was a chronic form [HCO_3^-] should be (36 × 0.35) = 12.6 mEq/L which added to reference bicarbonate (24 mEq/L) it gives 36.6 mEq/L, while actual bicarbonate is 32 mEq/L. If it was acute (36 × 0.1) = 3.1 mEq/L which added to reference bicarbonate it gives 27.1 mEq/L. Should be underlined the sensitive pH reduction, even in the presence of a high [HCO_3^-].

Final interpretation: acute respiratory acidosis superimposed on a chronic form.

Reasoned comment

The last and recent blood gas of the man was: pH 7.33, $PaCO_2$ 58 mmHg, HCO_3^- 31 mEq/L, PaO_2 64 mmHg, Na^+ 139 mEq/L, K^+ 4.1 mEq/L, Cl^- 92 mEq/L, anion gap 16 mEq/L, indicative for chronic respiratory acidosis.

The current values of blood gas during acute lung disease show, compared to the previous ones, a significant PaO_2 reduction, a clear $PaCO_2$ increase, a very modest rise in [HCO_3^-] and a pH significant reduction. Bicarbonate values are not consistent either with chronic respiratory acidosis (the expected is 36.6 mEq/L) or with the acute form (expected 27.1 mEq/L). In consideration of the clinical course and previous arterial blood gas values, we can assume that we are facing an acute hypercapnia condition superimposed on a chronic form.

Therefore, the clinical interpretation is of chronic respiratory acidosis with overlap of acute respiratory acidosis in a patient with acute hypoxemic and hypercapnic COPD.

NOTE

The clinical history and the comparison with the previous arterial blood gas are important tools for a correct diagnosis, as well as the pH reduction in the presence of a high [HCO_3^-].

Acute respiratory acidosis on chronic respiratory alkalosis

It is a disorder caused by acute hypoventilation following long lasting hyperventilation.

Clinical case A young 28-year-old male suffering from allergic bronchial asthma arrives in the emergency department due to a bronchial asthma attack lasted for several hours.

The patient is severely dyspniec, in orthopneic position. On physical examination, there are bronchial stenosis sounds, spread throughout the lung. Tachycardia on heart tones ausculation. The vital signs: BP 150/90 mmHg, HR 113 bpm, RR 31 bpm, T 36.4 °C, SpO_2 94% on room air, GCS 15.

ABG: pH 7.46, $PaCO_2$ 25 mmHg, HCO_3^- 17 mEq/L, PaO_2 73 mmHg, Na^+ 141 mEq/L, K^+ 3.3 mEq/L, Cl^- 109 mEq/L, anion gap 15 mEq/L.

In consideration of pH, PCO_2 decrease and bicarbonate reduction according to the expected adaptation, the correct interpretation is of chronic respiratory alkalosis. In the emergency department, aerosol therapy is performed with salbutamol associated with ipratropium bromide three times, parenteral methylprednisolone, oxygen with nasal cannula.

After an hour the clinical situation worsens and respiratory fatigue takes over.

ABG is performed again: pH 7.20, $PaCO_2$ 52 mmHg, HCO_3^- 20 mEq/L, PaO_2 55 mmHg, Na^+ 141 mEq/L, Cl^- 109 mEq/L, K^+ 3.4 mEq/L, anion gap 12, lactates 2.4 mmol/L.

ABG interpretation

pH	7.20	acidemia
$PaCO_2$	52 mmHg	elevated (respiratory acidosis)
HCO_3^-	20 mEq/L	reduced (metabolic acidosis?)
Anion gap	12 mEq/L	normal
Chloride	109 mEq/L	slightly increased
Na^+/Cl^-	1.29	normal

pH is acidic, PCO_2 is increased and bicarbonate is reduced. Anion gap is normal. *Therefore the interpretation, according to numbers, is of respiratory acidosis and metabolic acidosis with normal anion gap.*

Reasoned comment

Acid pH, PCO_2 increase and bicarbonate reduction (rule of the disregarded Kassirer-Bleich equation) point towards a mixed additive disorder. In reality, if we reflect, it is not so. We should start from the previous arterial blood gas that showed chronic respiratory alkalosis with an $[HCO_3^-]$ of 17 mEq/L.

The sudden deterioration, with acute ventilation reduction, brought PCO_2 from 25 mmHg to 52 mmHg. The $[HCO_3^-]$ had to rise by about 3 mEq/L ($52 - 25 = 27 \times 0.1 = 2.7$ mmHg), which occurred starting from the 17 mEq/L of the previous arterial blood gas. In conclusion: if we look at numbers, we are faced with a respiratory acidosis and a metabolic acidosis with normal anion gap, but if we consider the clinical history and the previous blood gas, the correct interpretation is of acute respiratory acidosis superimposed on chronic respiratory alkalosis in a patient with hyperventilation during bronchial asthma and subsequent acute hypoventilation due to respiratory failure.

NOTE

Also in this case the clinical history and the comparison with the previous ABG allows to make the correct diagnosis. Significant pH variation also helps.

Acute respiratory alkalosis on chronic respiratory alkalosis

It is a disorder characterized by an acute hyperventilation that is established on an already present hyperventilation.

Clinical case A 28-year-old pregnant woman, in the fourteenth week, with twins (a retained dead fetus and a living and vital fetus) arrives at the emergency department, for dyspnea that has arisen sharply. Fever for a few days. On physical examination she has difficulty to pronounce long sentences due to dyspnea onset. At chest auscultation expiratory rhonchi are present. Valid, frequent, rhythmic heart tones. She has always been well and does not take home therapy. Lack of familiarity with deep venous thrombosis/pulmonary embolism: The vital signs: BP 113/73 mmHg, HR 102 bpm, RR 32 bpm, SpO_2 96% on room air.

ABG: pH 7.54, $PaCO_2$ 20 mmHg, HCO_3^- 17 mEq/L, PaO_2 86 mmHg, Na^+ 134 mEq/L, Cl^- 107 mEq/L, K^+ 3,5 mEq/L, anion gap 10.

In the suspicion of pulmonary embolism some tests are performed. Chest X-ray: normal; ECG: sinus rhythm; incomplete right bundle branch block (IRBBB); CUS: negative; Chest ultrasound: normal; D-dimer: 1500 ng/mL; perfusion pulmonary scintigraphy: probable pulmonary embolism. Therapy with low molecular weight heparin (LMWH) is started.

ABG interpretation

pH	7.54	alkalemia
$PaCO_2$	20 mmHg	reduced (respiratory alkalosis)
HCO_3^-	17 mEq/L	reduced (adaptation mechanism)
Anion gap	10 mEq/L	normal
PaO_2	86 mmHg	reduced
$P(A-a)O_2$	37 mmHg	increased (intrapulmonary shunt)
Chloride	107	slightly increased
Na^+/Cl^-	1.25	reduced (but compatible with bicarbonate reduction)

Expected adaptation for acute respiratory alkalosis

Calculate $\Delta PaCO_2$ (40 – 20) = 20 mmHg. The $[HCO_3^-]$ for the expected adaptation rule (20 × 0.2) = 4 mmHg should be about (24 – 4) = 20 mEq/L.

The high pH gives evidence of an acute form.

Final interpretation: acute respiratory alkalosis (probable).

After 5 days from admission, the woman no longer has dyspnea, neither at rest nor during exertion.

Second ABG: pH 7.41, $PaCO_2$ 29 mmHg, HCO_3^- 18 mEq/L, PaO_2 102 mmHg, Na^+ 138 mEq/L, Cl^- 112 mEq/L, K^+ 4.2 mEq/L, anion gap 8.

ABG interpretation

pH	7.41	normal
$PaCO_2$	29 mmHg	reduced (respiratory alkalosis)
HCO_3^-	18 mEq/L	reduced (adaptation mechanism)
Anion gap	8 mEq/L	normal
PaO_2	102 mmHg	increased (hyperventilation)
$P(A-a)O_2$	13.8 mmHg	normal
Chloride	112 mEq/L	increased
Na^+/Cl^-	1.23	reduced (but compatible with HCO_3^- reduction)

Expected adaptation for chronic respiratory alkalosis

Calculate $\Delta PaCO_2$ (40 – 29) = 11. The $[HCO_3^-]$ for the expected adaptation rule (11 × 0.4) = 4.4 mEq/L should be about (24 – 4.4) = 19.6 (± 2).

Reasoned comment

Let's start with the second arterial blood gas, where the respiratory alkalosis shows the chronic form characteristics (normal pH, reduced PCO_2 and bicarbonate consistent with the expected adaptation rule for chronic respiratory alkalosis).

PaO_2 is increased with normality of $P(A-a)O_2$ and therefore is not the cause of hyperventilation and hypocapnia. Probably this is determined by progesterone increase, as observed in pregnancy, and the blood gas analysis values represent its steady state. Instead the first arterial blood gas values suggest an acute hypercapnia caused by an event that reduced PaO_2 with an increase in $P(A-a)O_2$ as from an intrapulmonary shunt (pulmonary embolism? other origin?). $[HCO_3^-]$ of 17 mEq/L is lower than the one we would expect (20 mEq/L) and is compatible with an acute respiratory alkalosis on a chronic one.

Therefore the most probable diagnosis of the first arterial blood gas analysis is of acute respiratory alkalosis caused by intrapulmonary shunt on chronic respiratory alkalosis secondary to progesterone increase in a pregnant woman.

Importance of serum albumin dosage in critically ill patients

Clinical case An 81-year-old woman arrives in the emergency department for fever and soft tissue infection.

The woman has a long history of high blood pressure and for three years has had a pacemaker.

On physical examination the patient appears to be suffering, pale, diaphoretic, with red and edematous skin on the chest and upper limbs. The vital signs: BP 80 /? mmHg, HR 60 bpm, RR 34 bpm, T 38.2 °C, SpO_2 91% on room air. Chest X-ray shows flow redistribution to the upper lung fields. The ECG highlights a pacemaker rhythm. Blood tests are required (WBC 19,000/μL, INR 13, creatinine 2.4 mg/dL, bilirubin 2.3 mg/dL, CRP 33 mg/L) and also arterial blood gas with electrolytes and lactic acid.

ABG: pH 7.44, $PaCO_2$ 30 mmHg, HCO_3^- 21 mEq/L, PO_2 62 mmHg, Na^+ 133 mEq/L, Cl^- 97 mEq/L, K^+ 3.9 mEq/L, lactic acid 6.1 mmol/L, anion gap 15 mEq/L.

ABG interpretation

pH	7.44	normal
$PaCO_2$	30 mmHg	reduced (respiratory alkalosis)
HCO_3^-	21 mEq/L	reduced (adaptation mechanism)
Anion gap	15 mEq/L	normal
Chloride	97 mEq/L	normal
Na^+/Cl^-	1.37	normal

Expected adaptation for chronic respiratory alkalosis

Calculate the $\Delta PaCO_2$ (reference $PaCO_2$ – actual $PaCO_2$) 40 – 30 = 10 mmHg.

Calculate the expected reduction of bicarbonate compared to reference value (24 mEq/L) in relation to $PaCO_2$ reduction, taking into account the expected adaptation rule during chronic respiratory alkalosis: 10 × 0.4 = 4 mEq/L; (reference bicarbonate) 24 – (bicarbonate reduction) 4 = 20 mEq/L (expected bicarbonate).

Final interpretation: chronic respiratory alkalosis.

First reasoned comment

The combination of a normal pH, a reduced $PaCO_2$ and bicarbonate decrease points towards a primary acid-base disorder such as chronic respiratory alkalosis.

Bicarbonate decrease is consistent with the expected adaptation rule for chronic respiratory alkalosis. Since $PaCO_2$ reduction is 10 mmHg, compared to reference value of 40 mmHg and since bicarbonate has to drop by 0.4 mEq/L for every mmHg of $PaCO_2$ decrease, the expected reduction is 10 × 0.4 = 4 mEq/L which after being subtracted from the reference value (24 mEq/L) gives 20 mEq/L. Since actual bicarbonate concentration (21 mEq/L) is almost equal to the expected one (20 mEq/L ± 2) we can speak of adaptation achieved. pH is normal as often happens in chronic respiratory alkalosis.

Reflections

The patient's general condition is severe and the clinical picture supported by blood tests indicates for septic shock and multi-organ failure in a framework of soft tissue infection.

Lactic acid is significantly increased (6.1 mmol/L), renal insufficiency is present and despite this anion gap is normal.

Since patients with sepsis often have a reduction in serum albumin, its serum concentration was determined, which turned out to be 2.3 g/dL (nv 4.5 g/dL). The discovery of this significant reduction in serum albumin raises the need to re-evaluate anion gap, knowing that the latter drops by 2.5 mEq/L for each g/dL of albumin concentration reduction, starting from the reference value of 4.5 g/dL. Applying the Figge formula for the correction of the anion gap for the actual value of albumin:

adjusted AG = actual AG + 2.5 x ([reference albumin] – [actual albumin])

which in our case becomes:

15 + 2.5 × (4.5 – 2.3) = 15 + (2.5 × 2.2) = 15 + 5.5 = 20.5 mEq/L adjusted AG

At this point everything is more clear.

ABG interpretation in the light of the adjusted anion gap

pH	7.44	normal
$PaCO_2$	30 mmHg	reduced (respiratory alkalosis)
HCO_3^-	21 mEq/L	reduced (metabolic acidosis)
Anion gap	20.5 mEq/L	increased (AG metabolic acidosis)
ΔAG	8.5 mEq/L	
ΔHCO_3^-	3 mEq/L	
Δgap	+5.5 mEq/L	normal
Chloride	97 mEq/L	normal
Na^+/Cl^-	1.37	normal

Correct and final interpretation: AG metabolic acidosis and respiratory alkalosis.

Second reasoned comment

Anion gap high value gives evidence of metabolic acidosis and bicarbonate reduction is consistent with this interpretation. The Δgap is normal as normal is the Na^+/Cl^- ratio, excluding the presence of a second metabolic disorder.

$PaCO_2$ is not consistent with bicarbonate reduction: in fact $(3 \times 1.2) = 3.6$ mmHg which subtracted from reference val ue (40 mmHg) gives 36.4 mmHg as the expected value.

Actual $PaCO_2$ is 30 mmHg and therefore much more reduced than the expected one, emphasizing the presence of respiratory alkalosis.

Therefore the final diagnosis is of AG metabolic acidosis with respiratory alkalosis in a patient with septic shock and multiple organ failure.

NOTE

Clinical reasoning is always very important.
In critically ill patients, especially septic ones, serum albumin concentration should be evaluated.

Triple mixed acid-base disorders

Definition

A triple mixed acid-base disorder is characterized by the simultaneous presence of three primary acid-base disorders.

The most common triple disorder consists of metabolic acidosis and metabolic alkalosis and the simultaneous presence of respiratory alkalosis or respiratory acidosis.

Another triple non-infrequent disorder is composed of metabolic alkalosis and chronic respiratory acidosis with subsequent overlap of acute respiratory acidosis.

Below we will discuss some triple acid-base disorders.

Causes

- *Severe hepatic failure*: patients with this disease may have metabolic alkalosis due to fluid gastric loss during nasogastric tube placement or due to diuretics use; respiratory alkalosis caused by hyperventilation secondary to liver failure; metabolic acidosis secondary to diarrhea, uremia or renal tubular acidosis.
- *Chronic obstructive pulmonary disease with hypercapnia*: patients have chronic hypercapnia and therefore chronic respiratory acidosis; they are often treated with diuretics (metabolic alkalosis) for concomitant congestive heart failure.

  During COPD exacerbation there is ventilation worsening which leads to a further $PaCO_2$ increase which in turn causes acute respiratory acidosis, overlapping and aggravating the previous chronic condition.
- *Complex onco-hematological diseases*: patients may develop metabolic alkalosis from vomiting during chemotherapy; respiratory alkalosis due to gram⁻ sepsis or respiratory acidosis due to alveolar ventilation failure secondary to pneumonia and metabolic acidosis due to lactic acid production secondary to cytolysis caused by chemotherapy or septic shock.

Clinical case 1 A 40-year-old man is taken to the emergency department for high fever and severe fatigue. Anamnesis reveals non-Hodgkin's lymphoma in relapse. Four days earlier he had undergone a cycle of chemotherapy, badly tolerated due to nausea and vomiting onset that persisted, although reduced in the number of episodes, at the emergency department access. On physical examination he appears to be suffering greatly with warm skin and mucosal xerosis.

Examination of the thorax shows on percussion modest right basal hypophonesis, while the abdomen is distended and at palpation hepatosplenomegaly is evident.

The vital signs: BP 85/55 mmHg, HR 130 bpm, RR 38 bpm, T 39.6 °C, SpO_2 89% on room air.

After the clinical examination, a chest radiograph is requested, blood culture and some blood tests are performed, including ABG.

ABG: pH 7.66, $PaCO_2$ 19 mmHg, HCO_3^- 21 mEq/L, PaO_2 58 mmHg, Na^+ 140 mEq/L, Cl^- 90 mEq/L, K^+ 3.3 mEq/L, anion gap 29 mEq/L, lactic acid 12 mmol/L.

The blood culture, three days after the collection, is positive for *Escherichia Coli.*

Chest X-ray shows pneumonia at the right lung base.

ABG interpretation

pH	7.66	alkalemia
$PaCO_2$	19 mmHg	reduced
HCO_3^-	21 mEq/L	reduced (metabolic acidosis)
Anion gap	29 mEq/L	increased
ΔAG	17 mEq/L	
ΔHCO_3^-	3 mEq/L	
Δgap	+14	increased
Chloride	90 mEq/L	reduced (for electroneutrality reasons related to $[HCO_3^-]$ increase)
Na^+/Cl^-	1.55	increased

Expected adaptation for metabolic acidosis

Calculate the expected reduction of $PaCO_2$ with respect to the reference value (40 mmHg) in relation to the reduction of bicarbonate, taking into account the adaptation rule: 1.2 × 3 (bicarbonate reduction) = 3.6 – reference $PaCO_2$) = 36.4 mmHg (expected $PaCO_2$). The actual $PaCO_2$ is 19 mmHg so there is a failure to comply with the adaptation rule.

Final interpretation: metabolic acidosis AG with metabolic alkalosis and respiratory alkalosis.

Reasoned comment

The clinical picture and laboratory tests point towards a septic shock.

The alkaline pH, the high anion gap (29 mEq/L), the modest bicarbonate reduction in relation to a high anion gap and the marked $PaCO_2$ reduction with respect to the modest bicarbonate reduction lead us to believe that we are faced with a really complex disorder.

Nothing is respected: neither the Kassirer-Bleich equation, nor the adaptation rule and moreover the Δgap is positive (> +6 mEq/L).

Discussing by order. pH is very alkaline, so surely we are dealing with a disorder referable to alkalosis. Anion gap is significantly increased and therefore AG metabolic acidosis is present; the increase in anion gap of 17 mEq/L was not followed by an equivalent reduction in bicarbonate which fell by only 3 mEq/L (Δgap +14), so we are dealing with metabolic alkalosis also confirmed by chloride reduction and Na^+/Cl^- ratio increase.

The actual $PaCO_2$ (19 mmHg) is much more reduced than the expected one (36.4 mmHg) which means that respiratory alkalosis is also present.

Therefore the diagnosis is of metabolic acidosis with high anion gap, metabolic alkalosis and respiratory alkalosis in a patient with gram negative septic shock and with vomiting secondary to chemotherapy.

NOTE

This clinical case teaches us that even in the presence of a very alkaline pH a metabolic acidosis is possible. The evaluation of electrolytes is fundamental, allowing us to calculate the anion gap and the Na^+/Cl^- ratio.

Clinical case 2 A 82-year-old woman arrives in the emergency department for vomiting, diarrhea (lasted for at least three days) and oliguria.

The woman suffers of hypertension, chronic heart disease, obesity and type 2 diabetes mellitus. She is on therapy with metformin 500 mg three times a day and irbesartan/hydroclortiazide 300 mg/12.5 mg once a day. On physical examination, she presents with a depressed state of consciousness, visible dehydrated skin and mucous membranes.

The vital signs: BP 150/90 mmHg, HR 75 bpm, RR 28 bpm, T 36 °C, SpO_2 97% on room air, GCS 12. Exams are requested including serum creatinine which resulted 7.7 mg/dL.

ABG: pH 6.92, $PaCO_2$ 27.6 mmHg, HCO_3^- 5.5 mEq/L, PaO_2 96 mmHg, Na^+ 140 mEq/L, Cl^- 87 mEq/L, K^+ 5.2 mEq/L, anion gap 47.5 mEq/L, lactic acid 18 mmol/L.

ABG interpretation

pH	6.92	acidemia
$PaCO_2$	27.6 mmHg	reduced
HCO_3^-	5.5 mEq/L	reduced (metabolic acidosis)
Anion gap	47.5 mEq/L	increased
ΔAG	35.5	
ΔHCO_3^-	18.5	
Δgap	+17	increased
Chloride	87 mEq/L	reduced (for electroneutrality reason)
Na^+/Cl^-	1.60	increased

Expected adaptation for metabolic acidosis

Calculate the expected $PaCO_2$ reduction compared to reference value (40 mmHg) in relation to bicarbonate reduction, taking into account the adaptation rule: 1.2 × 18.5 (bicarbonate reduction) = 22.2 – 40 (reference $PaCO_2$) = 17.8 mmHg (expected $PaCO_2$).

The actual PCO_2 is 27.6 mmHg so there is a failure to comply with the adaptation rule.

Final interpretation: AG metabolic acidosis with metabolic alkalosis and respiratory acidosis.

Reasoned comment

Acid pH, bicarbonate reduction and anion gap of 48 mEq/L indicate AG metabolic acidosis. The very positive Δgap (+17) indicates the presence of a second metabolic disorder such as metabolic alkalosis, confirmed by Na^+/Cl^- ratio increase. Verifying the respiratory component, it is evident that the adaptation rule during metabolic acidosis is not respected.

The expected $PaCO_2$ should be 17.8 mmHg, while the actual is 27.6 mmHg, which demonstrates the presence of respiratory acidosis.

Therefore the diagnosis is of metabolic acidosis with high anion gap with metabolic alkalosis and respiratory acidosis in a patient with metformin intoxication due to acute renal failure caused by hypovolemia secondary to vomiting and diarrhea.

NOTE

This clinical case teaches us that even with a very acid pH it is possible the presence of metabolic alkalosis. The electrolytes evaluation is fundamental, allowing us to calculate the anion gap and the Δgap, in addition to the Na^+/Cl^- ratio.

Clinical case 3 A 67-year-old man arrives in the emergency department for a sincopal episode occurred standing up to go to the bathroom, reporting a mild head injury. For about a month, he has had 4/5 diarrhea discharges a day.

Stools are watery without blood. He denies any fever. The vital signs: BP 130/83 mmHg; HR 102 bpm; RR 26 bpm; T 36.5 °C; SpO2 98% on room air; GCS 15. On physical examination skin and mucous membrane are dehydrated. Chest X-ray: normal; ECG: Q-Tc prolongation with presence of U waves; CT of the skull: normal. Some blood tests are required. Hb 18.7 g/dL, leukocytes 23,000/μL, serum creatinine 6.1 mg/dL, serum albumin 5.4 g/dL, blood glucose 279 mg/dL.

ABG: pH 7.49, $PaCO_2$ 19.6 mmHg, HCO_3^- 14.8 mEq/L, PaO_2 101 mmHg, SpO_2 98%, Na^+ 116 mEq/L, Cl^- 66 mEq/L, K^+ 3.0 mEq/L, anion gap 35.2 mEq/L.

ABG interpretation

pH	7.49	alcalemia
$PaCO_2$	19.6 mmHg	reduced
HCO_3^-	14.8 mEq/L	reduced (metabolic acidosis)
Anion gap	35.2 mEq/ L	increased
ΔAG	23.2 mEq/L	
ΔHCO_3^-	9.2 mEq/L	
Δgap	+14 mEq/L	increased
Chloride	66 mEq/L	reduced
Na^+/Cl^-	1.75	increased

Expected adaptation for metabolic acidosis

Calculate the expected $PaCO_2$ reduction with respect to reference value (40 mmHg) in relation to bicarbonate reduction, taking into account the adaptation rule: 1.2 × 9.2 (bicarbonate reduction) = 11 – 40 (reference $PaCO_2$) = 29 mmHg (expected $PaCO_2$). The actual PCO_2 is 19.6 mmHg, so there is a failure to comply with the adaptation rule.

Final interpretation: AG metabolic acidosis with metabolic alkalosis and respiratory alkalosis.

Reasoned comment

Bicarbonate reduction and anion gap of 35.2 mEq/L indicate for AG metabolic acidosis. The very positive Δgap (+14) indicates the presence of a second metabolic disorder such as metabolic alkalosis, confirmed by the increase in Na^+/Cl^- ratio.

Verifing $PaCO_2$, it is evident that the adaptation rule during metabolic acidosis has not been respected.

The expected $PaCO_2$ should be 29 mmHg, while the actual is 19.6 mmHg, which demonstrates the presence of respiratory alkalosis, thus it is clear that we are dealing with three disorders, two metabolic and one respiratory. At this point we will try to understand the genesis of acid-base and water-electrolyte disorders.

AG metabolic acidosis is very well explained by renal failure while the diarrhea that the patient is complaining about should cause hyperchloremic metabolic acidosis, but the Δgap gives evidence of metabolic alkalosis and so does the Na^+/Cl^- ratio, in the absence of vomiting and use of diuretics or steroids. At this point it is right to consider those cases of hypersecretive diarrhea caused by the villous adenoma of the colon-rectum, which by secreting mainly water and chloride as well as potassium, cause chloride-sensitive metabolic alkalosis and serious water-electrolyte disorders.

A rectal colonoscopy confirmed the suspicion, as well as the subsequent histological examination, allowing the diagnosis of McKittrick-Wheelock syndrome.

This syndrome is characterized by secretory diarrhea due to colorectal tumor, dehydration, renal failure and severe water-electrolyte and acid-base disorders.

The added respiratory alkalosis may be due, in our case, to hyperventilation caused by anxiety.

Therefore the final diagnosis is of metabolic acidosis with high anion gap and metabolic alkalosis, accompanied by respiratory alkalosis, in McKittrick-Wheelock syndrome.

Clinical case 4 A 76-year-old man known for heart failure and chronic hypoxemic and hypercapnic chronic obstructive pulmonary disease, with chronic respiratory acidosis, metabolic alkalosis and normal pH, is admitted to an internal medicine ward and subjected to oxygen therapy (3 liters per minute by nasal cannula).

About 6 hours after admission, the patient appears lethargic and cyanotic.

The arterial blood gas is repeated and shows the following values: pH 7.33, $PaCO_2$ 80 mmHg, 41 mEq/L, PaO_2 55 mmHg, Na^+ 140 mEq/L, Cl^- 88 mEq/L, K+ 4.0 mEq/L, anion gap 11 mEq/L.

ABG interpretation

pH	7.33	acidemia
$PaCO_2$	80 mmHg	elevated (respiratory acidosis)
HCO_3^-	41 mEq/L	increased (metabolic acidosis)
Anion gap	11 mEq/L	normal
Chloride	88 mEq/L	reduced (for electroneutrality reasons caused by HCO_3^- increase)
Na^+/Cl^-	1.59	increased

Expected adaptation for respiratory acidosis

Calculate the expected bicarbonate increase compared to reference value (24 mEq/L) in relation to $PaCO_2$ increase (80 mmHg) with respect to reference value (40 mmHg), taking into the adaptation rule for chronic respiratory acidosis: 40 × 0.35 = 14 mEq/L (increase of bicarbonate) + 24 (reference bicarbonate) = 38 mEq/L (expected bicarbonate).

The current bicarbonate concentration (41 mEq/L) is very close to the expected one (38 mEq/L ± 2/± 3).

Final interpretation: in the absence of clinical data: chronic respiratory acidosis. With the clinical data: metabolic alkalosis and chronic respiratory acidosis with overlap of acute respiratory acidosis.

Reasoned comment

The described patient had arrived in emergency department with chronic respiratory acidosis and metabolic alkalosis (pH 7.40, $PaCO_2$ 67 mmHg, HCO_3^- 40 mEq/L, Na^+ 140 mEq/L, Cl^- 88 mEq/L, K^+ 4.0 mEq/L, anion gap 12 mEq/L).

The subsequent O_2 administration, as often happens in hypercapnic patients, was the cause of hypoventilation which led to a considerable $PaCO_2$ increase from 67 to 80 mmHg and of acidemia with a pH reduction from 7.40 to 7.33.

Bicarbonate concentration is increased by only one mEq/L.

Examining the values of the last arterial blood gas without knowing the clinical history, we do not depart from a blood gas framework of chronic respiratory acidosis (even if the very high value of $PaCO_2$ is not compatible with a chronic situation).

Knowleage of clinical dynamic and of the previous ABG values leads us to correctly interpret the report: the overlap of an acute process (acute respiratory acidosis) to a pre-existing chronic respiratory acidosis and metabolic alkalosis.

Therefore the correct diagnosis is of metabolic alkalosis and chronic respiratory acidosis with overlapping of acute respiratory acidosis caused by the administration of oxygen in a hypercapnic patient.

NOTE

This clinical case underlines once again how fundamental it is to interpret the blood gas measurements in the light of clinical-anamnestic data.

Quadruple mixed acid-base disorders

A quadruple mixed acid-base disorder is due to the presence of four primary acid-base disorders.

A possible and not rare quadruple disorder consists of AG metabolic acidosis and metabolic alkalosis with chronic respiratory acidosis and overlapping of acute respiratory acidosis.

Clinical case This clinical case is the continuation of the previous number 4.

The man with chronic hypoxemic-hypercapnic chronic obstructive pulmonary disease and metabolic alkalosis caused by diuretics is discharged. The last morning, a further room air ABG, is comparable to his usual chronic condition: pH 7.40, $PaCO_2$ 67 mmHg, HCO_3^- 40 mEq/L, PaO_2 50 mmHg, Na^+ 140 mEq/L, Cl^- 88 mEq/L, K^+ 4.0 mEq/L, anion gap 13 mEq/L.

As soon as he arrives home he suffers sudden dyspnea, followed by a return to the local emergency department.

Upon arrival the patient is very dyspneic, agitated sweaty and cyanotic. On chest auscultation, rattling sounds spreading over the whole area are found. Chest ultrasound shows the presence of B lines spreading to both lungs.

The vital signs: BP 90/80 mmHg, HR 120 bpm, RR 36 bpm, T 37.4 °C, SpO_2 80% on room air.

ABG: pH 7.22, $PaCO_2$ 80 mmHg, HCO_3^- 32 mEq/L, PaO_2 44 mmHg, Na^+ 142 mEq/L, Cl^- 90, K^+ 4.3, anion gap 20 mEq/L, lactic acid 8 mmol/L.

ABG interpretation

pH	7.22	
$PaCO_2$	80 mmHg	elevated (respiratory acidosis)
HCO_3^-	32 mEq/L	increased
Anion gap	20 mEq/L	increased
Chloride	90 mEq/L	reduced
Na^+/Cl^-	1.57	increased

Calculation of the expected adaptation for metabolic acidosis

It makes no sense to do this calculation since compared to ΔAG of 8 mEq/L bicarbonate is much more increased and also there is no relationship between PCO_2 and $[HCO_3^-]$ in terms of adaptation.

Final interpretation: AG metabolic acidosis with metabolic alkalosis and acute respiratory acidosis superimposed on chronic respiratory acidosis.

Reasoned comment

The interpretation of this arterial blood gas out of context is really complex.

Acid pH and anion gap beyond normal values, point towards AG metabolic acidosis. Bicarbonate has not fallen as predicted by anion gap increase, which suggests a metabolic alkalosis, a data also confirmed by the Na^+/Cl^- ratio of 1.57. There is no adaptive relationship between $PaCO_2$ and $[HCO_3^-]$.

Everything becomes clearer if we compare this arterial blood gas with the previous one that presented a mixed respiratory acidosis and metabolic alkalosis and if we consider the clinical picture.

The patient arrives in the emergency department for acute pulmonary edema causing acute hypercapnia ($PaCO_2$ 80 mmHg) on a chronic condition (67 mmHg) and peripheral hypoperfusion with increased lactic acid and consequent metabolic acidosis (AG 20 mEq/L).

The latter determines a $[HCO_3^-]$ reduction of the previously documented (40 mEq/L) but which still remains high (32 mEq/L) while the metabolic alkalosis from the diuretics still remains. At this point the diagnosis is clear.

It is a quadruple acid-base disorder characterized by metabolic acidosis due to increased blood lactates with metabolic alkalosis caused by diuretics and acute respiratory acidosis caused by pulmonary edema superimposed on chronic respiratory acidosis due to chronic hypoxemic and hypercapnic COPD.

NOTE

Anion gap must always be calculated, because, as in this case, it allows us to correctly interpret the acid-base disorders. Also very useful is the evaluation of the chloride ion and the calculation of the Na^+/Cl^- ratio that allow us, immediately, to understand that metabolic alkalosis is present.

References

Relating to clinical interpretation

- Adrogué HJ. Mixed acid-base disturbances. J Nephrol 2006;19 Suppl 9:S97-103.
- Adrogué HJ, Gennari FJ, Galla JH et al. Assessing acid-base disorders. Kidney Int. 2009;76(12):1239-47.
- Adrogué HJ, Madias NE. Secondary responses to altered acid-base status: the rules of engagement. J Am Soc Nephrol 2010;21(6):920-3.
- Berend K, de Vries AP, Gans RO. Physiological approach to assessment of acid-base disturbances. N Engl J Med. 2014; 371(15):1434-45.
- Bia M, Thier SO. Mixed acid base disturbances: a clinical approach. Med Clin North Am. 1981;65(2):347-61.
- Dzierba AL, Abraham P. A practical approach to understanding acid-base abnormalities in critical illness. J Pharm Pract. 2011;24(1):17-26.
- Goodkin DA, Krishna GG, Narins RG. The role of anion gap in detecting and managing mixed metabolic acid-base disorders. Clin Endocrinol Metab. 1984;13(2):333-49.
- Kamel KS, Halperin ML. Fluid, electrolyte and acid-base physiology. A problem-based approach. 5th ed. Elsevier 2016.
- Martin L. All you really need to know to interpret arterial blood gases. Philadelphia. Lippincott Williams & Wilkins 1999.
- Maxwell & Kleemans. Clinical Disorders of fluid and electrolyte metabolism. 5th ed. New York. McGraw-Hill 1994.
- Narins RG, Emmett M. Simple and mixed acid-base disorders: a practical approach. Medicine (Baltimore). 1980;59 (3):161-87.

- Narins RG, Jones ER et al. Diagnostic strategies in disorders of fluid, electrolyte and acid-base homeostasis. Am J Med. 1982;72(3):496-450.
- Rastegar A. Use of the DeltaAG/DeltaHCO$_3^-$ ratio in the diagnosis of mixed acid-base disorders. J Am Soc Nephrol 2007;18(9):2429-31.
- Rose BD, Post TW. Clinical physiology of acid-base and electrolyte disorders. 5th ed. New York. McGraw-Hill 2001.
- Walmsley RN, White GH. Mixed acid-base disorders. Clin Chem. 1985;31(2):321-5.

Relating to the causes of mixed disorders

- Aberman A, Fulop M. The metabolic and respiratory acidosis of acute pulmonary edema. Ann Intern Med. 1972;76(2):173-84.
- Andersen LE, Heinrich WL. Alkalemia-associated morbidity and mortality in medical and surgical patients. South Med J. 1987;80(6):729-33.
- Elisaf M, Theodorou J, Pappas H et al. Acid-base and electrolyte abnormalities in febrile patients with bacteraemia. Eur J Med. 1993;2(7):404-7.
- Elisaf MS, Tsatsoulis AA, Katapodis KP et al. Acid-base and electrolyte disturbance in patients with diabetic ketoacidosis. Diabetes Res Clin Pract. 1996;34(1):23-7.
- Fencl V, Jabor A, Kazda A et al. Diagnosis of metabolic acid-base disturbances in critically ill patients. Am J Respir Crit Care Med. 2000;162(6):2246-51.
- Gabow PA, Anderson RJ, Potts DE et al. Acid-base disturbances in the salicylate-intoxicated adult. Arch Intern Med. 1978;138(10):1481-4.
- Gennari FJ, Weise WJ. Acid-base disturbances in gastrointestinal disease. Clin J Am Soc Nephrol. 2008; 3(6):1861-8.
- Holland AE, Wilson JW, Kotsimbos TC et al. Metabolic alkalosis contributes to acute hypercapnic respiratory failure in adult cystic fibrosis. Chest. 2003;124(2):490-3.
- Jammalamadaka D, Raissi S. Ethylene glycol, methanol and isopropyl alcohol intoxication. Am J Med Sci. 2010;339 (3):276-81.
- Kamel KS, Hlaperin ML. Acid-base problems in diabetic ketoacidosis. New Engl J Med. 2015;372(6):546-54.
- Kassirer JP, Madias NE. Respiratory acid-base disorders. Hosp Pract 1980;15(12):57-9, 65-71.
- McKurdy DK. Mixed metabolic and respiratory acid-base disturbances: diagnosis and treatment. Chest. 1972;62(2): 35S-44S.
- Meng QH, Adeli K, Zello GA et al. Elevated lactate in ethylene glycol poisoning: true or false? Clin Chim Acta. 2010;411(7-8):601-4.
- Mokhlesi B, Leiken JB, Murray P et al. Adult toxicology in critical care. Part I: general approach to the intoxicated patient. Chest. 2003;123(2):577-92.
- Mountain RD, Heffner JE, Brackett NC Jr et al. Acid-base disturbance in acute asthma. Chest 1990; 98(3):651-5.
- O'Donovan R, McGowan JA, Lupinacci L et al. Acid-base disturbances in cardiogenic pulmonary edema. Nephron. 1991;57(4):416-20.
- Oh YK. Acid-base disorders in ICU patients. Electrolyte Blood Press. 2010;8(2):66-71.
- Oster JR, Perez GO. Acid-base disturbances in liver disease. J Hepatol. 1986;2(2):299-306.
- Paulson WD, Gadallah MF. Diagnosis of mixed acid-base disorders in diabetic ketoacidosis. Am J Med Sci. 1993;306 (5):295-300.
- Perez GO, Oster JR, Rogers A. Acid-base disturbances in gastrointestinal diseases. Dig Dis Sci. 1987;32(9):1033-43.
- Taylor D, Durward A, Tibby SM et al. The influence of hyperchloraemia on acid base interpretation in diabetic ketoacidosis. Intensive Care Med. 2006;32(2):295-301.
- Ucgun I, Oztuna F, Dagli CE et al. Relationship of metabolic alkalosis, azotemia and morbidity in patients with chronic obstructive pulmonary disease and hypercapnia. Respiration. 2008; 76(3):270-4.
- Webster NR, Kulkarni U. Metabolic alkalosis in the critical ill. Crit Rev Clin Lab Sci 1999;36(5):497-510.
- Wiener SW. Toxicologic acid-base disorders. Emerg Med Clin North Am. 2014;32(1):149-65.

Management of acid-base disorders

Gaetano Esposito, Rodolfo Sbrojavacca, Nicolò Capsoni,
Giulio Cassano, Andrea Bellone

Premise

A brief premise. The treatment of acid-base disorders cannot be improvised and does not need to be implemented. Do not start the navigation without a route drawn on the relatively precise coordinates of the pathophysiology and without a goal to reach. Do not feel obliged to take off: the compulsion to act that often takes possession of the doctor can be very dangerous, especially if it pushes him or her uncritically to the normalization of the parameters. There is always time to think. Good navigation.

Treatment of respiratory acidosis

Introduction

Unlike metabolic acidosis which can be caused by different acidogenic mechanisms, respiratory acidosis is always determined by CO_2 accumulation due to reduced alveolar ventilation.

There is therefore always at the base a picture of type 2 respiratory insufficiency (hypoxic-hypercapnic) which can be acute, chronic or acute on chronic. The rationale of therapy is therefore to improve ventilation by increasing CO_2 pulmonary clearance.

Acute respiratory acidosis treatment

Patients with acute respiratory acidosis are usually critically ill patients with acute reduction of alveolar ventilation.

In the emergency approach it is essential on one hand to identify the underlying causes and the pathophysiological mechanisms [reduction of respiratory rate (RR), reduction of tidal volume (Vt), increase of the dead space volume (Vd)] and set a targeted etiological treatment. On the other hand it is important to assess the need for mechanical ventilation support (invasive or non-invasive) based on the severity of respiratory failure, the underlying disease and the patient's functional reserve. Unlike the two ventilation options, there is "palliative" support in selected patients who would not benefit from conventional treatment.

Among the causes that can produce a depression of the respiratory drive, some substances with central action (sedatives and opioids for pharmacological or recreational use) can be neutralized with the specific antidote; similarly, the modification of excessive oxygen therapy may be sufficient to gradually restore a normal respiratory drive in patients with chronic obstructive pulmonary disease (COPD) with hypercapnic response to oxygen (see Chapter 4).

It should be remembered that, in any case, the depression of respiratory centers induced by O_2 therapy at high flows is only partly responsible for the accumulation of CO_2.

The most significant causes are the effect of oxygen in displacing the hemoglobin linked to CO_2 and therefore increasing its circulating share (Haldane effect) and the opening of vessels that involve unventilated alveoli, followed by alteration of the ventilation/perfusion ratio.

The rapid unblocking of the upper airways with aspiration and extraction of foreign bodies and the prompt treatment of laryngeal spasms are often decisive maneuvers, as well as the drainage of pneumothorax and pleural effusions.

In case of an acute asthma attack or exacerbation of COPD, on the other hand, therapy with bronchodilators and steroids, reducing the lower airways ob-

struction and consequently the alveolar air trapping, can reduce the airway resistance portion and improve the $\dot{V}a/\dot{Q}$ ratio and the pulmonary compliance.
The genesis of acute respiratory acidosis is more complex, often accompanying a picture of acute cardiogenic pulmonary edema. In this case the presence of a low pulmonary compliance due to the diffuse alveolar transudate, determines a distribution of ventilation mostly in areas where the alveolar pressure is dominated by the intrathoracic pressure (respiration that occurs below the residual functional capacity). Therefore, the resultant is a prevalence of areas with low ventilation/perfusion ratio and therefore hypercapnia.
Treatment, for example, with positive airway pressure (CPAP – continuous positive airway pressure or BPAP – bilevel positive airway pressure) determines an immediate, dramatic, hemodynamic effect (reduction of the left ventricular pre- and after load) with consequent unloading of the small circle congestion and increasing pulmonary compliance. This effect translates into a rapid improvement in gas exchange (the oxygenation increases and the hypercapnia decreases) as well as in respiratory rate reduction.
The use of mechanical ventilation is often useful and sometimes unavoidable in hypercapnic respiratory failure treatment, especially in cases where the cause cannot be quickly resolved.
The inspiration pressure delivered by the ventilator supports or replaces the patient's respiratory musculature in conditions where, due to increased respiratory work (compliance deterioration and resistive forces increase) and/or due to muscle exhaustion, the latter is not able alone to perform adequate alveolar ventilation; the muscular work reduction also allows to decrease CO_2 metabolic production. The delivery of a positive end expiratory pressure (PEEP), on the other hand, determines alveolar recruitment, counterbalances the intrinsic PEEP typical of bronchial obstruction clinical conditions and stabilizes the peripheral airways by moving the point of equal pressure more proximally, thus reducing the early bronchiolar collapse at high lung volumes.
Non-invasive mechanical ventilation (NIMV) due to its practicality and lower complications is increasingly an alternative to invasive ventilation.
Ventilation treatment is now the first choice in respiratory failure due to exacerbated COPD and acute cardiogenic pulmonary edema (ACPE) (level of evidence A).
In COPD the presence of respiratory distress (with increased RR, use of accessory respiratory musculature and thoracoabdominal dyskinesia), a persistent pH < 7.35 and/or a $PaCO_2 > 50$ after bronchodilator therapy and O_2, are an indication for ventilatory support.
In the ACPE, the NIMV, due to its effect on alveolar recruitment and hemodynamics, is instead indicated during respiratory distress and $P/F < 250$.
NIMV is also indicated in the acute respiratory failure treatment in patients with neuromuscular disease, when an infectious episode or an exacerbation of the disease can reduce patient's functional capacity, increase the elastic load imposed on the respiratory muscles and produce an increase in the RR (> 20) which may precede an initial muscular fatigue.
In pneumonia respiratory failure, the presence of a respiratory acidosis is always an alarm sign and an indication not to further delay invasive ventilation (pneumonia in COPD patients is an exception).
While in cases of acute respiratory acidosis the therapeutic goal is to normalize $PaCO_2$ and therefore pH, in acute on chronic acidosis the goal remains the acute component resolution, with pH increase and a $PaCO_2$ reduction, as close as possible to patient's baseline values, so as to prevent the onset of post-hypercapnic alkalosis.
In correcting respiratory acidosis, alkalizing substances (i.e., THAM – tromethamine) are no longer indicated.
Bicarbonate use also contraindicated: dissociating to buffer H^+ ions can aggravate hypercapnia, increase the risk of post-hypercapnic alkalosis in the case of effective ventilation and has a negligible protective effect on the central nervous system (CNS) pH due to its poor diffusion through the blood-brain barrier.

Chronic respiratory acidosis treatment

Chronic respiratory acidosis can count on an effective renal compensation mechanism that can bring pH back to acceptable values.
Therapeutic approach must aim primarily to prevent

exacerbations and the onset of an acute over a chronic acidosis, and in the event of an appearance to treat it quickly. It is therefore essential to optimize chronic therapies of the underlying disease and favor an adequate patient compliance. In COPD patients, chronic therapy optimized with bronchodilators reduces the exacerbations number and their rapid treatment avoids the onset of an acute respiratory acidosis picture over a chronic one.

In patients with obesity-hypoventilation syndrome (OHS), characterized by chronic day and night hypercapnia, the weight loss, lifestyle changes and CPAP-BPAP would be sufficient to progressively improve ventilation.

NIMV use in the chronic hypercapnia treatment is strongly indicated only in patients with OHS; even in that small share without a concomitant nocturnal obstructive apnea syndrome (< 30%), chronic NIMV cycles improve blood gas analysis parameters, symptoms, quality of life and sleep.

In patients with COPD, although certainly indicated in cases of overlap with obstructive sleep apnea syndrome (OSAS), some recent studies on selected populations (GOLD IV stage patients with $PaCO_2$ persistence > 52-53 mmHg at 2-4 weeks after discharge for bronchitis exacerbation) have shown that NIMV cycles alternated with O_2 therapy can reduce the exacerbations number and mortality at 12 months.

Respiratory alkalosis treatment

Respiratory alkalosis rarely, in both acute and chronic forms, generates pH variations requiring urgent action. An urgent correction is necessary if the pH increase is followed by a reduction in the ionized proportion of Ca^{++} and Mg^{++} and a reduction in serum potassium such as to induce electrocardiographic alterations or muscular symptoms (spasms, paresthesia), or if the sharp CO_2 drop causes symptomatic cerebral vasoconstriction (drowsiness, coma, seizure).

Treatment almost always aims to correct the underlying disease, especially when hyperventilation is caused by hypoxia, fever, low flow state, hyperthyroidism.

It is appropriate to differentiate the respiratory alkalosis according to the shunt presence (pulmonary embolism, pneumonia, contusion, atelectasis) or shunt absence typically during pulmonary interstitial diseases, where oxygen therapy plays a fundamental role unlike pathologies causing intrapulmonary shunt (see Chapter 4).

A special case is represented by the anxiety-hyperventilation syndrome in which hypocapnia can arise abruptly and be critical and symptomatic. In these cases a mild sedation (usually with low doses of benzodiazepines) may be indicated to reduce the action of the respiratory drive; "rebreathing" techniques to increase CO_2 in the inhaled air and reduce hypocapnia (for example, breathing into a paper bag), are generally not recommended because of risk of generating important and sometimes symptomatic hypoxemia.

Metabolic acidosis: principles of treatment

Metabolic acidosis includes an extremely heterogeneous group of disorders, with therapeutic indications that, in most cases, differ in relation to etiology and severity.

However, it is possible to identify four general points to which every therapeutic decision must refer. Priority:

- identify emergency situations, potentially life-threatening, requiring immediate measures and eventually intensive care;
- identify the determining cause of acidosis;
- evaluate whether is indicated an alkali administration (intravenously or orally);
- estimate possible changes in potassium before starting the acidemia correction.

- **Identify emergency situations.** In emergency contexts, before the results of laboratory tests are available (including arterial blood gas), patients must always be approached according to the ABC scheme, to evaluate and maintain airway patency, ventilation and perfusion.
- **Identify the determining cause of acidosis.** Causes identification is important for at least three reasons. It allows, first of all, to start specific and etiopath-

ogenic therapeutic measures, which we will describe in detail below; but it also allows to intervene promptly on those conditions, which regardless of patient's state, represent by themselves a danger to life. In intoxications, for example, rapid diagnosis allows to implement immediately measures to counteract the toxic substance (gastric lavage, antidotes and urine alkalinization) even before the development of significant metabolic alterations.
Finally, identifying the cause, allows us to estimate the rate of hydrogen ion production, which in some cases can be particularly high (type A lactic acidosis) and sometimes rather restrained (alcoholic ketoacidosis and prolonged fasting, chronic renal failure, intoxication from toxic alcohols). In forms with a high production rate it is essential to quickly block the production of H^+ (restoration of perfusion in the case of lactic acidosis type A) in order to avoid a rapid decline in blood pH.

- **Evaluate whether there is an indication for alkali administration.** The indication for the use of alkali (sodium bicarbonate) in the metabolic acidosis treatment depends on the pathophysiological mechanism underlying the acidosis and should be evaluated in parallel with the potential adverse reactions of the alkalizing solutions. Oral alkali therapy in hyperchloremic metabolic acidosis with normal anion gap (renal insufficiency, renal tubular acidosis, diarrhea) is a consolidated treatment of undoubted benefit, because the primum movens (cause) of these conditions is bicarbonate loss, accompanied by the inability of the nephron to regenerate it. In particular, in chronic forms of renal origin (chronic renal failure, renal tubular acidosis), oral bicarbonate limits long-term complications: bone demineralization, growth retardation and perhaps even renal disease progression.
The use of intravenous bicarbonate solutions in the acute acidemia treatment is extremely controversial. In vitro and animal model studies have shown, on several occasions, the negative effects on the cellular function of the rapid lowering of arterial and intracellular pH. Enzyme activity and proteins three-dimensional structure are in fact both pH-dependent processes. pH drop in the extracellular fluid influences the binding of hormones to their receptors, increases the ionized calcium concentration and alters the flow through the potassium channels in the conduction tissues (heart, vascular musculature, nervous system).
The most susceptible tissue to rapid pH reduction is with no doubt the cardiac tissue: acute acidemia reduces cardiac contractility and catecholamine sensitivity, increases venous congestion and therefore the risk of pulmonary edema and has vasoplegic effects. Acute acidemia also has profound effects on oxygen transport; it shifts the dissociation curve of oxyhemoglobin (P50) to the right, increasing the oxygen transfer to the tissues, but this effect, potentially positive in hypoperfused patients or those with respiratory failure, can be reset by the concomitant reduction of erythrocyte 2, 3-diphosphoglycerate levels, which on the contrary moves the curve to the left. Although the experimental data, which show how damaging effects of acute acidemia are solid, it remains difficult to prove that the rapid therapeutic inversion of a low pH is really advantageous. First of all because the blood pH does not always correlate with intracellular pH, but above all because the therapy with intravenous bicarbonate solutions is not free from potentially dangerous adverse events, especially when used in bolus and high osmotic formulations (8.4% sodium bicarbonate solution).
The disadvantageous effects of bicarbonate solutions (summarized in **Table 6.1**) often nullify the

TABLE 6.1 Main side effects of sodium bicarbonate infusion.

Hypokalemia
Hypocalcemia
Prolonged Q-T interval
Hypercapnia
Hemodynamic instability

potential positive effects induced by blood pH normalization. For details, refer to the treatment of the individual forms of metabolic acidosis listed below in this chapter.

These considerations highlight the limits of sodium bicarbonate therapy, especially in the metabolic acidosis with high anion gap (ketoacidosis and lactic acidosis, in particular).

In fact, in these forms, acidosis is only one of the manifestations of a complex pathological process, but it does not in itself represent the disease. Therapy goal should therefore be to reverse the pathophysiological process, treating determinant and triggering causes. The effective treatment of the cause leads to a reduction in the production of organic acids (lactates and ketoacids), improves their clearance and regenerates bicarbonate within a few hours. Supplying the extracellular buffers is unlikely to provide the same benefit.

The situation is different in severe toxic alcohols intoxications (ethylene glycol and methanol).

These patients could benefit from therapy with exogenous alkali, because due to the same effect of the toxic substance retention, endogenous (renal) regeneration of bicarbonate occurs only slowly over several days.

NOTE

In common clinical practice when one decides to administer a bicarbonate solution, the following formula is often referred to, to calculate the bicarbonate deficit:

$$\Delta HCO_3^- = 0.5 \text{ (target serum bicarbonate – actual serum bicarbonate) x total body weight (Kg)}$$

This formula underestimates the actual deficit, because blood bicarbonate is not directly proportional to the total amount of body bicarbonate.

- **Estimate possible changes of potassium.** It must never be forgotten that quickly correcting acidemia can mean reducing potassium just as quickly.
  In fact, in order to mantain intracellular electroneutrality, the cell membranes exchange the hydrogen ion with potassium and, by the same principle, acidemia correction moves potassium from the extracellular fluid (ECF) to the intracellular fluid (ICF), with consequent hypokalemia. The increased renal potassium excretion induced by acidosis participates in the genesis of hypokalemia. Since the relationship between the intracellular and extracellular potassium concentration (K^+_{in}/k^+_{out}) is mainly responsible for the resting membrane potential (for details see the Nernst equation), it follows that any abrupt kalemia modification alters excitability in the conduction tissues. Rapidly established hypokalemia has two serious clinical consequences: malignant arrhythmia and respiratory failure due to muscular weakness.
  The problem is particularly relevant in metabolic acidosis forms that accompany a deficit of the intracellular potassium pool (diabetic ketoacidosis and metabolic acidosis due to diarrhea). In these cases administering potassium becomes a priority and it can be extremely dangerous to administer alkali or insulin before having corrected the kalemia (see below).

Treatment of anion gap metabolic acidosis

Lactic acidosis

Introduction

Lactic acidosis and hyperlactatemia are traditionally considered to be biological and prognostic markers of tissue hypoxia. However, this view is too simplistic and does not take into account the numerous causes of lactate increase, which may occur in absence of tissue hypoxia or in addition to hypoxia itself. Lactate is not just a metabolic "waste" deriving from anaerobic glycolysis; rather, it is an important energy "shuttle" whose production involves different metabolic pathways, activated in conditions of exalted cellular metabolism (sepsis in the first place). Identifying and controlling the triggering conditions of hyperlactatemia is currently the only meaningful therapeutic device.

Lactate is produced from pyruvate in the last stage of anaerobic glycolysis.

In physiological conditions blood lactate/pyruvate ratio is 10:1, but it can increase significantly in hypoperfusion contexts. Lactate is produced in all tissues, but the main ones are skeletal muscle and red blood cells. Its catabolism occurs mainly in the liver (around 70%) and only a small part in the kidney. In these organs lactate is a substrate of neoglucogenesis. The whole process that converts lactate into glucose is called the "Cori cycle" (**Figure 6.1**).

The renal excretion threshold for lactate is very high (around 6-10 mEq/L), therefore the kidney directly eliminates lactate only during severe hyperlactatemia.

As already mentioned in the premise, establishing the pathogenetic mechanism underlying hyperlactatemia is a necessary condition to face therapy. Cohen and Woods have historically classified lactic acidosis into two types: type A from tissue hypoxia and type B from mechanisms other than hypoxic.

Type B hyperlactatemia is further subdivided into B1, if associated with an underlying disease (i.e., liver failure); B2, when it is induced by drugs or toxic substances; B3, if caused by congenital defects of metabolism (**Table 6.2**).

Tissue hypoxia (global or district) occurs whenever there is a mismatch between oxygen supply (oxygen delivery – DO_2) and its use (oxygen consumption – VO_2). In this context, anaerobic glycolysis and therefore lactate production reach their maximum expression.

In type B forms the main pathophysiological mechanism is the exalted aerobic glycolysis.

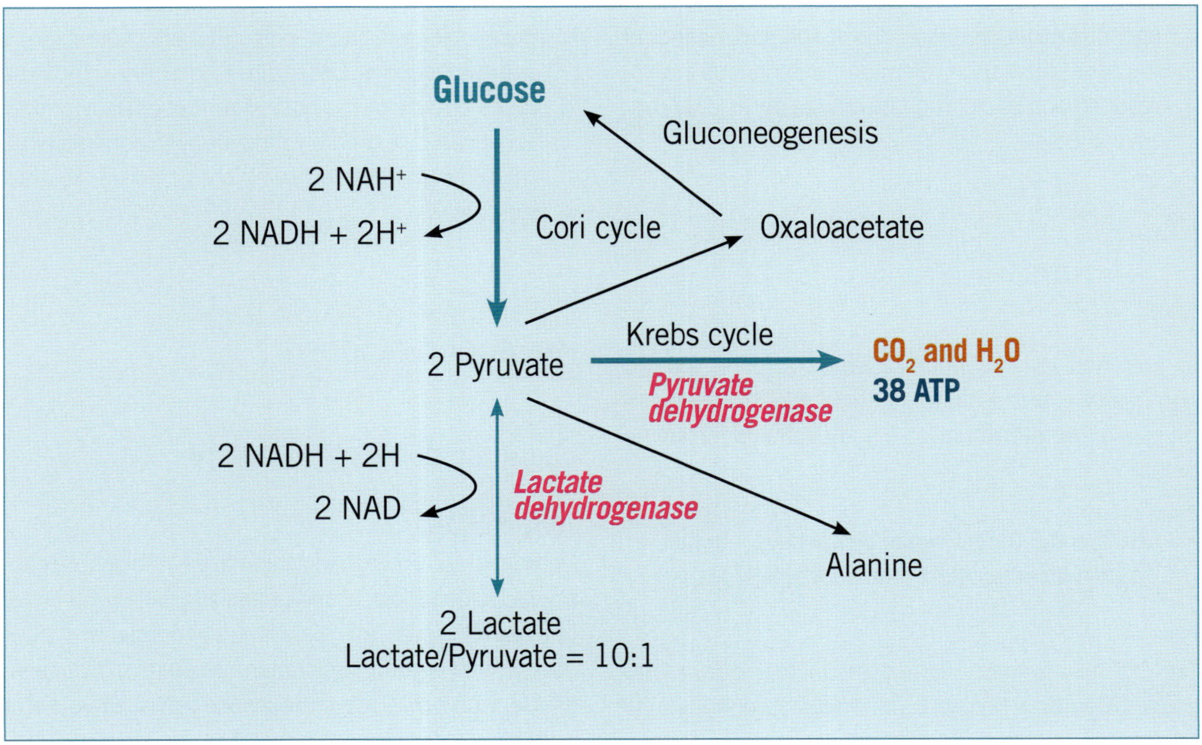

Figure 6.1 Lactate production.

In this scenario, glucose metabolism exceeds the oxidizing capacity of mitochondria and the increase in pyruvate concentration supports lactate production. Adrenergic (β_2) and cytokine hyperstimulation are most often the cause. This explains hyperlactatemia in the hyperdynamic state of sepsis, acute asthma attack, trauma, pheochromocytoma, diabetic ketoacidosis and AIDS.

Some drugs and toxic substances cause type B hyperlactatemia because they inhibit mitochondrial oxidative phosphorylation: it is the case of antiretrovirals, propofol, metformin and toxic alcohols.

NOTE

The mechanism that links liver failure to lactate production is complex. Cirrhosis, even severe, rarely generates significant hyperlactatemia and never acidosis. In contrast, in acute (fulminant) hepatitis, hyperlactatemia is common and reflects its prognosis. In septic patients (including hemodynamically stable) reduced hepatic metabolism (from pyruvate -dehydrogenase inhibition) participates together with the exalted production to the genesis of hyperlactatemia.

TABLE 6.2 Causes and classification of lactic acidosis. From Seheult J, Fitzpatrick G, Boran G. Lactic acidosis: an update. Clin Chem Lab Med. 2017; 55 (3): 322-33 (modified).

Type A Tissue hypoxia	Type B Mechanisms other than hypoxic
Shock (systemic hypoperfusion) • Hypovolemic • Cardiogenic • Maldistributive	**B1: associated with underlying diseases** • Diabetic ketoacidosis (DKA) • Leukemia/Lymphoma • Acquired immunodeficiency syndrome (AIDS) • Severe liver disease • Sepsis • Thiamine deficiency • Pheochromocytoma
Local hypoperfusion • Splanchnic ischemia • Aortic thromboembolism	**B2: associated with drugs and toxins** • Acetaminophen • β-agonists (including cocaine and adrenaline) • Cyanide • Insulin • Nitroprusside • Nucleoside reverse - transcriptase inhibitors • Phenformin • Propofol • Salicylates • Toxic alcohols: methanol, ethanol, ethylene glycol, diethylene glycol, propylene glycol
Other causes of tissue hypoxia • Severe hypoxemia (PaO_2 < 30-40 mmHg) • Severe euvolemic anemia • Carbon monoxide toxicity **Increased glycolysis** • Excessive muscle activity • Exercise • Trembling **Seizure**	**B3: associated with inborn errors of metabolism** • Mitochondrial myopathy • Pyruvate dehydrogenase deficiency **Miscellaneous** • Alkalosis/Hyperventilation • Hypoglycemia

General therapeutic approach

A high level of lactate should, for first instance, suggest an assessment of the causes of oxygen supply reduction (DO_2).

DO_2 is expressed by the product between cardiac output (CO) and arterial oxygen content (CaO_2). The content of arterial oxygen depends, in turn, on the quantity of hemoglobin (Hb), on its saturation in arterial blood (SaO_2) and on a minimal amount of oxygen dissolved in the blood (0.003 x PaO_2). All summarized in the following formula:

$$DO_2 = CO \times CaO_2$$

$$CaO_2 = (1.34 \times Hb \times SaO_2) + (0.003 \times PaO_2)$$

Therefore the causes of DO_2 reduction and hyperlactatemia due to tissue hypoxia (type A) are: systemic hypoperfusion status caused by reduced cardiac output (CO), severe anemia, respiratory failure with severe hypoxemia and regionally reduced perfusion (i.e., limb ischemia or mesenteric ischemia). In these forms the treatment consists in optimizing oxygen supply to the tissues.

Hemodynamics must be restored by administering the right amount of fluids and in selected cases with vasopressors and inotropes. Ventilation should be sustained (in an invasive or non-invasive manner) only when the oxygen saturation is less than 92%, due to the known vasoconstrictor effect that oxygen has on the cerebral and coronary circulation. Finally, in the case of severe anemia, recent evidence indicates the need to transfuse for hemoglobin concentrations below 7 g/dL.

If tissue hypoxia is excluded, after an exhaustive examination, the physician must consider the possibility of causes of hyperlactatemia without concomitant tissue hypoxia (type B forms).

Therapeutic approach in type A lactic acidosis

The basic principles of therapeutic treatment of type A lactic acidosis are: circulatory support, treatment of causes and, in some cases, containment of acidosis.

Circulatory support

Fluids – The fluids administration, aiming to cardiac output, remains the cornerstone of initial therapy for most hypoperfusion states. Regarding the choice of the solution to be administered, the dispute between colloids and crystalloids has enthralled intensivists for over twenty years (see Chapter 11).

Many studies (2012) (CHEST, CRYSTAL, 6S) have shown that colloids and in particular hydroxyethyl starch are not superior to crystalloids, indeed they are potentially dangerous especially in terms of developing acute renal failure; the only colloid that has any indication is albumin; two studies (SAFE – 2004 and ALBIOS – 2014) suggest the hemodynamic advantages (and potentially over the mortality) in patients with severe sepsis (according to the old definition) or septic shock. However, the role of albumin in patients with septic shock requires further study.

But even the crystalloids are not all the same. Normal saline solution, when used in large quantities, can generate or exacerbate hyperchloremic metabolic acidosis and cause renal vasoconstriction.

Crystalloids containing bicarbonate or its precursors (balanced saline solutions), such as Ringer's solutions with lactate and acetate, do not cause hyperchloremic metabolic acidosis, but may occasionally determine metabolic alkalosis.

Two recent (2018) RCTs (SMART and SALT-ED) have shown a significant superiority of balanced solutions (Ringer lactate and Plasma-Lyte A) in critically ill patients in intensive care and emergency areas, both in terms of mortality and acute kidney damage.

With regard to the method of administration, in recent years, the potential risk of fluid overload has been highlighted several times, with negative consequences also on septic patients mortality.

The pathophysiological assumption is the damage that the excess of liquids creates to endothelial glycocalyx which results in capillary rarefaction, interstitial edema and impairment of capillary-cell exchanges. Therefore, caution is advised on the amount of liquid to be administered.

Vasopressors and inotropes – In the case of septic patients in a state of hypoperfusion, unresponsive to fluids, there is an indication for the vasopressors administration.

Regarding the choice, a Cochrane meta-analysis (2016) on the use of vasopressors in shock, which compared six molecules (epinephrine, norepinephrine, dopamine, terlipressin, phenylephrine and vasopressin), did not show significant differences on mortality. However, the levels of evidence are low, except in the comparison between norepinephrine and epinephrine.
The expert opinion is to consider norepinephrine as the first choice drug. Norepinephrine is above all an α-agonist, with mild beta-stimulating properties, for this reason it is above all a vasoconstrictor, with little effect on the heart rate; a low dose is recommended (0.1-2 μg/Kg/min), to act only on the vasoplegic component of the shock.
At these dosages norepinephrine can be used safely even in peripheral vein.
Dopamine, used so much in the past, is associated with a greater risk of arrhythmias, has no protective effect on the splanchnic and renal circulation, if administered at low doses (study SOAP II – 2010) and seems to have immunosuppressive properties, therefore completely inappropriate in a septic context. Its only niche use is in patients in states of hypoperfusion and bradycardia.

NOTE

Recall that there is a complex relationship between catecholamines and lactic acidosis. Acidemia attenuates the catecholamines response, thus increasing the dose required. High doses of catecholamines can aggravate hyperlactatemia by reducing tissue perfusion and over stimulating β_2-receptors; therefore the doses must be regulated carefully.

The second vasopressor of choice is considered vasopressin, especially after the results of the VASST study (2008), which showed that adding vasopressin to norepinephrine in patients with septic shock is safe and effective, particularly in moderate forms and in patients using glucocorticoids; the recommended dosage is 0.03-0.04 U/min.

Inotrope drugs play a very limited role in the treatment of hyperlactatemia and lactic acidosis.
In extremely selected cases, the only indication drug is dobutamine. Its role is limited to transient use, in case of left ventricular dysfunction (acute heart failure and sepsis); however, the evidence is rather weak and the risk of ischemic cardiac complications are instead relevant.
Greater benefits are not obtained even with the other inotropes (phosphodiesterase III inhibitors, e.g. milrinone and levosimendan); these drugs are in fact potent vasodilators and therefore potentially hypotensive, they also have a strong proarrhythmic action and a long duration of action, in particular the levosimendan (LEOPARDS study – 2017).

Containment of acidosis

Role of bicarbonate and bases – Given the potentially harmful effects of an acid environment, some clinicians recommend intravenous sodium bicarbonate therapy in severe acidemia (pH < 7.2).
However, the role of bicarbonate therapy in reducing mortality or improving hemodynamics remains without evidence.
Bicarbonate in fact determines two main adverse events that compromise its effectiveness even at very low pH: the intracellular acidification due to the enzymatic transformation of bicarbonate into carbon dioxide and the reduction of ionized calcium levels, which depress cardiac contractility much more than acidosis itself. Intracellular acidification is assumed to be more frequent and severe, when large amounts of bicarbonate are rapidly administered in patients with severe hypoperfusion, because hypoperfusion prevents CO_2 removal first from the tissues and then from the lungs.
The results of the recent BICAR-ICU study (2018) seem to be in line with these assumptions. The study evaluated the effects of bicarbonate administration in intensive care patients for severe non-ketoacidotic metabolic acidosis (pH < 7.2). In these patients bicarbonate infusion reduces neither the mortality nor the organ dysfunction, with the sole exception of those with severe renal failure (stage 2 and 3 according to AKIN classification).

Dialysis can provide bicarbonate, countering the potential complications: decrease in ionized calcium, volume overload and hyperosmolality. Dialysis can also directly remove some substances responsible for lactic acidosis, such as metformin.
Continuous dialysis is often favored over intermittent dialysis, since it provides bicarbonate at a slower rate and is associated with fewer adverse events in patients with hemodynamic instability.
Other non-bicarbonate buffers have been developed to minimize carbon dioxide generation.
THAM alone (tris-hydroxymethylaminomethane) is currently available for clinical use, but there is little evidence of its real effectiveness.

Therapeutic approach in type B lactic acidosis

The treatment of type B lactic acidosis is very different because the goal is not to correct the mismatch between DO_2 (oxygen delivery) and VO_2 (oxygen consumption).
Since most cases are due to neoplastic conditions, drugs or toxic substances, treatment must focus on eliminating the determining cause.
The treatment main objective is to limit the harmful effects of acidosis, in particular the inhibition of myocardial contractility. Sodium bicarbonate, dichloroacetate, carbicarb and tromethamine have been studied for the management of type B lactic acidosis, but with little success.
In contrast, hemodialysis and continuous dialysis techniques play an important role in drug-induced lactic acidosis and in particular the one caused by metformin.
L-carnitine has shown promising results in the patients with AIDS treatment, since the latter often develop carnitine deficiency and the molecule plays an important role in mitochondrial function.
Thiamine and biotin deficiencies are common in patients with lactic acidosis due to total parenteral nutrition and chronic alcoholism. These nutrients should be integrated accordingly.
Mitochondrial disorders treatment involves the use of antioxidant molecules (coenzyme Q10, vitamin C, vitamin E) and amino acids (L-arginine), although there is not a good level of evidence.

Ketoacidosis

Introduction

Clinically relevant ketoacidosis includes:
- diabetic ketoacidosis;
- alcoholic ketoacidosis;
- prolonged fasting ketoacidosis.

The common denominator of the three forms is the establishment of a "hepatic ketogenic state", sustained from a bio-humoral point of view by low levels of insulin as opposed to enhanced secretion of counter-regulatory hormones (glucagon, epinephrine, cortisol, growth hormone). This peculiar hormonal arrangement generates uncontrolled lipolysis in the adipose tissue; the fatty acids thus released arrive in large quantities to the liver and by the mitochondria are oxidized into ketone bodies (acetoacetate and beta-hydroxybutyrate). The ketone bodies are strong acids, therefore they consume bicarbonate, determining metabolic acidosis and increase of the anion gap.

Diabetic ketoacidosis

DKA (Diabetic Ketoacidosis) is one of the acute complications of diabetes mellitus, in which insulin deficiency and elevated glucagon levels create a metabolic paradox: a large glucose availability is opposed to an almost impossible utilization.
The body, therefore, to get alternative fuel to glucose, uses other metabolic pathways, overlapping those activated in fasting, first of all lipolysis with consequent ketogenesis. Ketone bodies, it is worth remembering, are the only energy substrate of the neuron in the absence of glucose (**Figure 6.2**).

Identification and treatment of triggering causes

The DKA is in some cases the initial clinical presentation of an unknown diabetes, but more frequently it occurs in conjunction with physiological or pathological stressful events (pregnancy, infections, ischemia, trauma, inadequate compliance with insulin therapy, glucocorticoid therapy).
Regardless of the context, the identification and treatment of triggering factors is an integral part of the diabetic ketoacidosis therapy.

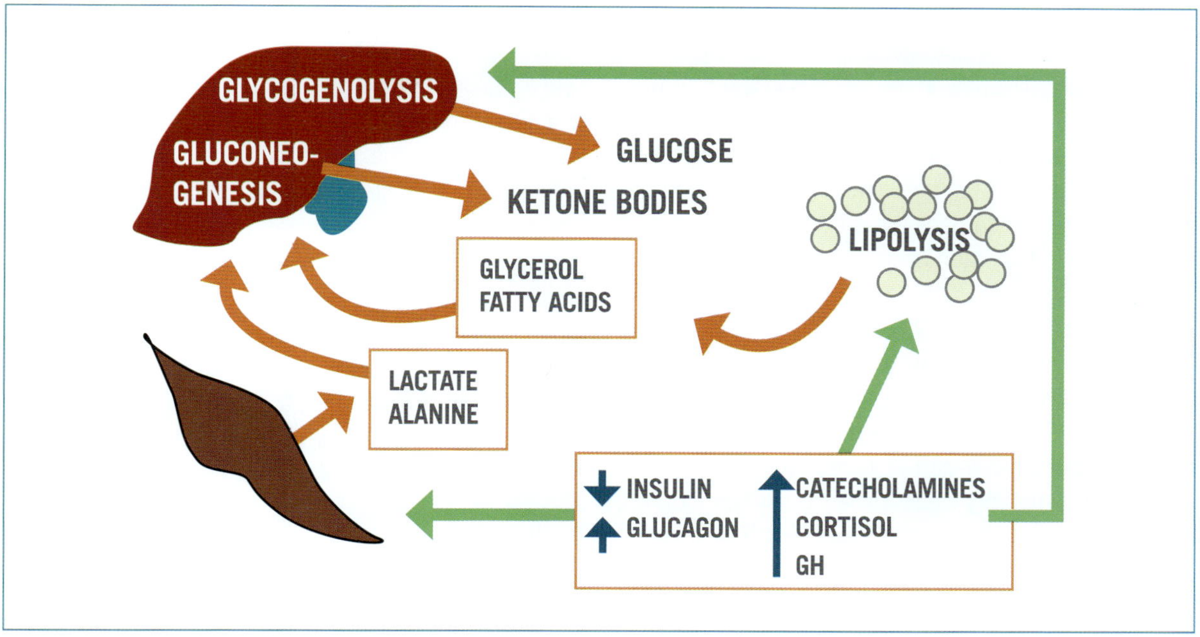

Figure 6.2 Diabetic ketoacidosis pathogenesis.

NOTE

About 10% of patients with DKA are surprisingly euglycemic (blood glucose level < 200 mg/dL). The euglycemic DKA (EDKA) occurs when one of the causes triggering ketoacidosis acts in the presence of reduced caloric intake. In these cases prolonged fasting and concomitant insulin therapy end up depleting glycogen storages and therefore also glucose, while lipolysis continues to support ketogenesis. The most common EDKA causes reported in literature are pregnancy, pancreatitis, cocaine overdose, prolonged vomiting or diarrhea, insulin pump malfunction and a new class of oral hypoglycemic agents, the sodium-glucose cotransporter 2 inhibitors (SGLT2) empagliflozin, canagliflozin.

The three phases of DKA and therapeutic implications

It is very important to remember, for therapeutic implications, that in diabetic ketoacidosis the anion gap is not increased at all stages of the disorder. There are in fact at least two phases in which the anion gap is normal and the acidosis has the characteristics of a hyperchloremic form: the "early phase" in which the circulating blood volume is still preserved and the "late phase" in which the blood volume was restored by saline solution administration.

In the "early phase", in fact, most of the ketone bodies are not held in plasma, but buffered and eliminated by the kidney in the form of sodium and potassium salts. Net this condition generates an indirect bicarbonate loss and therefore a hyperchloremic metabolic acidosis.

When the ketogenic process accelerates and volume depletion becomes more severe, the generated ketoacids concentrate to a greater extent in plasma and increase the anion gap. It is at this stage that ketoacidosis usually becomes symptomatic.

In the course of treatment ("late phase"), the metabolic acidosis is transformed once again into a hyperchloremic form. In fact, by ceasing ketoacids and restoring the extracellular volume, a structure very similar to the early one is recreated, in which the remaining ketoacids resume their urinary elimination. Fluids administered in this phase participate in the genesis of the disorder. The solutions containing chloride and in particular the normal saline solution, acidify when administered in large volumes (see Chapter 11) and potassium and sodium ions that accompany the chloride enter the cells in exchange to hydrogen ions.

Therapeutic approach

The order of priority in diabetic ketoacidosis treatment is as follows: volume restoration, potassium deficiency correction, insulin administration.

Although these three cornerstones (volume, electrolytes, insulin) are very clear, there are few randomized studies able to guide doctors towards the best management of the disorder; in particular the questions on "quantity" and "rate" of liquids and insulin to be administered remain open.

NOTE

Once the appropriate treatment has been started, the average resolution time for acidosis is 10-18 hours. During treatment, vital signs, diuresis, water-electrolyte balance and the dose of insulin administered should be monitored. After the initial arterial blood gas analysis, a venous blood gas with glucose and electrolytes should be performed every 2-4 hours. Patients with severe forms or potentially dangerous triggers ($pH < 7.0$, serum bicarbonate < 10 mEq/L, altered mental status, sepsis, gastrointestinal bleeding, myocardial infarction) should be admitted to an intensive care unit.

Fluid replacement

In DKA the osmotic diuresis induced by hyperglycemia is the cause of intracellular dehydration and ECF (extracellular fluid) reduction.

Water deficit can be considerable, up to 10% of the total body weight. Rapid replacement with fluids is essential to maintain tissue perfusion and eliminate ketone bodies.

Regardless of insulin therapy, fluid intake alone improves glycemic control, corrects acidosis and electrolyte imbalances, and reduces the level of counter-regulatory hormones.

Crystalloids are the fluids to be used even if among these it is not yet clear which is the best choice.

Normal saline solution, when used in large volumes, may worsen the hyperchloremic metabolic acidosis, which marks the terminal phase of diabetic ketoacidosis. Balanced solutions have less impact on hyperchloremic acidosis although this does not result in a reduction in mortality or outcomes.

Furthermore, the use of lactated Ringer's solution is associated with a significant delay in hyperglycemia correction. In summary, it is the experts opinion that the normal saline solution, economic and familiar, premixed with potassium, still remains the fluid of choice in the initial therapy of DKA.

The American Diabetes Association (ADA) guidelines suggest a dosage of 15-20 mL/Kg in the first hour. Once the hemodynamics has been restored, the choice of the infused solution depends on the natremia: the NaCl 0.9% saline solution in case of hyponatremia, the hypotonic (NaCl 0.45%) in the case of normal or hypernatremia at a rate of 250-500 mL/h. As soon as the glycemia levels have reached 200 mg/dL, the recommendation is to start 5-10% dextrose solution, to prevent hypoglycemia from occurring before the final correction of blood ketosis. The British guidelines [Joint British Diabetes Societies (JBDS), 2013] merely suggest the use of isotonic NaCl at a "not too rapid" rate with the sole exception of hypoperfusioned patients.

However, half of the water deficit should be corrected in the first 12 hours.

Another open question is the infusion rate for fluids after the first volume recovery phase; physicians have always been warned about the need to limit the infusion rate in this phase, to avoid a too rapid reduction in effective plasma osmolality (tonicity).

The risk is in fact the onset of the most threated ketoacidosis complication: cerebral edema. Cerebral edema develops in approximately 0.5-1% of patients with diabetic ketoacidosis during volume recovery. It is quite typical in childhood, very rare in adults.

The risk of death and sequelae is quite high, between 30% and 50%.

NOTE

Although there are studies (PERCAN DKA FLUID – 2013) suggesting that the rapid correction of plasma tonicity can only play a marginal role in determining neurological damage, giving more credit to alternative pathogenetic hypotheses, such as ischemia-reperfusion and neuroinflammatory damage, both correlated to the severity of underlying disease, rather than to the aggressiveness of reperfusion, it is still good practice to use hypotonic solutions only in strictly selected cases of high plasma tonicity, in conditions of restored perfusion.

Correction of potassium deficiency

DKA is characterized by a significant potassium deficiency (up to 3-5 mEq/Kg of body weight). Osmotic diuresis, elimination of ketoacids that bind opposite charge ions, metabolic acidosis and losses with vomiting are responsible.

However, despite the deficit, many patients with DKA appear with normal or even high levels of serum potassium, because the concentration of serum potassium does not reflect the total body content of the ion, due to its prevalent intracellular distribution (only 2% of the total potassium is found in circulating form in the blood).

During DKA the dehydration increases the concentration of serum potassium, despite the total deficit, and the acidosis favors the potassium passage from the intracellular to the extracellular space for the electroneutrality maintenance.

The presence of normal and reduced kalemia during DKA is a sign of a significant potassium loss and its administration, prior to any other therapeutic intervention, becomes a priority to avoid severe arrhythmic complications.

Insulin therapy and acidosis correction, in fact, favor potassium passage inside the cell, contributing to the kalemia reduction and increasing the risk of arrhythmias. For this reason in all hypokalemic patients the insulin administration should not be started before the correction of the electrolyte disorder.

The infusion rate should range between 10 and 40 mEq/h, because according to the experts opinion, at this rate, adverse cardiovascular and muscular events are minimal.

For pragmatic purposes we report the following indications from ADA:

- if kalemia > 5.2 mEq/L do not administer intravenous potassium, start insulin infusion and monitor the kalemia every 2 hours;
- if kalemia < 3.3 mEq/L do not administer insulin, start potassium infusion at 20-30 mEq/h until a value greater than 3.3 mEq/L is reached;
- if kalemia is between 3.3 and 5.2 mEq/L, add 20-30 mEq of potassium to each liter of infused fluid, with the aim of maintaining a kalemia between 4 and 5 mEq/L.

Insulin administration

Once the hypokalemia is corrected and the administration of fluids has begun, it is necessary to administer rapid acting insulin, aiming to correct the hyperglycemia, but above all to stop the lipolysis and consequently the ketogenesis.

Continuous intravenous infusion is preferred due to short latency and easy dose titration.

The main protocols (ADA and JBDS) suggest an insuline infusion rate of 0.1 IU/Kg/h until a blood glucose of 200 mg/dL is reached; at this point the dose should be halved (0.05 IU/Kg/h), parallel to the glucose infusion.

NOTE

For practical purpose we suggest to dilute 50 UI of rapid acting insulin in 500 mL of normal saline solution and infuse at a rate in mL/h equal to the patient's estimated body weight.

For non-severe forms in a non-monitored environment, subcutaneous administration is feasible.
In these cases it is recommended to perform a subcutaneous bolus of rapid acting insulin at a dose of 0.2-0.3 UI/Kg (twice or triple the recommended intravenous doses), followed by 0.1-0.2 UI/Kg every 1-2 hours until upon reaching a blood glucose of 250 mg/dL.

NOTE

Patients with type 1 diabetes mellitus often use continuous subcutaneous infusion pumps and it is well known that their malfunction can be the cause of DKA; in these cases, although not supported by any evidence, the current recommendations suggest the interruption of the subcutaneous infusion and the transition to intravenous infusion.

Controversies in the DKA treatment

Sodium bicarbonate administration
The current guidelines trend is to recommend the administration of sodium bicarbonate for arterial pH < 6.9.
Small randomized controlled studies show that administering bicarbonate for pH between 6.9 and 7.1, improves blood pH rapidly, albeit transiently. However, the effect on pH does not translate into a reduction in mortality or a faster resolution of ketosis and hyperglycemia, nor does it reduce the risk of neurological and cardiac damage.
On the contrary, complications from bicarbonate solutions in patients with acidemia are now well known (see also section on lactic acidosis): intracellular acidosis and paradoxical respiratory acidosis, increased plasma tonicity (especially when the 1 molar at 8.4% solution is used), worsening of kalemia and calcemia. At these blood pH values, therefore, bicarbonate would have only a cosmetic effect and its use is not recommended.

NOTE

Some experts (Kamel S, Halperin M, NEJM 2015) propose not to use pH as a parameter to assess bicarbonate indication, but rather to identify those subgroups of patients that would benefit the most. The first category is made up of subjects who are unable to adequately remove ketone bodies. Since the oxidative catabolism of ketone bodies occurs mainly in the cerebral glia and at renal level, patients with altered state of consciousness (diabetic coma, pharmacological sedation) or with severe renal failure (glomerular filtrate less than 30 mL/min) could benefit from the early administration of bicarbonate. A second category of patients are those that develop hyperchloremic acidosis after the first fluid replacement phase. The latter in fact may have insufficient circulating anions to metabolize and produce bicarbonate ions and the acidemia may rapidly deteriorate with a rapid infusion of normal saline solution, which, as written before, acidifies if infused at large volume.

Bolus insulin administration
The ADA suggests administering a bolus of intravenous insulin, at a dosage of 0.1 UI/kg, before starting the continuous infusion.
Numerous studies have shown that with an infusion regimen of at least 0.1 UI/Kg/h there is no advantage in terms of ketosis resolution, in a hospital lenght of stay and mortality.
It is also the experts opinion that bolus should be avoided in children to prevent a sharp reduction in plasma tonicity resulting in an increased risk of cerebral edema.

Subcutaneous insulin administration
One of the most difficult problems to solve in the DKA treatment is the transition to subcutaneous insulin administration once the ketoacidosis has resolved and the patient has resumed eating.
In fact, once intravenous administration of insulin is interrupted, its effect ends in a few minutes, while the

latency period of a basal (long-acting) insulin can be 1-2 hours: it follows that overlapping of the two administrations is absolutely necessary. There is currently solid evidence to recommend an insulin glargine dose of 80% of the insulin requirement at least two hours before discontinuing intravenous administration.

Potassium phosphate administration

As for potassium, in DKA, serum phosphate often appears normal or even increased, although there is a total body phosphate deficiency, generally up to 1.0 mmol/Kg of body weight. Phosphate levels further decrease with insulin therapy. Randomized prospective studies have shown that phosphate replacement offers no improvement in outcomes.

Nevertheless, the ADA suggests the administration of potassium phosphate (20-30 mmol) in patients with cardiac dysfunction, anemia, respiratory failure or with phosphate levels < 3.2 mmol/L.

Alcoholic ketoacidosis

Chronic alcoholism is accompanied by a variety of acid-base and water-electrolyte disorders. Isolated alcoholic ketoacidosis is rare, most often it occurs together with other acid-base alterations (up to 78% of cases according to one study). Metabolic acidosis (lactic acidosis and ketoacidosis) can coexist with metabolic alkalosis (vomiting) and respiratory alkalosis (liver failure).

Acid pH is found in about half of the cases. AKA (Alcoholic Ketoacidosis) is more frequent in subjects with discontinuous alcohol abuse, who experience dyspepsia, abdominal pain or vomiting induced by another alcohol related pathology (gastritis and pancreatitis, for example).

Reduced food intake indeed determines the characteristic hormonal structure (low levels of insulin, high levels of counter-regulatory hormones) that activates hepatic ketogenesis.

The ketogenesis is also supported by the same hepatic metabolism of ethanol: conversion of ethanol to acetaldehyde and acetate increases NADH/NAD ratio favoring the preferential formation of beta hydroxybutyrate. The high NADH/NAD ratio also explains the lactate increased synthesis, which however is always rather limited; on the contrary, severe lactic acidosis should lead to suspect thiamine deficiency or hypoperfusion (**Figure 6.3**).

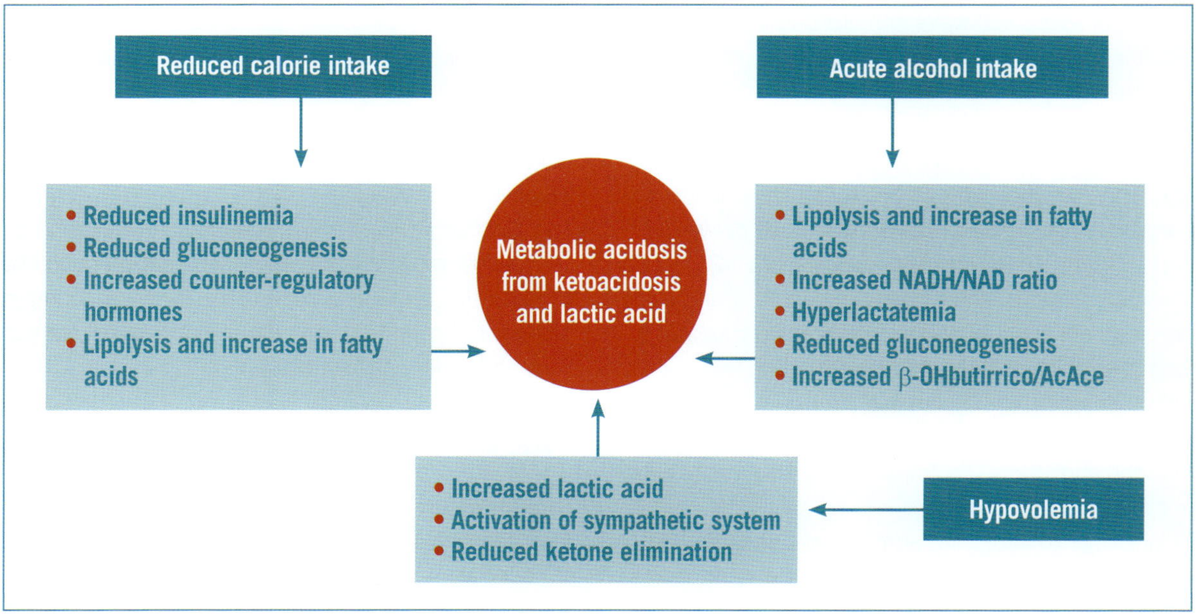

Figure 6.3 Alcoholic ketoacidosis pathogenesis.

Hypoglycemia accompanies AKA in about a quarter of cases and usually occurs after 14-24 hours of fasting, because the metabolism of ethyl alcohol inhibits the glucose synthesis (neoglucogenesis), but has no effect on the glucose mobilization by glycogen deposits (glycogenolysis).
Hypoglycemia is a potentially fatal event, because the transition from the alcoholic drowsiness to a hypoglycemic coma can be imperceptible and may escape to the physician evaluating the patient.

NOTE

Test stripes measuring urine ketones are sensitive to acetoacetate and not to hydroxybutyrate, with high risk of false negatives.

Therapy principles
The therapeutic goals in the treatment of AKA are:

- supporting hemodynamics and blocking ketogenesis;
- prevent neurological damage;
- control the symptoms of alcohol withdrawal;
- correct associated water and electrolyte disorders.

The first objective is pursued by administering crystalloids (normal saline solution) and dextrose 5-10% solution. The glucose administered, in fact, increases the insulin release and blocks the glucagon one, while volume recovery decreases the levels of circulating catecholamines. Intravenous glucose administered at a rate between 7.0 and 7.5 g/h usually reverses acidosis in 12-24 hours. Thiamine administration is very important to avoid the development of acute Wernike-type encephalopathy.
Traditionally it was believed that administering glucose before thiamine could increase the risk of neurological damage. According to some studies, this fear is unfounded and, on the contrary, it is essential not to delay of hypoglycemia correction.
Finally, benzodiazepine administration controls the symptoms of alcohol dependence.There is no indication for bicarbonate administration, due to the potential harmful effects, already mentioned in the paragraph on DKA, but above all because the kidney maintains unchanged the ability to "regenerate" bicarbonates. Attention should also be paid to the correction of electrolyte alterations, which are very frequent in these patients, in particular hypomagnesemia. Finally, remember that chronic alcoholics look for other alcohols to satisfy their dependence, in particular isopropyl alcohol (used as a skin disinfectant and as a detergent). Doctors must therefore be aware of the clinical effects and treatment following their voluntary ingestion (see below).

Starvation ketoacidosis

Starvation ketoacidosis is nothing but the extreme phase of a physiological process.
In fact, hepatic ketogenesis is essential for the production of alternative energy sources, when glucose is no longer available.
It usually begins after at least two or three days of fasting, but in patients with increased caloric needs (pregnancy, lactation) or depletion of the muscular mass (dystrophies) the process appears more rapid and severe. Treatment involves fluid replacement and administration of 5-10% dextrose solution, in relation to the same pathophysiological assumptions already described for the AKA.
Caloric intake is then gradually reintroduced to avoid the so-called refeeding syndrome (hyperalimentation syndrome). The rapid transition from a catabolic metabolism to an anabolic one can in fact have several negative consequences.
The glucose increased synthesis and the resumption of protein synthesis consumes ATP and reduces the levels of different ions, in particular phosphate, magnesium and potassium with the risk of organ complications and severe arrhythmias.

Toxic alcohols

Introduction

Toxic alcohols are intoxicating psychotropic substances, but they are not directly responsible for metabolic acidosis. The effects on the acid-base balance derive from their hepatic metabolism. The two key enzymes are alcohol-dehydrogenase and aldehyde-dehydrogenase (the same as in ethanol metabolism); the first enzyme catalyzes the alcohol oxidation into aldehyde while the second aldehyde oxidation into carboxylic acid which is then responsible for hig anion gap metabolic acidosis. Specifically, methanol is oxidized into formic acid and ethylene glycol into glycolic acid and oxalic acid.

Alcohol-dehydrogenase represents the main target on which antidotes act.

Toxic alcohol intoxications are characterized, not only by an anion gap increase but also by an osmolal gap increase because alcohols are small (low molecular weight) molecules and therefore able to significantly increase plasma osmolality.

During intoxication the anion gap and the osmolal gap do not change in parallel, but tend to have opposite trends. Both are then influenced by the start time of antidote therapy.

A high osmolal gap and a low anion gap are in fact characteristic of the first phase of intoxication, when the alcohol level is high and the carboxylic acid level is low. With the gradual transformation of alcohol into acid, the relationships are reversed. Antidotes block the alcohols metabolism, slowing the formation of toxic acids.

NOTE

It is worth remembering, in order to avoid misunderstanding, that many forms of metabolic acidosis caused by organic acids are accompanied by an osmolal gap increase (lactic acidosis, ketoacidosis, chronic renal failure). Therefore, the only increase of the osmolal gap in the presence of a high anion gap metabolic acidosis is not sufficient to diagnose alcohol intoxication without a history of ingestion.

Methanol and ethylene glycol intoxication

The two most frequent forms of alcohol intoxication are those from methanol and ethylene glycol.

Methanol is currently used in windshield detergents and fuels and as a solvent in chemical industry. It causes depression of the central nervous system, abdominal pain, reduction of visual acuity up to blindness and parkinsonism.

Ethylene glycol is used widely, as an engine coolant, in antifreeze and in brake fluid. Because of its sweet taste, accidental ingestion it is often in children and animals: the reason why products containing it are most often added with bitter agents.

Ethylene glycol toxicity typically evolves in three stages. A first stage (first 12 hours) in which neurological symptoms prevail (from intoxication to coma); a second stage (from 12 to 48 hours) characterized by cardiac toxicity (arrhythmia, acute pulmonary edema) and lung damage (ARDS); a third stage called "renal" (after 48 hours) in which acute renal failure develops, from tubular-interstitial damage, induced by the deposition of calcium oxalate.

Treatment principles

The treatment includes:

- inhibition of metabolism of the two alcohols with the use of antidotes;
- removal of alcohol and its metabolites.

The gastrointestinal absorption of methanol or ethylene glycol is fast, so the gastric lavage is worthless.

In accordance with the American Academy of Clinical Toxicology (AACT) guidelines, antidote treatment is indicated for:

- concentration of methanol or ethylene glycol greater than 20 mg/dL;
- documented ingestion of toxic quantities of methanol or ethylene glycol and an osmolal gap > 10 mOsm/Kg;
- strong clinical suspicion of poisoning and at least two of the following criteria: arterial pH < 7.3; $[HCO_3^-]$ < 20 mEq/L; osmolal gap > 10 mOsm/Kg.

The first choice antidote (absolute choice in children) is fomepizole (or 4-methylpyrazole), a strong alcohol dehydrogenase inhibitor (with an affinity 8,000 times higher than that of ethanol), which has received FDA approval for poisoning treatment with methanol and ethylene glycol, but it is not approved for the treatment of other poisonings with toxic alcohols. Fomepizole is effective at low concentrations, has minimal side effects and does not require monitoring in intensive care units. For patients who are not on dialysis, the loading dose is 15 mg/Kg, followed by a maintenance dose of 10 mg/Kg administered every 12 hours.

Since fomepizole is an inducer of its own metabolism by cytochrome P-450 enzymes, after 48 hours the maintenance dose should be increased to 15 mg/Kg every 12 hours.

The drug is removed by dialysis, so it should be administered immediately after the dialysis session. An alternative antidote to fomepizole, although not approved by the FDA, is ethanol.

Ethanol is in fact an alcohol with greater affinity for alcohol dehydrogenase (about 10 times higher than others) and when administered together with another alcohol it competitively blocks the enzyme, preventing its metabolism. The inhibitory effect is obtained with serum ethanol concentrations of at least 100 mg/dL.

The advantages of ethanol are its easy availability and low cost.

The disadvantages include the need to monitor serum concentrations, its effect on the sensory (which overlaps that of the alcohol taken), the risk of adverse reactions from ethanol administration (hypoglycemia, ion imbalances) and the need for hospitalization in intensive or intermediate care unit.

Ethanol can be administered intravenously in a 10% dilution or alternatively orally or by a nasogastric tube.

Toxic alcohols and their metabolites are small and water-soluble molecules, therefore easily removable by hemodialysis.

The indications for hemodialysis are well defined in the guidelines (AACT – American Academy of Clinical Toxicology and EXTRIP – EXtracorporeal TReatments In Poisoning); in general there is absolute indication in case of severe metabolic acidosis, concentrations of methanol and ethylene glycol greater than 50 mg/dL, deterioration of vital signs despite supportive care, visual disturbances or acute kidney damage. Intermittent hemodialysis removes toxic alcohols more rapidly than the continuous forms (CVVH – continuous veno-venous hemofiltration and CVVHD – continuous veno-venous hemodiafiltration).

Many experts promote the use of dialysis in association with antidotes, beyond the stringent indications dictated by the guidelines, because the use of antidotes alone greatly increases the elimination half-life of toxic substances, consequently increasing hospitalization duration.

There is indication for intravenous administration of sodium bicarbonate in methanol intoxication. Bicarbonate, in fact, increases the transformation of formic acid into formate, facilitating urinary excretion and preventing its diffusion into the optic nerve. In methanol poisoning, 1 mg per kilogram of folic acid every 4-6 hours promotes the conversion of formic acid to carbon dioxide and water.

In poisoning with ethylene glycol, pyridoxine and thiamine promote the metabolism of glycolic acid in less toxic compounds.

Salicylates intoxication

Acetylsalicylic acid is rapidly transformed in the body into salicylic acid. Although there is no correlation between plasma salicylates concentration and symptoms, most patients show signs of intoxication when plasma levels are above 40-50 mg/dL. A fatal overdose can occur with doses of 10-30 grams in adults and even only 3 grams in children.

The first symptoms, into which intoxication is suspected, are oto-vestibular (vertigo, dizziness, tinnitus) and neurovegetative (nausea, vomiting, diarrhea). More severe intoxications determine alterations in the state of consciousness (from headedness to coma), non cardiogenic pulmonary edema, hypoglycemia. During salicylates intoxication various acid-base disorders may occur.

The most common is respiratory alkalosis, due to the salicylates ability to directly stimulate the breath center. Metabolic acidosis is more frequent in children: the smaller they are, the more probable and serious the disorder is.

Metabolic acidosis is only minimally linked to the pres-

duce intraluminal electroneutrality and consequently inhibit the excretion of hydrogen ion and potassium. Hypokalemia is characteristic of all the conditions in which there is an excess of mineralocorticoids, on the contrary water retention is rather modest. This is because the increased absorption of sodium in distal nephron is compensated by an almost equal reduction in the other tubule segments (aldosterone escaping phenomenon). Correction of hypokalemia contributes to the alkalosis correction with two mechanisms: intracellular exchange between potassium and hydrogen ion to maintain electroneutrality and increased tubular bicarbonate excretion.

Severe hypokalemia

In patients with hypovolemia and severe hypokalemia (less than 2 mEq/L), the correction of volume depletion alone may not be sufficient to resolve alkalosis and surprisingly the urinary chloride appears high (above 20 mEq/L), despite the sodium retention. This phenomenon is the consequence of an increased excretion of chloride induced by severe potassium deficiency. In these cases an aggressive kalemia correction is necessary to resolve the alkalosis.

Bartter syndrome and Gitelman syndrome

Nephrologists know very well that, among all the metabolic alkalosis causes, these two syndromes represent the greatest therapeutic challenge. As with all other forms of chloride-resistant metabolic alkalosis, the treatment mainstay, for both disorders, is the administration of potassium chloride. Being chronic forms, they should be administered orally at extremely high doses (sometimes up to 500 mEq/day) and magnesium should always be associated with potassium supplementation. Although potassium and magnesium supplements reduce the severity of the respective deficits (thus avoiding the most severe arrhythmic complications), unfortunately they almost never completely correct hypokalemia and metabolic alkalosis. Prostaglandin inhibitors (NSAIDs) are therefore often used in combination, acting with a dual mechanism: lowering renin levels and reducing the glomerular filtrate, thus limiting the losses of different ions (chloride, potassium and sodium) by glomerular-tubular feedback. Less frequently, potassium-sparing agents (aldosterone antagonists and inhibitors of potassium channels) and ACE inhibitors are used. These latter treatments have limited usefulness due to their hypotensive effects and reduction in the extracellular volume; the consequence is that, unfortunately, patients continue to have hypokalemia and metabolic alkalosis, despite all these interventions.

Mixed acid-base disorders treatment

Introduction

The mixed disorders of acid-base balance are extremely frequent and in some contexts they are much more frequent than simple disorders.

Most of the time they are found in critically ill patients arriving in the emergency department or in those admitted to intensive care units. It is not infrequent, however, to find mixed disorders even in the elderly multipathological population (diabetic patients, patients with liver disease, kidney disease, or bronchial pulmonary disease), which mainly occupies ordinary hospitalizations in medical or specialized departments. For example, in sepsis as in hepatic failure hyperventilating respiratory alkalosis is frequent at onset; as the underlying disease progresses, lactic acidosis may develop due to hypoperfusion (type A) or hyperactivation of aerobic glycolysis (type B).

Similarly, the post-hypercapnic metabolic alkalosis is a typical example of a mixed disorder in the elderly with bronchial pulmonary disease and with chronic pulmonary heart disease.

Formally, mixed disorders can be divided into two categories: additives, if they determine pH changes in the same direction (double acidosis or double alkalosis), and counterbalancing, if they cause pH changes in the opposite direction (acidosis with alkalosis); it is evident that additive disorders are responsible for important clinical consequences, due to the greater impact that profound alterations of blood pH have on cellular function. As a result, pH extremes impose appropriate therapeutic interventions. The approach to mixed disorders necessarily requires a more in-depth pathophysiological knowledge and a further diagnostic effort, which is never an end in itself. To use the previous example (post-hypercapnic metabolic alkalosis), not recognizing a metabolic alkalosis overlapped on a chronic respiratory acidosis can aggravate hypoxia, because both disorders increase PCO_2 and at the same time, a vigorous administration of a saline solution could improve the metabolic disorder, but also bring blood pH back to too low levels. To avoid such consequences, it is extremely important to recognize both disorders, clarify which of the two is the dominant one and treat them simultaneously, paying particular attention to the consequences of pH changes.

Treatment of the main mixed disorders

Counterbalancing disorders

Respiratory acidosis and metabolic alkalosis
This combination is common in COPD complicated by chronic pulmonary heart disease and congestive heart failure during treatment with loop diuretics and thiazides or, more rarely, during vomiting or NGT use. Occasionally patients with metabolic alkalosis at onset may develop respiratory acidosis if airway infections occur. Post-hypercapnic metabolic alkalosis has already been extensively discussed in the paragraph on metabolic alkalosis.
In this disorder, alkalosis tends to reduce the acidemia degree, which would seem apparently advantageous; but as already mentioned in the introduction, clinical studies have shown that the overlap of metabolic alkalosis on a stable respiratory acidosis can worsen the CO_2 retention degree, because these patients use mild acidemia as a respiratory drive. For this reason, it is essential to also correct the metabolic alkalosis to obtain a benefit on lung function. Since the forms of metabolic alkalosis from diuretics and vomiting are chloride-responsive, administration of NaCl and KCl is effective in reducing plasma bicarbonate levels and lowering blood pH.
In plethoric patients with congestive heart failure or chronic renal failure, in whom the administration of sodium chloride is not indicated and it is not possible to reduce the diuretic dosage, the administration of carbonic anhydrase inhibitors (acetazolamide) will increase renal bicarbonate excretion. Another option is dialysis with a low bicarbonate bath.

Metabolic acidosis and respiratory alkalosis
This mixed disorder occurs in septic patients who develop renal failure, lactic acidosis or ketoacidosis, in hypotensive patients with decompensated cirrhosis, in salicylates intoxication, and in high-risk pulmonary embolism (with unstable hemodynamics).
In all conditions the onset disorder is respiratory alkalosis, induced by cytokines (in the case of sepsis and hepatic failure), by metabolites in salicylates intoxication, by hypoxemia and by direct receptor stimulation in the case of pulmonary embolism. However, the dominant disorder is almost always metabolic acidosis. All these conditions require first and foremost immediate interventions on the pathological basis.
Skipping the specific actions to be taken during sepsis or pulmonary embolism, we recall that in the salicylates intoxication, there is indication to use bases only if the dominant disorder is metabolic acidosis. In the most severe forms, with a concentration of salicylates greater than 60 mEq/L, hemodialysis should be considered.
More generally, since respiratory alkalosis can cause a significant increase in intracellular pH, the clinician should always be very cautious in administering bases to patients with this combination of acid-base disorders. Similarly, some patients may benefit from hypocapnia induced by metabolic acidosis. In fact, some studies have shown that in intubated patients, in whom hypocapnia had been reduced by the sodium bicarbonate infusion, an important exacerbation of respiratory acidosis was often observed.

Metabolic acidosis and metabolic alkalosis
The condition that most frequently causes this disorder is diabetic ketoacidosis complicated by protracted vomiting.
In general, there are two contexts in which this disorder can occur:

- a metabolic acidosis with high anion gap (ketoacidosis, lactic acidosis, advanced chronic renal failure) with overlapping metabolic alkalosis induced by vomiting or by the placement of a nasogastric tube;
- a metabolic alkalosis from loop diuretics or thiazides, to which a renal failure caused by dehydration or a lactic acidosis due to hypoperfusion overlaps.

Adequate volume recovery with normal saline solution and possible supplementation with potassium chloride are able to correct both disorders.

Additive disorders

Mixed acidosis (metabolic acidosis and respiratory acidosis)

Mixed acidosis is the typical disorder of patients with cardio-respiratory failure who have previously undergone cardio-pulmonary resuscitation, but it is also very frequent in critically ill patients admitted to intensive care units, in whom lactic acidosis is accompanied by respiratory failure.

At other times it is accompanied by advanced heart failure. The mixed acidosis poses first of all a diagnostic problem: it is not always easy to distinguish an acute respiratory acidosis on chronic respiratory acidosis from a chronic respiratory acidosis with overlapped metabolic acidosis being the anion gap a very specific but not very sensitive parameter. A correct anamnesis that allows to determine the chronology of the events is essential to correctly classify the disorder.

The combination of metabolic and respiratory acidosis produces the most severe degree of acidemia and intracellular acidosis.

Studies conducted both in vitro and in vivo have shown that both alterations are the main cause of cellular dysfunction.

Although to a lesser extent also changes in plasma CO_2, regardless of their effects on pH, can have negative effects on the cellular function. Therefore, it appears evident that during severe acidemia the main therapeutic goal remains to quickly correct blood and intracellular pH.

The optimal value of blood pH to be reached is still the subject of discussion among experts. Maintaining the pH around 7.2 seems a reasonable goal, because in animal models, below these values, there is a significant reduction of cardiac contractility and cardiac output.

Unfortunately, short-term human studies have not shown these beneficial effects, probably due to the adverse effects of administering bicarbonate solutions. In particular, intravenous bicarbonate is rapidly converted into CO_2, which crosses cell membranes and exacerbates intracellular acidosis (phenomenon of intracellular paradoxical acidosis).

This complication appears to be more likely when sodium bicarbonate is administered as a bolus, in the presence of tissue hypoperfusion or respiratory dysfunction.

Plasma alkalinization also reduces the amount of ionized calcium, with a negative inotrope effect greater than that of mild acidemia.

Finally, the increase in plasma osmolality, with consequent volume overload, induced by the more concentrated solutions (8.4% sodium bicarbonate), can further aggravate respiratory failure.

For all these reasons, some clinicians avoid the administration of bicarbonate in patients with metabolic acidosis, especially in the presence of respiratory failure.

The most consistent advantages in mixed acidosis treatment come however from dialysis; today, different dialysis methods are available to stabilize the extracellular ionized calcium and to prevent the volume overload induced by hypertonic solutions. Large but uncontrolled studies have shown benefits on mortality in patients with lactic and respiratory acidosis when treated with ultra filtration (CVVH).

$PaCO_2$ lowering in patients with combined metabolic and respiratory acidosis attenuates acidemia and presumably also decreases the degree of intracellular acidosis.

On the basis of this pathophysiological assumption, controlled hyperventilation is proposed.

Mixed alkalosis (metabolic alkalosis and respiratory alkalosis)

The combination of respiratory and metabolic alkalosis is often present in patients with chronic infections or liver disease (responsible for respiratory alkalosis) who use diuretics, who have vomiting or a nasogastric tube, or if they are poly-transfused (all factors responsible for metabolic alkalosis).

Another category at risk are pregnant women. Progesterone is able to stimulate the breath centers and gravidic emesis are often the cause of metabolic alkalosis. It is the acid-base disorder with the worst prognosis. In a study of more than 300 patients, the overall mortality reached 44%, with a direct correlation between the magnitude of alkalemia and mortality: mortality approaches 49% when the pH exceeds 7.60.

These data justify the aggressive treatment.

In principle, the intervention on the metabolic component is easier to carry out and foresees the same measures already mentioned in the simple disorder discussion (saline solution, KCl, dialysis with a bath at low bicarbonate concentrations).

In intubated patients, increasing the dead space or reducing the respiratory rate can increase the CO_2 to bring the pH below 7.5, a value considered safe.

References

Treatment of respiratory acidosis

- Bellone A, Vettorello M, Monari A et al. Noninvasive pressure support ventilation vs. continuous positive airway pressure in acute hypercapnic pulmonary edema. Intensive Care Med. 2005;31(6):807-11.
- Bersten AD, Holt AW, Vedig AE et al. Treatment of severe cardiogenic pulmonary edema with continuous positive airway pressure delivered by face mask. New Engl J Med. 1991;325(26):1825-30.
- Bott J, Carroll MP, Conway JH et al. Randomized controlled trial of nasal ventilation in acute ventilatory failure due to chronic obstructive airways disease. Lancet. 1993;341 (8860):1555-7.
- Brochard L, Mancebo J, Wysocki M et al. Noninvasive ventilation for acute exacerbation of chronic obstructive pulmonary disease. N Engl J Med. 1995;333(13):817-22.
- Comellini V, Pacilli AMG, Nava S. Benefits of non-invasive ventilation in acute hypercapnic respiratory failure. Respirology. 2019;24(4):308-17.
- Confalonieri M, Garuti G, Cattaruzza MS et al. A chart of failure risk for noninvasive in patients with COPD exacerbation. Eur Respir J. 2005;25(2):348-55.
- Davidson AC, Banham S, Elliott M et al. BTS/ICS guideline for the ventilatory management of acute hypercapnic respiratory failure in adults. Thorax. 2016;71 Suppl 2:ii1-35.
- Dunn WF, Nelson SB, Hubmayr RD. Oxygen-induced hypercapnia in obstructive pulmonary disease. Am Rev Respir Dis. 1991;144(3 Pt 1):526-30.
- Kelly CR, Higgins AR, Chandra S. Noninvasive Positive-Pressure Ventilation. N Engl J Med. 2015;373(13):1279.
- Masa JF, Pépin JL, Borel JC et al. Obesity hypoventilation syndrome. Eur Respir Rev. 2019;28(151). pii:180097.
- Masip J, Roque M, Sanchez B et al. Noninvasive ventilation in acute cardiogenic pulmonary edema: systematic review and meta-analysis. JAMA. 2005;294(24):3124-30.
- Murphy PB, Rehal S, Arbane G et al. Effect of Home Noninvasive Ventilation with Oxygen Therapy vs Oxygen Therapy Alone on Hospital Readmission or Death After an Acute COPD Exacerbation: A Randomized Clinical Trial. JAMA. 2017;317(21):2177-86.
- O'Driscoll BR, Howard LS, Davison AG et al. BTS guideline for emergency oxygen use in adult patients. Thorax. 2008;63 Suppl 6:vi1-68.
- Peter JV, Moran JI, Phillips-Huges J et al. Effects of non-invasive positive pressure ventilation (NIPPV) on mortality in patients with acute cardiogenic pulmonary edema: a meta-analysis. Lancet. 2006; 367(9517):1155-63.
- Pfeffer G, Povitz M. Respiratory management of patients with neuromuscular disease: current perspectives. Degener Neurol Neuromuscul Dis. 2016;6:111-18.
- Rochwerg B, Brochard L, Elliott MW et al. Official ERS/ATS clinical practice guidelines: noninvasive ventilation for acute respiratory failure. Eur Respir J. 2017;50(2).pii: 1602426.
- Rose BD, Post TW. Clinical physiology of acid-base and electrolyte disorders. New York, McGraw-Hill 2011, pp. 673-81.
- Singh D, Agusti A, Anzueto A et al. Global Strategy for the Diagnosis, Management, and Prevention of Chronic Obstructive Lung Disease: the GOLD science committee report 2019. Eur Respir J. 2019;53(5). pii: 1900164.

Treatment of respiratory alkalosis

- Callaham M. Hypoxic hazards of traditional paper bag rebreathing in hyperventilating patients. Ann Emerg Med. 1989;18(6):622-8.

Treatment of respiratory metabolic acidosis

- Adeva-Andany MM, Fernández-Fernández C, Mouriño-Bayolo D et al. Sodium bicarbonate therapy in patients with metabolic acidosis. The Scientific World Journal. 2014;2014: 627673.
- Halperin ML, Goldstein MB. Fluid, Electrolyte, and Acid-Base Physiology. 3rd Ed. Toronto. WB Saunders 1999.
- Mount DB, Sayegh MH, Singh AK. Core Concepts in the Disorders of Fluid, Electrolytes and Acid-Base Balance. Springer 2013.

Lactic acidosis

- Bentzer P, Griesdale DE, Boyd J et al. Will this hemodinamically unstable patient respond to a bolus of intravenous fluids? JAMA. 2016;316(12)1298-309.
- Jaber S, Paugam C, Futier E et al. Sodium bicarbonate therapy

for patients with severe metabolic acidaemia in the intensive care unit (BICAR-ICU): a multicentre, open-label, randomised contolled, phase 3 trial. Lancet. 2018;392(10141):31-40.
- Kraut JA, Madias NE, Lactis Acidosis. N Engl J Med. 2014; 371(24):2309-19.
- Monnet X, Marik PE, Teboul JL. Prediction of fluid responsiveness: an update. Ann. Intensive Care. 2016;6(1):111.
- Reddy AJ, Lam SW, Bauer SR et al. Lactis acidosis: clinical implications and management strategies. Cleve Clin J Med. 2015;82(9):615-24.
- Seheult J, Fitzpatrick G, Boran G. Lactis acidosis: an update. Clin Chem Lab Med. 2017;55(3):322-33.
- Suetrong B, Walley KR. Lactis acidosi in sepsis: it's not all anaerobic: implications for diagnosis and management. CHEST. 2016;149(1):252-61.
- Semler MW, Self WH, Wanderer JP, et al. Balanced crystalloids versus saline in critically Ill adults. N Engl J Med. 2018 Mar 1;378(9):829-839.
- Guidet B, Martinet O, Boulain T, Philippart F, Poussel JF, Maizel J, Forceville X, Feissel M, Hasselmann M, Heininger A, Van Aken H. Assessment of hemodynamic efficacy and safety of 6% hydroxyethylstarch 130/0.4 vs. 0.9% NaCl fluid replacement in patients with severe sepsis: The CRYSTMAS study. Crit Care. 2012;17:R94.
- Myburgh JA, Finfer S, Bellomo R, Billot L, Cass A, Gattas D, Glass P, Lipman J, Liu B, McArthur C, McGuinness S, Rajbhandari D, Taylor CB, Webb SA. CHEST Investigators; Australian and New Zealand Intensive Care Society Clinical Trials Group. Hydroxyethyl starch or saline for fluid resuscitation in intensive care. N Engl J Med. 2012.
- Perner A, Haase N, Guttormsen AB, et al. for the 6S Trial Group and the Scandinavian Critical Care Trials GroupHydroxyethyl starch 130/0.4 versus Ringer's acetate in severe sepsis, N Engl J Med , 2012, vol. 367 (pg. 124-34).
- Russell JA1, Walley KR, Singer J, et al; VASST Investigators-Vasopressin versus norepinephrine infusion in patients with septic shock. N Engl J Med. 2008 Feb 28;358(9):877-87.
- Gordon AC, Perkins GD, Singer M, et al. Levosimendan to prevent acute organ dysfunction in sepsis: the LeoPARDS RCT. N Engl J Med 2016; 375:1638-1648.
- Finfer S, Bellomo R, Boyce N, French J, Myburgh J, Norton R; SAFE Study Investigators. A comparison of albumin and saline for fluid resuscitation in the intensive care unit. N Engl J Med 2004; 350:2247-2256.
- Caironi P, Tognoni G, Masson S, et al., for the ALBIOS for the ALBIOS Study Investigators. Albumin replacement in patients with severe sepsis or septic shock. N Engl J Med 2014; 370:1412-1421.

Diabetic ketoacidosis

- Dhatariya KK, Vellanki P. Treatment of diabetic ketoacidosis (DKA)/hyperglicemic hyperosmolar state (HSS): novel advances in the management of hyperglicemic crises (UK versus USA). Curr Diab Rep. 2017;17(5):33.
- Fayfman M, Pasquel FJ, Umpierezz GE. Management of hyperglycemic crises: diabetic ketoacidosis and hyperglycemic hyperosmolar state. Med Clin North Am. 2017;101(3): 587-606.
- Kamel SK, Halperin ML. Acid-Base problems in diabetic ketoacidosis. N Engl J Med. 2015;372(6):546-54.
- Kuppermann N, Ghetti S, Schunk JE et al. Clinical trial of fluid infusion rates for pediatric diabetic ketoacidosis. N Engl J Med. 2018;378(24):2275-87.
- Nyce LA, Lubkin CL, Chansky ME. Diabetic Ketoacidosis. In Tintinalli JE. Tintinalli's Emergency Medicine. A Comprehensive Study Guide. 2015. Chapter 225.
- Palmer BF, Clegg DJ. Electrolyte and acid-base disturbances in patients with diabetes mellitus. N Engl J Med. 2015;373(6):548-59.
- Tran TT, Paese A, wood AJ et al. Review of evidence for adult diabetic ketoacidosis. Front Endocrinol (Lausanne). 2017;8:106.

Alcoholic ketoacidosis

- Frise CJ, Mackillop L. Starvation ketoacidosis. J Intensive Care Soc. 2016;17(4):356.
- Hammerbeck H, Holland MR. Starvation ketoacidosis: Treatment pitfalls. J. Intensive Care Soc. 2017,18(3):265.
- Palmer BF, Clegg DJ. Electrolyte disturbances in patients with chronic alcohol-use disorder. N Engl J Med. 2017;377 (14):1368-77.
- Schabelman E, Kuo D. Glucose before thiamine for Wernicke encephalopathy: a literature review. J Emerg Med. 2012; 42(4):488-94.
- Svart MV, Voss TS, Bayat M et al. Rare Presentations of ketoacidosis: diabetic ketoalkalosis and ketoacidosis secondary to fasting and muscular dystrophy. Clin Diabetes. 2015; 33(1):37-9.
- Wrenn KD, Slovis CM, Minion GE et al. The syndrome of alcoholic ketoacidosis. Am J Med. 1991;91(2):119-28.

Salicylates intoxication

- Halperin ML, Goldstein MB. Fluid, Electrolyte, and Acid-Base Physiology. 3rd Ed. Toronto. WB Saunders 1999.
- Rose BD. Clinical Physiology of Acid-Base and Electrolyte Disorders. New York. McGraw-Hill 2001.
- Skorecki K, Chertow GM, Marsden PA et al. Brenner & Rector The Kidney. 10th ed. Philadelphia, Elsevier 2015.
- Juurlink DN, Gosselin S, Kielstein JT, et al. Extracorporeal Treatment for Salicylate Poisoning: Systematic Review and Recommendations From the EXTRIP Workgroup. Ann Emerg Med. 2015 Aug;66(2):165-81.

Toxic alcohols

- Beatty L, Green R, Magee K et al. A systematic review of ethanol and fomepizole use in toxic alcohol ingestions. Emerg Med Int. 2013;2013:638057.
- Beauchamp GA, Valento M, Kim J. Toxic alcohol ingestion: prompt recognition and management in the emergency department. Emerg Med Pract. 2016;18(9 Suppl Points & Pearls):S1-S2.
- Kraut JA, Mullins ME. Toxic alcohols. N Engl J Med. 2018; 378(3):270-80.

- Lavergne V, Nolin TD, Hoffman RS, et al. The EXTRIP (EXtracorporeal TReatments In Poisoning) workgroup: guideline methodology Clin Toxicol (Phila). 2012 Jun;50(5):403-13.
- Roberts DM, Yates C, Megarbane B, et al ; EXTRIP Work Group. Recommendations for the role of extracorporeal treatments in the management of acute methanol poisoning: a systematic review and consensus statement. Crit Care Med. 2015 Feb;43(2):461-72.

Treatment of hyperchloremic metabolic acidosis

- Mount DB, Sayegh MH, Singh AK. Core Concepts in the Disorders of Fluid, Electrolytes and Acid-Base Balance. Springer 2013.
- Reddi AS. Fluid, Elettrolyte and Acid-Base Disorders: Clinical Evaluation and Management. 2nd Ed. Springer 2018.
- Rose BD. Clinical Physiology of Acid-Base and Electrolyte Disorders. New York, McGraw-Hill 2001.
- Skorecki K, Chertow GM, Marsden PA et al. Brenner & Rector The Kidney. 10th ed. Philadelphia, Elsevier 2015.

Metabolic alkalosis

- Adamson R, Swenson ER. Acetazolamide use in severe chronic obstructive pulmonary disease. Pros and cons. Ann Am Thorac Soc. 2017;14(7):1086-93.
- Mount DB, Sayegh MH, Singh AK. Core Concepts in the Disorders of Fluid, Electrolytes and Acid-Base Balance. Springer 2013.
- Reddi AS. Fluid, Elettrolyte and Acid-Base Disorders: Clinical Evaluation and Management. 2nd Ed. Springer 2018.
- Rose BD. Clinical Physiology of Acid-Base and Electrolyte Disorders. New York, McGraw-Hill 2001.
- Skorecki K, Chertow GM, Marsden PA et al. Brenner & Rector The Kidney. 10th ed. Philadelphia, Elsevier 2015.
- Tanios BY, Omran MO, Noujeim C et al. Carbonic anhydrase inhibitors in patients with respiratory failure and metabolic alkalosis: a systematic review and meta-analysis of randomized controlled trials. Critical Care. 2018;22(1):275.
- Van Berkel MA, Elefritz JL. Evaluating off-label uses of acetazolamide. Am J Health Syst Pharm. 2018;75(8):524-31.

Treatment of mixed disorders

- Adroguè HJ, Madias NE. Respiratory acidosis, respiratory alcalosis, mixed disorders. In Feehally J, Floege J, Johnson R et al. Comprehensive Clinical Nephrology. 6th Ed. Elsevier 2018.
- Kallet RH, Liu K, Tang J. Management of acidosis during lung-protective ventilation in acute respiratory distress syndrome. Respir Care Clin N Am. 2003;9(4):437-56.
- Mount DB, Sayegh MH, Singh AK. Core Concepts in the Disorders of Fluid, Electrolytes and Acid-Base Balance. Springer 2013.
- Reddi AS. Fluid, Elettrolyte and Acid-Base Disorders: Clinical Evaluation and Management. 2nd Ed. Springer 2018.

SECTION II

SODIUM AND WATER

anisms responsible for constancy maintaining of the milieu interieur, but also because it brought out the primary importance of the renal function in the regulation of body fluids homeostasis. In his book *From Fish to Philosopher*, which demonstrates the close relationship between the evolution of the species and the progressive improvement of renal function, Homer William Smith (1895-1962) concluded: "If at first it can be said that the function of the kidney is to produce urine, looking deeper it must be said that kidney is the essence of philosophy".

Osmosis as a fundamental mechanism of regulation and exchanges between body fluids through blood vessels and cell membranes was proposed in 1883 by Hartog Jacob Hamburger (**Figure 7.3**), professor of physiology at Groningen in the Netherlands, who had observed how the red cells are shrinked in sodium chloride solutions with a concentration higher than 0.9%, while at lower concentrations they swell up to hemolysis, confirming the term "physiological solution" for the 0.9% concentration. Hamburger exploited these results by creating a method for analyzing the osmotic resistance of red blood cells, which spread particularly in France as the "methode de l'echelle chromatique". Indeed, osmosis has long been known. The search for the responsible mechanism interested many reserchers including Justus von Liebig (1803-1873), the school of Dorpat, and in particular Thomas Graham (1805-1869) who devoted himself to study the diffusion of high molecular weight solutions, which he called "colloids", as opposed to saline solutions called "crystalloids", emphasizing that the basic of osmotic pressure lies in the membranes properties. Despite this the mechanism remained obscure for a long time, until a reliable semi-permeable membrane was made available in 1877 by Wilhelm Friedrich Philipp Pfeffer (1845-1920). These advances allowed Jacobus Henricus van 't Hoff (1852-1911) to investigate the physical-chemical principles on which osmosis is based, and above all to express in his well-known equation the relationship between osmotic pressure and solute concentration.

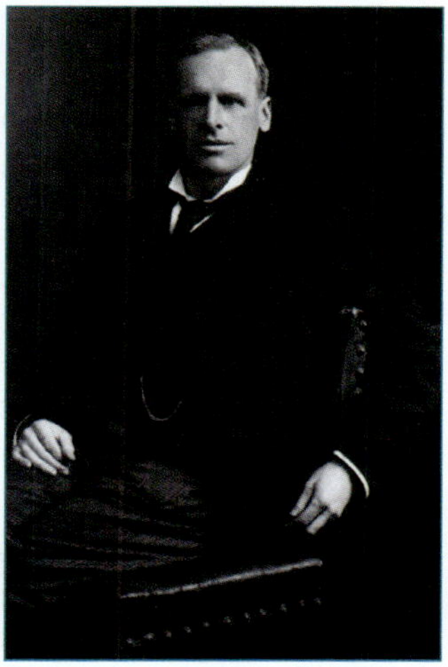

Figure 7.2 Ernest Henry Starling (1866-1927).

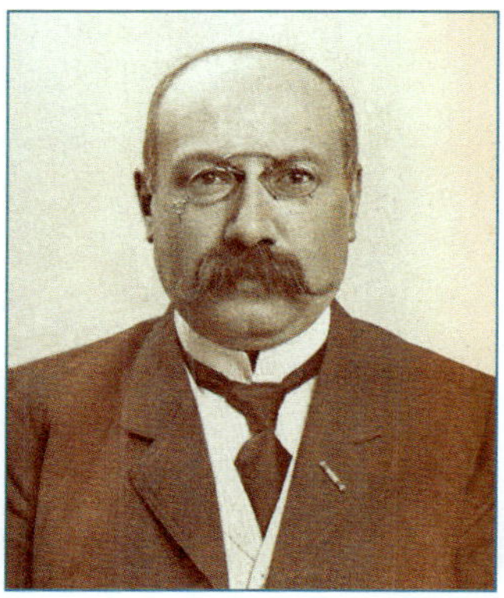

Figure 7.3 Hartog Jacob Hamburger (1856-1924).

As, or even more relevant, for physiology was the study of Ernest Henry Starling, professor at the University College of London, since he developed the principles of osmotic pressure by applying them to the physiology of blood circulation. In 1896 he obtained the measurement of blood colloid-osmotic pressure, 30-40 mmHg, due to plasma proteins; later he clarified the mechanism of pericapillary circulation. These principles are summarized in the laws and formulations elaborated by Starling, which still retain their validity, without new important concepts to be added, despite the progress of knowledge in recent decades. Starling also extended his studies to the clinical field, in particular to edema pathogenesis.

In the same years, towards the end of the XIX century, another discovery came to enrich the knowledge in body fluids physiology and in regulation of exchanges by means of osmosis, clarifying the meaning of proteins in the distribution of ions in solutions separated by a semi-permeable membrane. The theory in question, proposed and elaborated by Josiah Willard Gibbs (1839-1903), was later studied in depth by Frederick George Donnan (1870 1956) (**Figure 7.4**).

These two contributions were of great importance in the development of chemistry in the following century, so much so that they were considered by Henri Louis Le-Chatelier (1850-1936) to be of the same magnitude as those of Lavoisier a century earlier. van 't Hoff understood its meaning in reference to osmotic pressure, publishing in 1911, *The theory of membrane equilibrium in the presence of a non-dialyzable electrolyte*, where he highlighted the importance of the presence in solution of non-dialyzable substances such as proteins upon the distribution of dialyzable components such as electrolytes.

As we have mentioned, although the process of osmosis had been known for a long time, the physical-chemical mechanism underlying this exchange process remained uncertain for a long time. We need to reach the years closest to us to witness the definitive clarification of this mechanism. In fact, the importance of transporting water and solutes through cellular membranes has always been one of the topics of greatest interest in research, but only in the 1950s and 1960s did the studies show that, at least in certain types of cells, this process could not be attributed only to a diffusion-partition mechanism. The existence of pores or water channels in the cell membranes of many organs and tissues, including erythrocytes and renal tubules, was envisaged.

The search for the water channel ended in the early 1990s, thanks to the studies of Peter Agre (1949) and his Baltimore group.

During the process of isolating the Rh protein, a second protein appeared, distinguished with the abbreviation 28K based on its molecular size, unknown and not reported before.

Erythrocytes and renal tubules were rich in it, but also many other organs and tissues, from the nervous tissue of vinegar flies to bacterial species, the lens of the eye, and also plant tissues. This variegated diffusion suggested that it could be the much sought after, the water channel-protein and, given the interest of this perspective, Agre and his group concentrated their efforts in this direction. They cloned the 28K cDNA and obtained a polypeptide of 269 amino acids which they called CHIP28 (CHannel forming Integral membrane Protein 28 kDa).

But the decisive proof was the demonstration of the osmotic permeability of CHIP28: the water channel, later named "aquaporin", had been discovered. Thus, a finding that initially appeared as a laboratory interference turned out to be one of the most important discoveries of the century, worthy of the Nobel Prize that Peter Agre received in 2003.

But this story does not end here. Among the many who, as we have already mentioned, dedicated them-

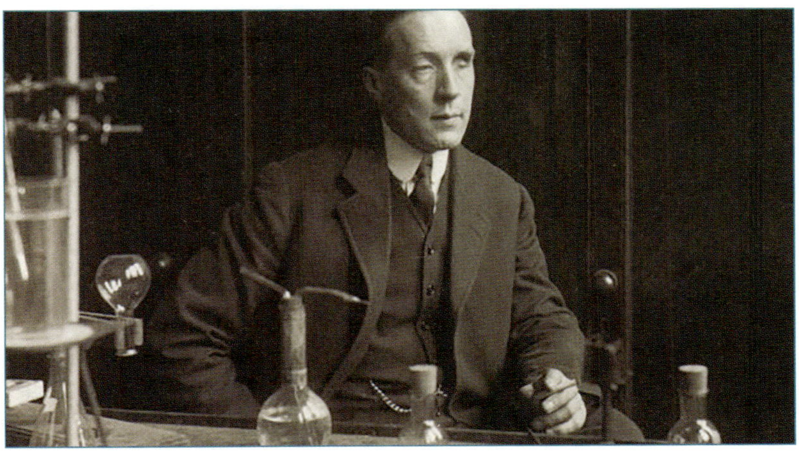

Figure 7.4 Frederick George Donnan (1870-1956)

selves to the research of the water channel-protein is also Gheorghe Benga (1944), of the Department of Molecular Cell Biology of Cluj-Napoca, Romania.
Already in 1986 he published the identification of a water protein-channel in the erythrocytes, thus claiming priority in the discovery of aquaporins; just scroll through the literature to see the outcry of the Romanian medical world in defense of their colleague. Thus, the story of one of the greatest advances in the knowledge of the physiology of body fluids and cell biology, which deserves the Nobel Prize, remains veiled by a paternity dispute that does not obscure its scientific importance.

Salt and water balance regulation

Although the physiological importance of water and salt had long been taken for granted, the knowledge of sodium-water homeostasis regulation had a slow evolution, especially in relation to the development and availability of the means of investigation. Thus, at the end of the nineteenth century, although it was clear to everyone that salt and water were variables that had to be carefully controlled, the mechanisms were completely unknown, except for thirst and diuresis. Between 1920 and 1930 it was known that in Addison's disease the salt content was very low, and that it was possible to control hypertension with a low sodium diet, but the mechanisms of regulation of the salt-water balance were not focused until during the years immediately after the Second World War, thanks above all to the development of adequate investigation techniques: the osmometry for the measurement of the osmolarity, the flame photometer for the sodium and potassium measurement, the isolation and the characterization of hormones.

Water regulation

Because of the striking symptoms, diabetes insipidus was known for a long time. Already in 1794, in the treatise *Decurandis Hominum Morbis Epitome*, Johann Peter Frank (1745-1821) observed that the taste of urine was not as sweet as in the analogous polyuria of diabetes mellitus. Apart from this difference between the two types of diabetes, the etiology of diabetes insipidus remained completely unknown until the beginning of the 20th century.
The hypertensive effect of the pituitary extracts was discovered in 1895 by George Oliver (1841-1915) and Eduard Albert Sharpey-Schäfer (1850-1935)
Three years later William Henry Howell (1860-1945) surprisingly ascertained that the pressure effect was due not to the glandular segment (adenohypophysis), but was only found in extracts of the neurogenic segment, thus identifying the neurohypophysis as an endocrine organ – it was a novelty for the time that the nervous tissue carried out such activity.
The relationship with renal function came out in 1901 when Rudolf Magnus (1873-1927) and Schäfer described that the pituitary extract caused an increase in the volume of the kidneys and diuresis (sic!). However, later, in 1909, Schäfer corrected these statements by claiming that the pituitary produces not one but two substances that act on the kidney, since the increase in diuresis is preceded by a decrease or even an arrest in the elimination of urine. As can be seen, the first report of an antidiuretic effect of the pituitary gland occurred fourteen years after the discovery of the pressure effect. Despite this, the opinion continued to prevail that diabetes insipidus was due to the hyperfunction of neurohypophysis secretion. It therefore aroused a certain surprise when in 1913 two independent publications, one by F. Farini of Venice, and one by R. van der Velden from Düsseldorf, showed with convincing documentation that the administration of pituitary extract to patients with diabetes insipidus causes no increase but a decrease if not an arrest of the diuresis in a reproducible and reversible way. However the confirmation remained uncertain, with confusing and contradictory experimental results, above all because in the meantime the possibility emerged that the hypothalamus, instead of the pituitary gland, was the real seat of the endocrine activity, a completely new perspective because until then the humoral regulation and the neurogenic regulation were considered two completely distinct and not overlapping activities, so much so that two schools were formed, the pituitary and hypothalamic, among them in antithesis.

To compose this antithesis and to clarify the nature of the neurohypophysis secretion, numerous and complex studies were needed on the consequences of degenerative or experimental lesions of the hypothalamus and pituitary peduncle – thanks above all to the studies of Stephen Walter Ranson (1880-1942) – as well as on the relationships between these lesions and the changes in renal function, which were concluded only in the 1930s, distinguishing two hormonal principles, antidiuretic and uterotonic based on their effects, but the nature and chemical composition still remained unknown. This was defined by the studies of Vincent du Vigneaud (1901-1978) and his collaborators, who isolated them, characterized and synthesized them with such precision that they deserved the Nobel for the first synthesis of a peptide hormone.

These advances were important not only for the physiology, but also for the clinic practice and above all the therapy of water balance disorders. Until then, the pharmacology of diuretics was limited to digitalis for cardiac edema and organic mercury compounds for other diuresis disorders; this therapy remained in use until the early decades of the 20th century.

Only after the end of the Second World War were carbonic anhydrase inhibitors introduced. Hamilton Southworth (1907-1994) demonstrated in 1937 that sulfanilamide causes a large increase in diuresis due to the excessive loss of bicarbonate, the cause of metabolic acidosis.

In 1950 Richard Roblin (1907-1985) and James Clapp synthesized acetazolamide, and introduced it in the treatment of diuresis in 1954. In 1958 thiazide diuretics were proposed, studied in particular by Karl Beyer (1914-1996), but the treatment in the long term with these drugs caused metabolic alkalosis with hypokalemia. Finally, in the early 1960s the powerful loop diuretics were available, put on the market simultaneously by Hoechst in Germany (furosemide) and Merck – Sharp & Dohme in the United States (etacrinic acid). In more recent years, as is known, other types of drugs with activity on diuresis have been marketed, such as aldosterone inhibitors, triamterene, amiloride, drugs that act on the distal part of the tubular nephron with relatively limited toxicity.

Salt regulation

Until the mid-nineteenth century the physiological significance of the adrenal glands – described by Bartolomeo Eustachio (1520-1574) in his text *Opuscula Anatomica* of 1563 – remained unknown. For about three hundred years the most disparate functions were attributed to these organs without a concrete conclusion, until 1855 when Thomas Addison (**Figure 7.5**) described the disease that would later take his name, Addison's disease.

Attributed initially to an idiopathic anemia, due to the hematological alteration associated with a progressive dark pigmentation of the skin, Addison subsequently found that this disease was associated with profound alterations of the adrenal glands – to which it therefore attributed the cause of the disease –, whose most significant manifestations were, in addition to those mentioned above, the loss of sodium with urine and the decrease in glycogen stores.

A year after Addison's original description, the French physiologist Charles-Édouard Brown-Sequard (1817-1894) reported that the ablation of the adrenal glands caused the death of the animals within a few hours or a few days, demonstrating the physiological essentiality of these organs, even if the function remained unknown for years.

Around the 1920s it became evident that the cortical part of the gland, and not the medulla, was the physiologically essential portion. It was clear, however, that two classes of hormones could be distinguished: those active on carbohydrate metabolism, or glycoactives

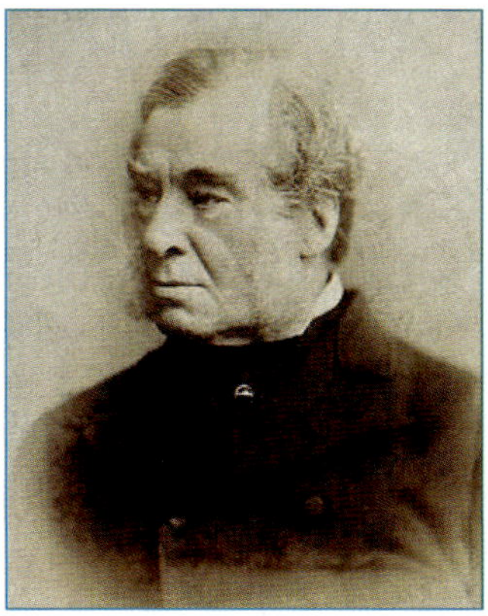

Figure 7.5 Thomas Addison (1793-1860).

corticoids or glucocorticoids, and those with activity on the electrolyte homeostasis or mineralocorticoids.

In the years of the Second World War it was possible to isolate, crystallize and determine the structure of five biologically active substances, among which the most important of the glucocorticoids: hydrocortisone. For the discovery of the main mineralocorticoid it was necessary to wait another decade, when Aaron Simpson and his collaborators isolated aldosterone in 1953 and defined its structure the following year. Furthermore the studies dating back to 1895, made by Robert Adolph Armand Tigerstedt (1853-1923) and Per Gustaf Bergman (1874 1955), had demonstrated the effect of kidney extracts on blood pressure, giving the name renin to the substance with this activity. However, these studies were long forgotten, and were taken up by Harry Goldblatt (1891-1977) only in 1930, confirming the hypertensive effect of partial renal artery constriction. This result stimulated further research that allowed two scientific groups around 1940 – one from Cleveland, Ohio, directed by Irvin Page (1901-1988), and the other from Buenos Aires, directed by Eduardo Braun-Menendez (1903-1959) –, to isolate and identify the same substance, a peptide of eight amino acids with pressure activity, produced by renin on a plasmatic substrate, which was given the name of angiotensin. The influence of these substances on aldosterone secretion was eventually demonstrated after more than ten years both for the complexity of the experiments, due to the extreme sensitivity of the pressure substances to numerous stimulation spurious sources, and for the analytical difficulty of individual steroids without incurring interference, both for the numerous and varied activities, more than twenty, demonstrated by angiotensin. Finally, towards the end of the 1950s, the renin-angiotensin-aldosterone system (RAAS) was definitively demonstrated.

However, it soon became clear that, although important in different pathological conditions, the RAAS could not be the only controller of the mineralocorticoid regulation of electrolyte homeostasis under physiological conditions. In 1983 Adolfo de Bold (1942) together with Geoffrey Flynn (1937) presented the isolation and identification of a biologically active peptide of 28 amino acids, called atrial natriuretic peptide (ANP).

Salt and water in clinical medicine and therapy

As it is easy to understand, the interest in salt and water in medicine has very ancient origins. Paracelsus considered salt one of the three elementary principles of the human body. Mattias Untzer's treatise *Physiologia Salis* dates from 1624 and the *Tractatus Medicus de Sale* by Johannes Saphronius Kozak (1602-1685) from 1663. Carl von Linné (1707-1778) stated in his Readings of 1770 that salt had not only an external function, but also an internal function: it was important for growth, for physical prowess, for sexual activity but, singular affirmation, was the cause of scurvy[2]. Given the authority of Linnaeus, many clinicians of the time shared this opinion, contributing to its spread in the clinical practice and in therapy.

Water disorders, on the other hand, received less attention, above all due to the important regulatory intervention of thirst.

However, edema was considered a manifestation of heart failure, and was treated with strict water restriction and, in the late eighteenth century, with digitalis leaves introduced by William Withering (1741-1799) in 1778 in England. Subsequently the mercurial diuretics spread, which remained in therapy until the first decades of the twentieth century, as we have seen previously.

With the increase of knowledge on renal physiology in the nineteenth century, a form of edema of renal origin was also distinguished in the clinical medicine, whose pathogenesis was recognized not by the cardio-circulatory function, but by the decrease in plasma proteins resulting from proteinuria, as was discovered by Rich-

[2] "Defectus vegetabilium, som andre medici halla före. Det ses klart af ware lappar og hoffolk; ty ingen af dem hafwa scorbutum, emedan de ei ata salt" "Not a vegetable deficiency, as other doctors believe: it is evident in our Lapponi farmers, none of whom suffer from scurvy, because they do not consume salt".

ard Bright (1789-1858) with his studies on chronic nephropathy, and by Johann Florian Heller (1813-1871) with his studies on proteinuria and nitric acid test to reveal it.

In 1902 Hermann Strauss (1868-1944) showed that an increase in serum osmotic pressure is due almost exclusively to the increase in low molecular weight nitrogenous substances, and introduced the method for the determination of non-protein nitrogen (blood urea). The progress of knowledge on the ability of the kidney to cope with a water load suggested to Strauss the preparation of a urine concentration and dilution test for the assessment of renal function, a test further modified in 1922 by Thomas Addis (1881-1949), worldwide known as the test of Addis, which has survived in the practice of routine up to the present day.

But the disorders of the salt-water balance, whose study and treatment accelerated the progress of clinical and therapeutic knowledge of salt-water balance disorders, but also of the physiology of salt and water, were severe gastrointestinal disorders caused by cholera epidemics and infectious childhood enteritis.

Cholera epidemics

Cholera was an important problem mainly due to the relationships between the British and their colonies in India and Africa, which facilitated their spread in Europe. An epidemic in Jessore, Bangladesh, in 1817 had caused more than 10,000 deaths in just two months. The following epidemic in 1826 along the Ganges spread through Afghanistan and Persia to Russia and from there to Western Europe, reaching Great Britain in 1831.

The disease, of sudden onset, affected thousands of people every day, with a mortality rate of 30%-50%. The lack of water in the body was evident. Blood tests were difficult and unreliable on this material, especially because at that time they were conducted on whole blood and the methods involved the previous incineration of the sample.

However, tests were carried out on the material emitted with the feces, demonstrating a sodium chloride content of 13 g/L. William Brooke O'Shaughnessy (1804-1889), an Irish clinician, had proposed with great insistence and documented conviction the venous treatment for a disease of the severity of cholera, reporting in 1831 the first results of the blood analysis, which showed extreme deficiency of salt and water (neutral saline ingredients) as well as sodium bicarbonate (free alkali).

Shortly thereafter, William Reid Clanny (1776-1850), also an Irishman, reported similar results, using a venous sample collection method which can be considered the anticipation of the vacutainer, since a vacuum container was used with a valve that was open after being inserted into the vein to let the sample flow into the container.

Both the results of O'Shaughnessy and those of Clanny, however, did not attract the attention of the medical class in general, but a young general practitioner of Scottish origin, Thomas Aitchison Latta (1796-1833), was interested instead, deciding to adopt venous infusions of sodium chloride and sodium bicarbonate in cholera patients.

The results were obviously encouraging, and by adequately adjusting the volumes of the infusions, Latta obtained the healing of a patient: "In forty-eight hours she smoked her pipe free from distemper".

The courageous replacement treatment undertaken by Latta immediately received the approval of the medical class and from there a few letters appeared in "The Lancet" which confirmed similar results with the venous infusion therapy, including an enthusiastic comment by O'Shaughnessy. Among others of great importance was the contribution of William Stevens (1786-1868), who had gathered a particularly thorough experience during a long stay in the West Indies, then a Danish dominion, where he had been able to face not only cholera, but numerous other tropical diseases, reaching the belief that the cause was not in the "solid ingredients of the blood", but in the lack of "saline fluids" that kept those "solid ingredients" in solution.

Hence the need for the replacement of lost fluids and salts through the vein, the most appropriate route of administration given the rapidity of the course of most of these diseases.

This therapeutic approach naturally contrasted with

the then current measures, largely of a galenic nature, above all bloodletting, which Stevens struggled to prove to be the exact intervention contrary to the necessary one.

Stevens collected his experiences in the book *Observations on the Healthy and Diseased Properties of the Blood* (1832) dedicated "*to his Majesty Frederick the Sixth, King of Denmark*".

Driven by Stevens' insistence, and by the reports that increasingly appeared in "The Lancet" on the cholera salt deficit, the British Central Board of Health promoted a survey among health care professionals to compare the new therapeutic methods suggested by Stevens with the traditional ones such as bloodletting, opium, calomel as a diuretic, and distilled spirits. Unexpectedly, this confrontation turned out to be uncertain and contradictory, so as to induce the Central Board to reject Stevens' proposal, who was not surprised but convinced that every new initiative would be contested and eventually not accepted[3].

In 1840 the blood analysis of cholera patients was renewed by Carl Schmidt of the Dorpat school, which we have already met in the previous pages, who measured in the serum a decrease in sodium and chloride of 20 mmol/L, and a bicarbonate concentration of 5 mmol/L. However, there is no documentation of the venous replacement treatment in the subsequent epidemics of Riga in 1848 or in Copenhagen in 1853, but only of oral treatments with water and/or salt.

The treatment with salt infusions was used only sporadically in Great Britain, and in continental Europe it was introduced only in 1884 by Arnoldo Cantani (1837-1893) from Naples who used subcutaneous infusions of sodium chloride 0.4% and sodium bicarbonate 0.3%.

It can therefore be concluded that the victory over cholera infection at the beginning of the 1900s, rather than the progress of therapy, was due to the improvement and modernization of the hygienic-sanitary conditions and to preventive measures, aimed in particular at the decontamination of streams and waterworks.

Enteritis in childhood

We have already discussed childhood enteritis in the notes of the history of acid-base balance (Chapter 1) which we therefore refer to, limiting ourselves here to mention more closely the water-saline component of these disorders.

Naturally the problems of salt-water homeostasis are certainly not due only to pediatric gastroenterology and even less were so in the past, but this pathology is of particular historical interest because it has represented one of the experimental fields where most have developed, clarified, perfected the most important modern knowledge on salt-water exchange and on the role of the kidney in the homeostasis of physiological fluids and their disorders.

As we described in the chapter on the history of blood gas analysis, the merit of progress in the first decades of the twentieth century is due first of all to the founder of the Pediatric School of Johns Hopkins Hospital in Baltimore, John Howland (**Figure 7.6**), who promoted in particular the development of laboratory investigations with methods and procedures for blood sampling suitable for pediatrics. This was a priceless progress, because the control of blood values allowed the adaptation of the replacement therapy.

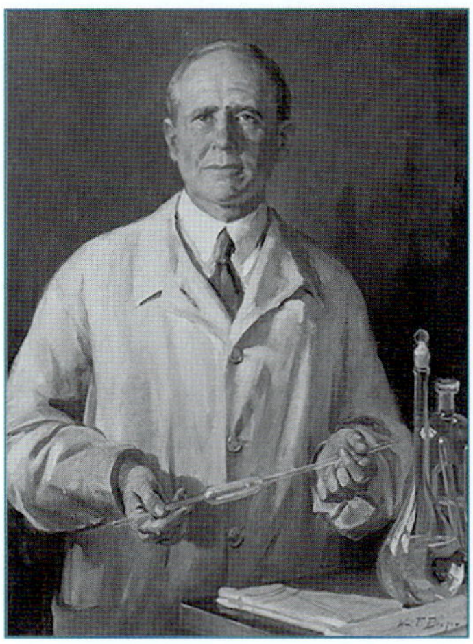

Figure 7.6 John Howland (1873-1926).

[3] "The experience... shows that any improvement opposing the established articles is certain to encounter opposition. If salt treatment were to prove an efficient remedy... this would contradict the principles of the prevailing solidary pathology and... the new treatment would probably... find no recognition at all".

Until then, in fact, the treatment was kept within ridiculously ineffective volumes, both because of the difficulty in ascertaining its extent and because of the fear of complications (for example, the hyperpyretic reactions that invariably accompanied vein therapy), and especially because there was no clarity about the composition and dosages to be prescribed.
James Lawder Gamble (1883-1959) was the component of that school that gained greater fame, due to the importance of the new criteria of interpretation of the plasmatic electrolyte framework (the Gamble-grams). But we cannot omit mentioning among the members of the Baltimore school also Daniel Darrow (1885-1965), who established the principle that water is freely permeable through cellular membranes, and that osmotic variations are due to the increase in cell volume resulting from hyponatremia, as well as cellular shrinkage resulting from hypernatremia.
But even more decisive were his studies on potassium metabolism and the determination of blood potassium. Fearing the risks of an excess of potassium, especially cardiac arrest, this electrolyte was excluded from the therapeutic regimens of childhood enteritis. Darrow showed that in this disorder the potassium deficit could reach ¼ of the total patrimony, and that with appropriately prepared solutions, and with the control of the potassium (the flame photometry was available in the 40s), the reintegration of the deficit could be obtained safely.
The introduction of these therapeutic measures, as we have described in the history of blood gas analysis, drastically reduced the mortality rate of childhood enteritis which went from 12%-20% to about 5%.

The replacement venous treatment

Until the last decades of the nineteenth century, while blood transfusion was employed – even though it was considered a resource only in extreme conditions, due to the risk of often fatal complications – the replacement therapy with other fluids was rarely used, because it was considered ineffective as it lacked vital oxygen.
Around the 1980s, however, proposals began to appear in literature for a re-use of the replacement therapies that had been successful in cholera epidemics.
In 1881 Emil Schwarz (1852-1918) showed that the circulatory deficiency in animals after hemorrhage is not the result of the loss of the corpuscular part of the blood, but of the imbalance between the dimensions of the circulatory system and its content. These experimental indications soon aroused the interest of the scientific world, in particular of surgery. Already shortly after the publication of Schwarz's experiments, Johann Bischoff (1841-1892) reported the result of an alkaline solution of common intra-arterial salt, decisive in a woman with severe post-partum hemorrhage. Hermann Kümmell (1852-1937), while also approving the treatment with saline solutions, recommended the venous route instead of the arterial one.
Treatment with saline solutions soon spread not only to surgical specialties but also to medical ones, despite the risk of complications, in particular of febrile reactions attributed to non-sterile infusion materials, which however persisted even with the use of distilled or boiled water. This complication was resolved only in 1923, when Florence Barbara Seibert (1897-1991) isolated a bacterium that survived in distilled water and produced stable filterable pyrogenic substances, so that it was possible to provide for decontamination.
In those years the saline treatment was not only difficult but also often disappointing, especially in acute conditions, mainly due to incorrect methods of administration, too short or occasional; but there were also cases in which the treatment was not effective in promoting diuresis and the patient was suffering from pulmonary edema.
Thus researches for alternatives to the so called physiological solution were made, and Ringer's solutions made their appearance on the market: these were complex solutions composed of different salts in appropriate combination, which took their name from their creator, Sidney Ringer (1835-1910).
However, as a result of the clinical application, they proved inferior to expectations. Of greater interest were the dextrose solutions, introduced for the first time in 1897 by Fritz Voit (1863) and by Wilhelm von Leube (1842-1912) in the form of subcutaneous infusions composed of carbohydrates, fats and proteins for nutritional purposes. These first solutions contained

10%-20% dextrose, and because they caused local irritation, they were soon abandoned in favor of isotonic dextrose solutions, introduced in 1904 by Paul Leopold Friederich, surgeon in Greifswald, which could be used subcutaneously without harmful effects. In the first decades of the last century the most used solutions were therefore the physiological NaCl solutions, perfected at 0.9%, as well as different variants of the Ringer solution.

The major obstacle of these therapies were the unpredictable hyper pyretic reactions which, as we mentioned, could become problematic for critically ill patients. As a result, the rectal route gained favor, especially in surgical wards.

The progressive development and modernization of clinical chemistry laboratory services contributed decisively to improving and making more precise the replacement treatments of salt and water.

In particular, the introduction of the analysis by means of radioactive isotopes allowed more in-depth research on the metabolism of water and salt in normal and pathological conditions, as well as on the mechanisms of physiological regulation as described in the previous pages; among the studies, those of Francis Daniels Moore (1913-2001) and his group of the Peter Bent Brigham Hospital in Boston should be mentioned.

In the years in which the First World War broke out, the knowledge on water, salt, blood volume and their role in the pathogenesis of shock were not yet defined. In times of peace, as we have mentioned, the physiological solution was administered after surgery to patients in severe conditions, usually via the rectum, sometimes subcutaneously, rarely via the vein, reserved only for gastric, pulmonary, or postpartum hemorrhages of serious entity if blood transfusion was not available (few hospitals were organized for transfusion purposes).

During the four years of war these treatment modalities obviously proved to be utterly derisory, and in England in August 1917 the Medical Research Committee promoted a commission led by Ernest Henry Starling for the study of the relationships between blood loss and fluids and the onset of shock after trauma or surgery, as well as the appropriate therapeutic measures.

One can imagine the difficulties that this study had to face, given the context of war, and also given the limited knowledge of the time on the physiology and physiopathology of the regulation of body fluids. It is also easy to understand how the war pathology had drastically imposed an adjustment of the replacement therapeutic treatments, not only by enhancing the transfusion therapy to cope with the massive loss of blood, but also above all by developing and differentiating the replacement treatments with saline solutions, for a rapid correction of volume losses, increasingly adopting the venous route of administration, more suited to the needs of urgency than the rectal and subcutaneous routes in use up until then. Also the composition of the solutions underwent modifications in line with the different therapeutic requirements.

One of the most important advances, if not the most important with regard to transfusion therapy during war years, was the realization, for the first time, of blood preserved for transfusion, an initiative that would have started the development of blood transfusion services. Pressed by the difficulty of procuring fresh donor blood, especially during war actions at the front, P. Rous and J.R. Turner of the Rockefeller Institute of Medical Research in 1916 undertook a study on the preservation of blood, demonstrating erythrocyte viability for up to four weeks. Following this indication, shortly after, Oswald Hope Robertson was the first to put into practice the clinical utility of "blood preserved for transfusion".

The erythrocyte suspension was prepared from 500 mL of blood collected in a glass bottle with 350 mL of isosmotic sodium citrate solution, and 850 mL of isosmotic dextrose solution. This suspension could be stored at a low temperature for three weeks, but was usually used within 10-15 days.

During storage the erythrocytes sedimented: at the time of use the overlying liquid was removed, and the erythrocytes were re-suspended in a 2.6% gelatin solution in 0.9% saline solution.

In the years following the First World War, despite the experience acquired with venous infusions, this route of administration returned to being used rarely, even if there were further evolutions.

Rudolph Matas (1860-1957), professor of surgery at Tulane, adopted the venous infusion of normal saline or dextrose solutions in each operation, and even once it was finished as needed.

Of primary importance was the appearance in the literature of Gamble's work, *Chemical Anatomy, Physiology and Pathology of extracellular fluid*, as we have already mentioned above, especially for the quantitative information on the composition and volume of water compartments, in particular the extracellular compartment, whose constancy and composition stability conditions were a prerequisite for the maintenance of all life processes.

To obtain these conditions, Gamble assured, only three components are needed: water, sodium and chloride. Of equal importance were the studies of Francis Daniels Moore (1913-2001) and of his group at the Massachusetts General Hospital, which by means of radioactive isotope techniques obtained the measurements of the extracellular compartment and of the electrolytes that compose it.

The results of the research were collected in the work *The Metabolic Response to Surgery* by Francis Moore and Margaret Ball, published in 1952, indispensable in cultural background for anyone in those years wanting to learn about the physiology and pathophysiology of body fluids.

While taking into account these advances, the therapeutic treatments of body fluid disorders did not improve until the hormonal regulation of salt-water homeostasis was clarified, as described above.

The discovery in the 50s of the last century of the mineral-active secretion of aldosterone, previously known as electrocortin, and the definition of its specific activity on the regulation of renal elimination of sodium, were decisive steps in advancing the knowledge on body fluid homeostasis.

Two further steps that quickly led to our current knowledge concerned the study of renal mechanisms of urine formation, that is the mechanism of countercurrent concentration, and the progress of clinical chemistry laboratories in determining electrolytes with the introduction of the flame photometer and then of the electrometric technique.

References

- Allen JG. O. H. Robertson--an inquiring mind: from blood bank to cutthroat trout. Pharos Alpha Omega Alpha Honor Med Soc. 1985;48(2):25-7.
- Alleva K, Chara O, Amodeo G. Aquaporins: another piece in the osmotic puzzle. FEBS Lett. 2012;586(19):2991-9.
- Astrup P, Bie P, Hengell HC. Salt and water in culture and medicine. Munksgaard International Publishers, 1994.
- Awad S, Allison SP, Lobo DN. The history of 0.9% saline. Clin Nutr. 2008;27(2):179-88.
- Basso N, Terragno NA. History about the discovery of the renin-angiotensin system. Hypertension. 2001;38(6):1246-9.
- Berman LB. Harry Goldblatt: 1891-1977. JAMA. 1977;238 (17):1846.
- Beyer KH. Chlorothiazide. How the thiazides evolved as antihypertensive therapy. Hypertension. 1993;22(3):388-91.
- Bhave G, Neilson EG. Body fluid dynamics: back to the future. J Am Soc Nephrol. 2011. 22(12):2166-81.
- Cannon WB. The Wisdom of the Body. New York, W.W. Norton 1932.
- Dantzler WH, Layton AT, Layton HE et al. Urine-concentrating mechanism in the inner medulla: function of the thin limbs of the loop of Henle. Clin J Am Soc Nephrol. 2014;9(10):1781-9.
- Du Pont JJ, Hill MA, Bender SB et al. Aldosterone and vascular mineralocorticoid receptors: regulators of ion channels beyond the kidney. Hypertension. 2014;63(4):632-7.
- Ellis H. Sydney Ringer: physician, physiologist and pharmacologist. Br J Hosp Med (Lond). 2010;71(11):645.
- Fine LG. Ernest Henry Starling (1866-1927) on the formation and reabsorption of lymph. Nephron Physiol. 2014; 126(3):9-17.
- Frøkiaer J, Nielsen S, Knepper MA. Molecular physiology of renal aquaporins and sodium transporters: exciting approaches to understand regulation of renal water handling. J Am Soc Nephrol. 2005;16(10):2827-9.
- Gamble JL. Early history of fluid replacement therapy. Pediatrics. 1953;11(5):554-67.
- Harvey AM. Classics in clinical science: James L. Gamble and "Gamblegrams". Am J Med. 1979;66(6):904-6.
- Henriksen JH. Ernest Henry Starling (1866-1927): the scientist and the man. J Med Biogr. 2005;13(1):22-30.
- Hoenig MP, Zeidel ML. Homeostasis, the milieu intérieur, and the wisdom of the nephron. Clin J Am Soc Nephrol. 2014;9(7):1272-81.
- Holmes F. The milieu interieur and the cell theory. Bull Hist Med. 1963;37:315-35.
- Houssay BA. Eduardo Braun Menendez (1903-1959). Rev Soc Argent Biol. 1959;35:1-4.
- Janakan G, Ellis H. Dr Thomas Aitchison Latta (c1796-1833): pioneer of intravenous fluid replacement in the treatment of cholera. J Med Biogr. 2013;21(2):70-4.
- Kinder CH. Richard Bright (1789-1858). Invest Urol. 1966;4(3):288-90.
- Klimpel V. Our surgical heritage. Hermann Kümmell (1852-1937). Zentralbl Chir. 1987;112(9):589-92.

- MacGillivray N. Sir William Brooke O'Shaughnessy (1808-1889), MD, FRS, LRCS Ed: Chemical pathologist, pharmacologist and pioneer in electric telegraphy. J Med Biogr. 2017;25(3):186-96.
- Mandler O. Johann Jacob Bischoff (1841-1892) and the beginnings of modern obstetrics in Basel. Praxis. 1960;4 9:995-1001.
- O'Shaughnessy WB. Proposal of a new method of treating the blue epidemic cholera by the injection of highly-oxygenised salts into the venous system: Read before the Westminster Medical Society. The Lancet. 1831;17:366-71.
- Parisi M, Dorr RA, Ozu M et al. From membrane pores to aquaporins: 50 years measuring water fluxes. J Biol Phys. 2007;33(5-6):331-43.
- Peitzman SJ. The flame photometer as engine of nephrology: a biography. Am J Kidney Dis. 2010. 56(2):379-86.
- Robertson OH. A method of citrated blood transfusion. Br Med J. 1918;1(2991):477-9.
- Roblin RO, Clapp JW. The preparation of heterocyclic sulfonamides. J Am Chem Soc. 1950;11:4890.
- Rossier BC, Baker ME, Studer RA. Epithelial sodium transport and its control by aldosterone: the story of our internal environment revisited. Physiol Rev. 2015;95(1):297-340.
- Rous P, Turner JR. The preservation of living red blood cells in vitro: I. Methods of preservation. J Exp Med. 1916;23 (2):219-37.
- Singh D. Rudolph Matas (1860-1957): father of vascular surgery. Indian J Surg. 2007;69(6):270-1.
- Smith HW. The fate of sodium and water in the renal tubules. Bull N Y Acad Med. 1959;35(5):293-316.
- Van den Velden, R. Die Nierenwirkung von Hypophysenextrakten beim Menschen. Berl Klin Wochenschr. 1913;50:2083-86.

Homeostasis of body fluids Fundamentals of physiology

Mario Tarantino

Introduction

A 60-year-old man with a small cell lung cancer has been admitted to hospital because his level of consciousness was worsening for two weeks. The physical examination does not reveal abnormalities beyond those already known except the patient's mental state. The laboratory tests give the following results:

Plasma		*Urine*	
Na^+	105 mEq/L	Na^+	78 mEq/L
K^+	4 mEq/L	Uosm	604 mOsm/Kg
Cl^-	72 mEq/L		
HCO_3^-	21 mEq/L		
Posm	222 mOsm/Kg		

Anticipating clinical contents of the subsequent chapters, let's open these introductory physiological notes with a hypothetical case study: a severe hyponatremia in apparent contrast with renal elimination of sodium and with high urine osmolality which reveals the inability of the kidney to eliminate excess free water so as to correct hyponatremia. To understand the pathophysiological alterations and to interpret them correctly for diagnostic and therapeutic purposes, it is essential to clear the physiological fundamentals of the homeostatic regulation of body fluids.

Anatomy of body fluids

Water constitutes about 60% of total body weight in adult men and around 50% in adult women; in the first years of life the percentage of water present is between 65% and 75% while it tends to decrease with age.
Total body water is divided into two main compartments: 2/3 in the intracellular space (intracellular fluid, ICF) and 1/3 in the extracellular (extracellular fluid, ECF). The latter in turn divides into two subcompartments, extravascular (or interstitial), which occupy 75%-80%, and intravascular, the plasma, for the remaining 20% (**Figure 8.1**).
The most important feature is the different composition of the two compartments. In particular, each one is characterized by a cation: sodium in the ECF and potassium in the ICF.
A small fraction of the ECF, about 5%, is the trans-cellular or third space fluid, which includes the one enclosed in cavities covered by epithelia, such as synovial, peritoneal and cerebrospinal fluid.
In the ECF the main anions that accompany sodium are chloride and bicarbonate; in the ICF, potassium is accompanied by multiple anionic charges of protein macromolecules and cellular organic phosphates.
The differences in the concentration of electrolytes in the various sectors of the extracellular compartment (Figure 8.1) are mainly caused by proteins, due to both size and charge, and to their different distribution in plasma and in the interstitial fluid, occupying in the first a space of about 7%.
The proteins in the extracellular compartment have a total anionic charge with a concentration of 12-14 mEq/L, so they participate in electroneutrality, and being confined to intravascular sector they behave like non-permeable anions, influencing the distribution of the other ions between the two extracellular sectors.
As we will see later, plasma proteins, in particular al-

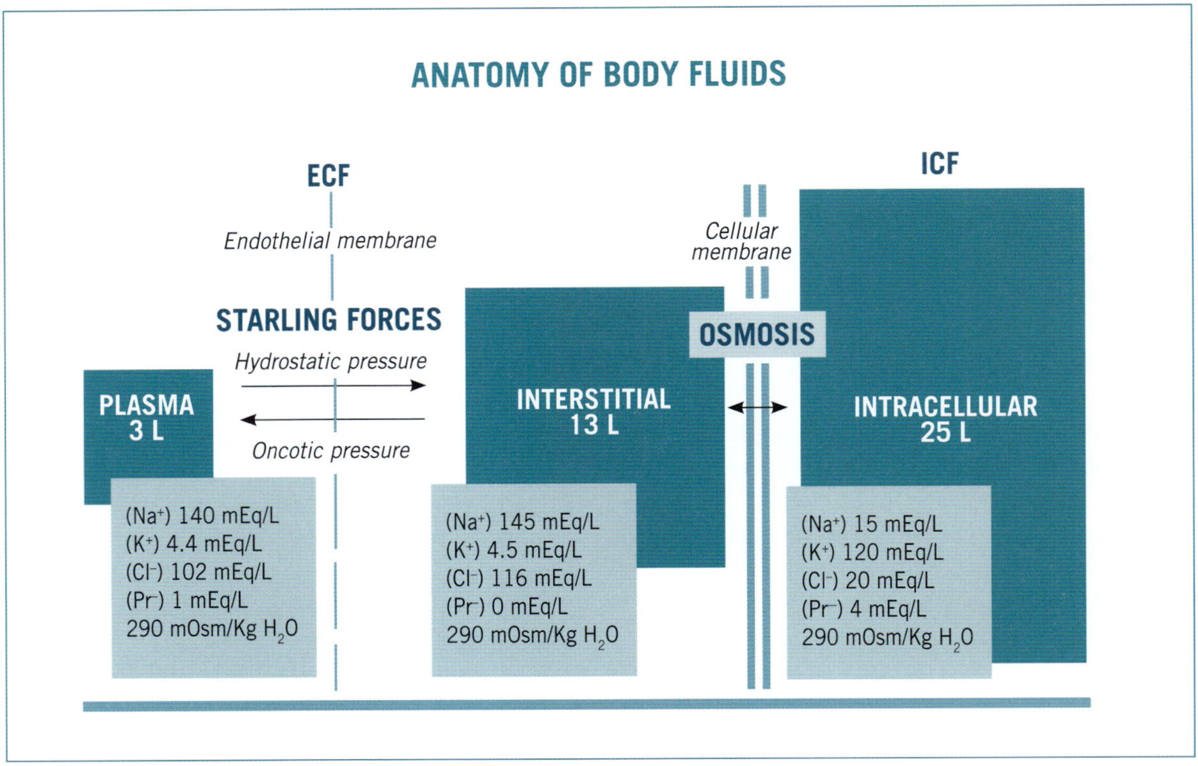

Figure 8.1 Distribution and composition of body fluids.

bumin, perform in the intravascular sector of the ECF the important function of osmotic pressure, one of the fundamental forces in the regulation of fluid exchange between the two sectors of the ECF.

Fluid movement among compartments

Osmosis, osmolality and tonicity

The ECF and the ICF communicate with each other through the cell membrane.

As shown in Figure 8.1 this membrane has the properties of semi-permeability, i.e. it is permeable to the solvent, the water, but impermeable to most solutes, including electrolytes, creating the premises for the osmosis mechanism as an exchange system between the two compartments.

According to this mechanism, if such a membrane separates two solutions of different concentrations, the solvent passes from the most diluted compartment to the more concentrated one until the concentration in the two compartments equals: the pressure that must be opposed to counteract this passage of the solvent is called osmotic pressure. Obviously, once the equilibrium is reached, the volume of the two solutions also varies, in particular it is increased in the more concentrated solution and decreased in the more diluted one. The essential condition for osmosis is therefore the impermeability to solutes and the solvent permeability of the membrane that separates the two solutions: in this case the osmotic pressure depends only on the number of particles not further dissociable of dissolved solutes, called osmols, while the size, charge, or other structural characteristics do not count.

The overall osmotic concentration is called osmolarity, expressed in milliosmole (mOsm)/L, or rather osmolality in milliosmole (mOsm)/Kg H_2O to avoid temperature

interference, the latter definition will be used in this textbook. Osmolality can be measured by a direct method using osmometry, or by indirect methods by resorting to one of the colligative properties of osmolality such as lowering the freezing point or increasing the boiling point which, like osmosis, depend on number of particles in solution. Both the direct and indirect methods, however, measure all the particles in solution, without distinguishing between membrane permeable or impermeable solutes.
However, it is important to distinguish effective osmoles, i.e. those that are effectively impermeable to the membrane, from the ineffective osmoles, those that are permeable to the membrane and therefore ineffective for osmosis purposes: in plasma, for example, urea is an ineffective osmole. The effective osmoles are those that determine the tonicity.
Therefore osmolality is determined by the total concentration of solutes in a fluid compartment, while tonicity refers to the ability that all solutes together have to generate an osmotic force capable of causing the displacement of water from a fluid compartment to another. Under normal conditions it is the sodium that determines the plasmatic tonicity, the effective osmolality can therefore be calculated: $2 \times [Na^+]$ if blood glucose is normal, otherwise $2 \times [Na^+]$ + glucose (mg/dL)/18.

NOTE

The electrolytes would be per se permeable to biological membranes, but they are actively rendered impermeable, through the intervention of the enzyme Na^+K^+ATPase (pump) which, with energy consumption, actively confines sodium in the extracellular space and potassium in the intracellular compartment, together with the anions that accompany them.

Starling forces: hydrostatic pressure and oncotic pressure

Although the exchanges between the extra- and intracellular can also take place directly, at the level of the cellular membrane, more commonly they occur through another exchange system interposed between the capillary network and the interstitial space, which provides with blood nutriens supply to peripheral tissues and catabolites removal produced by cellular metabolism. Exchange takes place through the membrane of the capillary endothelium, whose permeability depends on molecular size, especially excluding protein macromolecules (only albumin is partly permeable).
Two forces govern this exchange, called "Starling forc-

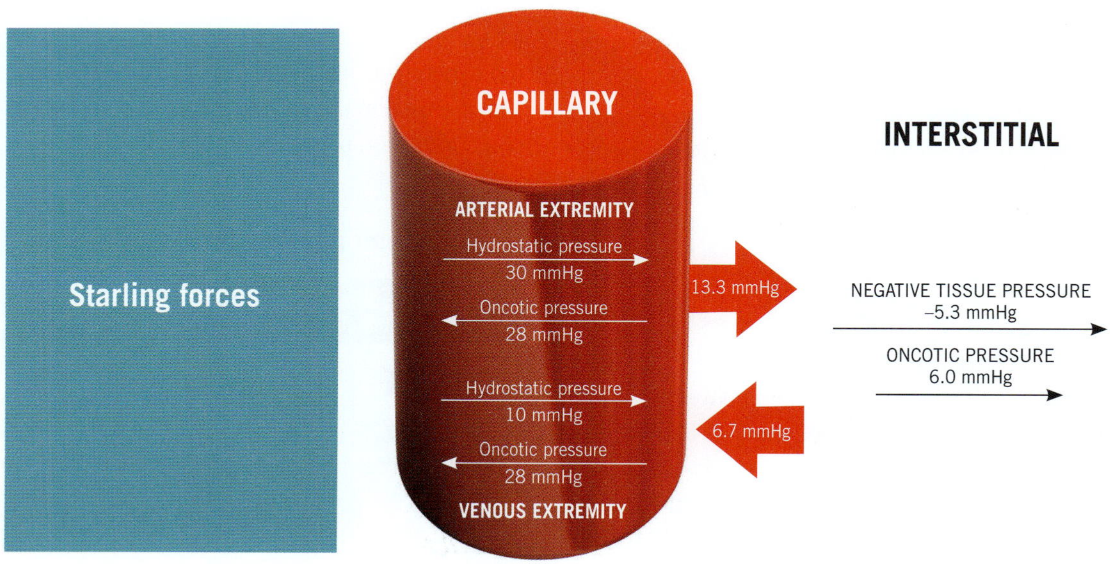

Figure 8.2 Starling's forces in the exchange between blood and interstitial space.

es" by the physiologist who investigated the physiological function (**Figure 8.2**): hydrostatic pressure that comes from the arterial pressure in the capillaries, and which promotes the diffusion of solutes from the bloodstream in the interstitial space, and osmotic pressure of plasma proteins (called oncotic pressure) which, remaining confined in the capillaries, recall fluid from the interstitial space in the blood. The tissue pressure and the osmotic pressure of the interstitial space contribute to the exchange to a lesser extent. The hydrostatic pressure prevails at the arteriolar end of the capillary, favoring in particular the diffusion of nutrients from the blood to the interstitial fluid and from here to the cells, while the oncotic pressure of the plasma proteins prevails at the venular end, favoring above all the recall of catabolic products from cells in the venular circulation of the capillary bed.

Sodium physiological significance

Sodium has two important fundamental significances in the physiology of body fluids, both linked to its function as an extracellular osmole.

The first one is related to its plasma concentration also referred to as natremia.

Thanks to the osmotic exchange of water between ECF and ICF, the concentration of sodium with its anions is crucial in the regulation of osmolality and the volume of the intracellular compartment.

The second significance is related to total body quantity or total body content of sodium ($TBNa^+$): as the main osmole in extracellular compartment, sodium is crucial in maintaining and regulating the volume of the extracellular compartment.

Plasma sodium concentration and intracellular volume

Plasma osmolality, P_{osm} is maintained between 275 and 290 mOsm/Kg with an average value of 280 mOsm/Kg, and is almost entirely due to sodium and anions that accompany it, mainly chloride: in fact the average normal concentration of plasma sodium is 140 mEq/L, therefore:

$$P_{osm} \cong 2 \times [Na^+]p \quad (1)$$

Since ECF and ICF are among them in osmotic equilibrium, the P_{osm}, and therefore plasma concentration of sodium or natremia, is representative not only of the osmolality of the ECF but also of the osmolality of the ICF. Since the exchangeable sodium (Na^+_e) with its extracellular anions, and the exchangeable potassium (K^+_e) with its intracellular anions are the main effective osmoles of body fluids,

$$P_{osm} \cong \frac{2 \times Na^+_e + 2 \times K^+_e}{\text{total body } H_2O} \quad (2)$$

And therefore, from (2) and (3)

$$[Na^+]p \cong \frac{Na^+_e + K^+_e}{\text{total body } H_2O} \quad (3)$$

it follows that alterations in natremia and, therefore, in extracellular osmolality, result in alterations of intracellular osmolality and intracellular volume.

Figure 8.3 illustrates these important relationships between ECF and ICF.

An increase in natremia, or in extracellular osmolality, causes by osmosis the shift of water from the less concentrated ICF to the more concentrated ECF, until a new equilibrium. This shift of water partially corrects the hyperosmolality of the ECF and the hypernatremia, with increase in the volume of the ECF, at the expense of a contraction of the ICF.

Sodium physiological significance

Added substance	Plasmatic osmolality	(Na^+)p	ECF	ICF	Urine sodium
NaCl	▲	▲	▲	▼	▲
H_2O	▼	▼	▲	▲	▲
Isotonic NaCl	0	0	▲	0	▲

Figure 8.3 Relationship between osmolality and volume (ECF and ICF) increased ▲ decreased ▼ unchanged 0

Alterations in the opposite direction are observed if natremia, and therefore the osmolality of the ECF, decreases due to an excess of water in the ECF. The hyposmolality of the ECF is followed by the passage of water from this compartment to the ICF, so that at equilibrium achieved, hyponatremia is accompanied by an increase in ICF.

To conclude, hyponatremia, or extracellular hyposmolality, indicates cellular hyperhydration, as hypernatremia, or extracellular hyperosmolality, means cellular dehydration.

Finally, isotonic modifications of the ECF, which do not alter either osmolality or sodium, merely change the ECF, leaving both extracellular osmolality and intracellular osmolality and volume unchanged.

What has just been described illustrates two principles of fundamental importance in the physiology of salt-water balance:

1) Natremia does not give any information either on the total body sodium content or on the fluid volume of the extracellular compartment. In the experiments of Figure 8.3 the ECF is always increased, but natremia one time is increased, one it is decreased, and another time remains unchanged. This can be explained because natremia is a concentration, that is a relative entity expressing the relationship between quantity and volume.
2) The regulation of osmolality, that is plasma concentration of sodium, is obtained through the regulation of water. The change in sodium may in some cases be due to a change in the total sodium content, but it is almost always due to a change in water volume, regardless of the changes in the total sodium content. Equation (3) displays the concept.

NOTE

As we shall see in the clinical chapters, hyponatremia is classified in the forms with normal, increased or decreased ECF and normal, increased, or decreased total sodium content. What needs to be reaffirmed is that in any case there is an excess of total body water compared to the total body sodium. Differentiation is important for therapeutic purposes, because the treatment is different in the three groups. In the case of hypernatremia the ECF can be reduced (very often), normal or increased and there is a total body water deficit compared to the total body sodium. In conclusion, when we talk about hyper- or hyponatremia everything must be seen through the lens of water.

At the conclusion of the paragraph, it is clear that the osmolality of the ECF, and therefore natremia, must be the object of a very sensitive and precise regulation. As we will see, this regulation is a renal function and occurs through the regulation of water balance.

Total body sodium content and extracellular fluid volume

As we mentioned earlier, sodium has also another physiological significance no less important in the regulation of body fluids, this time not in the form of plasma concentration, but in that of total body content ($TBNa^+$). Being the main osmole in the extracellular compartment, together with the anions that accompany it, it is essential in determining the ECF. An increase in the total sodium content increases the ECF, and an opposite effect follows its decrease. Maintaining the extracellular volume, or rather the portion of ECF defined as an effective circulating blood volume (ECBV), is essential to support adequate tissue perfusion. Hence the importance of the homeostatic regulation of $TBNa^+$.

In the following paragraphs we will see how the regulation of sodium balance acts precisely on its renal elimination, in response to changes in the volume of extracellular compartment, as also shown in column 6 of Figure 8.3.

The regulation of osmolality

Water regulation

In physiological conditions the plasma osmolality (and therefore the extracellular) is maintained between 275 and 290 mOsm/Kg, with an average value of 280 mOsm/Kg.

As we mentioned earlier, these values correspond in practice to concentration of sodium and the anions that accompany it, so that osmolality and plasma sodium concentration are closely related to each other. However, the regulation of osmolality does not occur through the regulation of sodium metabolism, but through the regulation of body water.

The importance of this regulation can be seen in the double control that concerns both input of water into the organism, through the stimulation of thirst, and its output, with the regulation of urinary elimination (**Figure 8.4**).

Table 8.1 shows the daily balance of water in adults in physiological conditions.

Only the intake in the form of fluids and urinary elimination are widely variable and in function of the homeostatic maintenance of water exchange. It is on these components that the mechanisms that provide for the regulation of osmolality and the volume of the water compartments act, while the other sources of supply or elimination are part of functions beyond the maintenance of water compartments, such as thermoregulation and the digestive function.

Water regulates plasma osmolality	
Sensors	Hypothalamic osmoceptors
Effectors	Thirst and ADH
Action	Water excretion Water intake (thirst)

Figure 8.4 Water balance.

TABLE 8.1. Daily water balance.

Input		Output	
Fluids	1,200	Urine	1,500
Solid foods	1,000	Feces	100
Metabolism	300	Skin	550
		Breathing	350
Total	2,500	Total	2,500

Thirst

The main receptors (osmoceptors) for thirst are located in hypothalamus, in the anteroventral area of the third ventricle, near the centers where the receptors for the antidiuretic hormone vasopressin (ADH) are located. It is important that these nuclei are external to the blood-brain barrier, because in this way they are not affected by any influences of the cerebral circulation, ensuring a rapid and sensitive response.

Osmolality is the fundamental stimulus for thirst, which is however also sensitive to a deficit of the extracellular volume, in particular of the ECBV.

The renal regulation of water

The renal regulation of water, with the concentration or dilution of urine, as we shall see, is performed in the most distal tract of tubular nephron, the collecting tubule.

However this regulation would not be possible without the important preparation processes in the previous sections of tubular nephron.

Faithful to its main functional characteristic, receiving the glomerular filtrate (about 200 liters in the 24 h in physiological conditions) the proximal tubule is essentially concerned with the recovery of the quantity or, in the case of water, the volume, rather than the need to dilute or to concentrate: more than 60% of the glomerular filtrate is in fact reabsorbed in an isosmotic form with the plasma. The solute that drives this recovery is sodium, facilitated by a favorable electrochemical gradient and by aquaporin 1 (AQP1), the water channel whose tubular cells in this section of the nephron are provided.

The loop of Henle is of particular importance in the regulation of water, and it is the tract of the tubular nephron where the countercurrent concentration mechanism takes place creating the stratification of osmolality in the interstitial space, laying the foundations for the regulation of osmolality and of urine volume according to the needs of water balance. The factors that initiate the creation of the countercurrent concentration mechanism are both anatomical and physiological in nature (**Figure 8.5**).

The loop arrangement with countercurrent flow is the essential premise, but of no less importance are the different permeability and transport properties in the two descending and ascending limbs of the loop: water permeability in the first and impermeability in the second; the active transport of NaCl in the thick tract of ascending limb, which starts the countercurrent mechanism; the relative impermeability to urea in the more cortical tracts, which determine a progressive concentration of urea in the tubular lumen, with subsequent greater permeability in the medullar tract. The starting mechanism of the concentration process is the active transport of sodium chloride from the ascending limb of the loop into the interstitial tissue, increasing its osmolal concentration. The descending limb is permeable to water and therefore this diffuses into the interstitial space with higher osmolality. This leakage of water does not dilute the interstitial space, because meanwhile active transport of sodium that started the process continues, multiplying the interstitial osmolality.

The continuation of the mechanisms and processes now described multiplies the countercurrent concentration, which progressively stratifies, reaching the

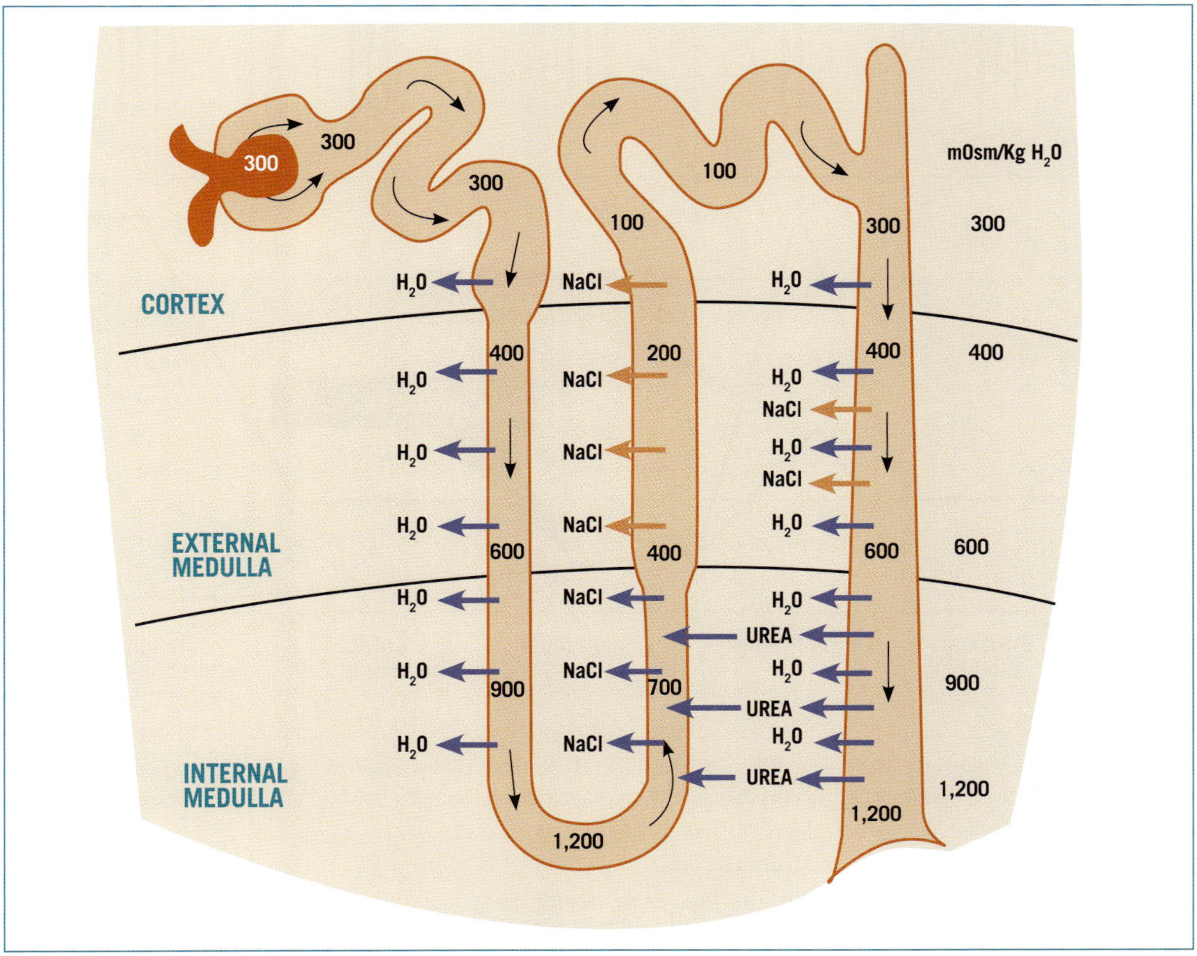

Figure 8.5 Countercurrent concentration mechanism (modified from the web).

highest osmolality levels around 1200 -1400 mOsm/Kg H_2O in the medullar areas.
Urea plays an important role. Only about 50% of this metabolite is reabsorbed in proximal tubule, the remainder persists to the most distal medullar zones in tubular lumen, which becomes progressively more permeable to urea, which then diffuses copiously into the interstitial tissue to form most of the interstitial osmolality.

However, it must be clear that the process described so far does not concentrate urine, which leaves diluted from the loop of Henle (**Figure 8.6**): this section of the nephron is in fact called the diluent tract[1]. Countercurrent concentration mechanism is however of fundamental importance, preparing with stratification of interstitial osmolality the conditions for the concentration of urine according to the needs of salt-water balance.

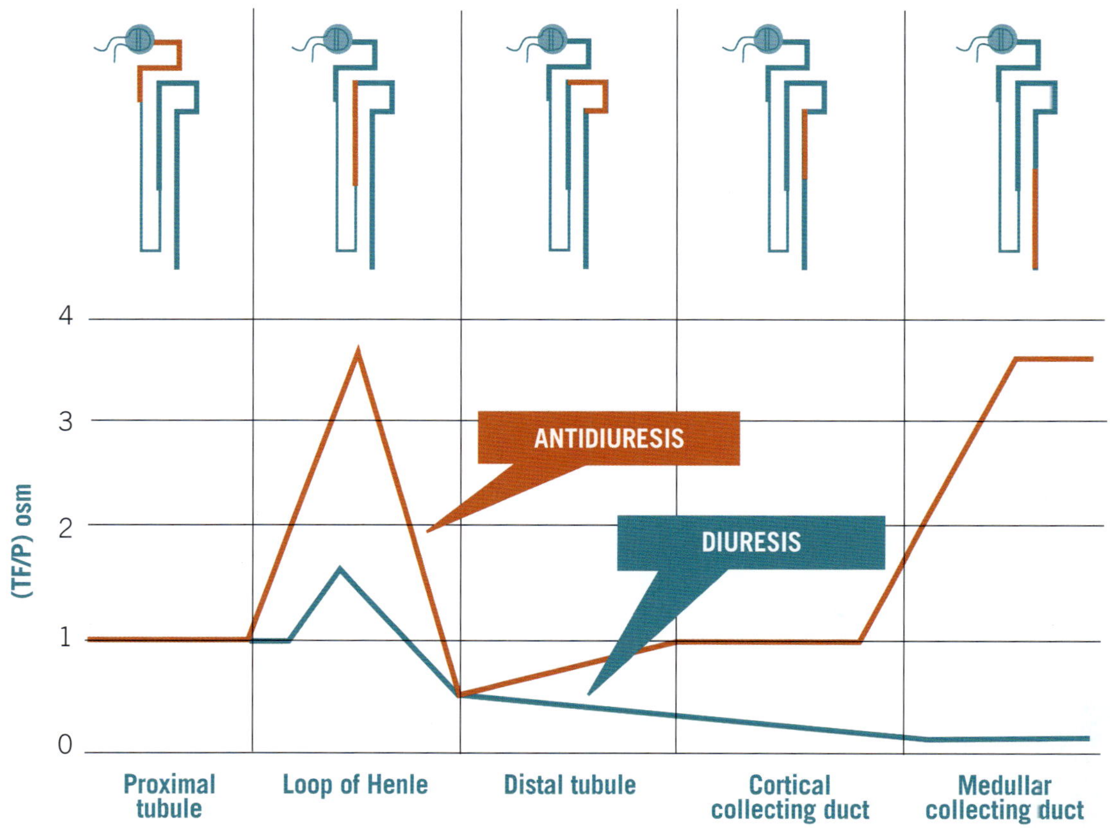

Figure 8.6 The renal regulation of water (from Boron WF, Boulpaep EL. Textbook of Medical Physiology. 2005, modified). TF/P: the ratio between tubular and plasma fluid (function of concentration and amount of solutes in the tubular fluid).

[1] As shown by H. Smith in his book *From Fish to the Philosopher*, the migration of animal species from the marine environment to dry land brought with it settling in fresh water of rivers and lakes, with the risk of excessive dilution of physiological fluids, from which we defended ourselves by developing an excretory apparatus capable of effectively diluting body fluids. By default, therefore, the kidney dilutes the urine: concentration is optional.

NOTE

Loop diuretics interfere with this process by inhibiting the reabsorption of NaCl at the level of the thick segment of the ascending limb that is located in the medullar part, thus reducing the interstitium osmolality of the latter. In this way the loop diuretics determine volume losses (Na^+ + water) followed by ADH increase and water reabsorption, which however is limited by the reduction of the interstitial osmolality and this means that hyponatremia from loop diuretics is rare. Thiazide diuretics, on the other hand, act at the distal tubules level, in the cortex, and therefore do not interfere with medullar osmolality. Following the loss of sodium and water the action of ADH can be expressed and the passage of water at the collecting ducts level, through the osmotic gradient, is not reduced. Therefore there is an effective loss of sodium and potassium in excess to water which is instead reabsorbed following the action of ADH (**Figure 8.7**).

The ultimate water regulation is decided in the last part of the tubular nephron, precisely in the distal tubule and especially in the collecting duct.

As we have mentioned, this section of the tubular nephron passes through the osmolal stratification up to the deepest levels of the medullar area where the interstitium is more concentrated thanks to the accumulation of urea. By itself the distal tubule and the collecting duct are almost impermeable to water, so if no other factors intervene the urine is eliminated diluted. The factor that gives the collecting duct the capability to change the osmolality and the volume of urine according to the needs of salt-water balance is the anti-diuretic hormone ADH.

Physiological function of ADH

ADH is a nonapeptide produced in the form of a precursor (pre-pro-ADH) in hypothalamic supraoptic (SON) and paraventricular nuclei (PVN) located adjacent to the nuclei that provide stimulation of thirst.

Post-translational modifications lead to the definitive

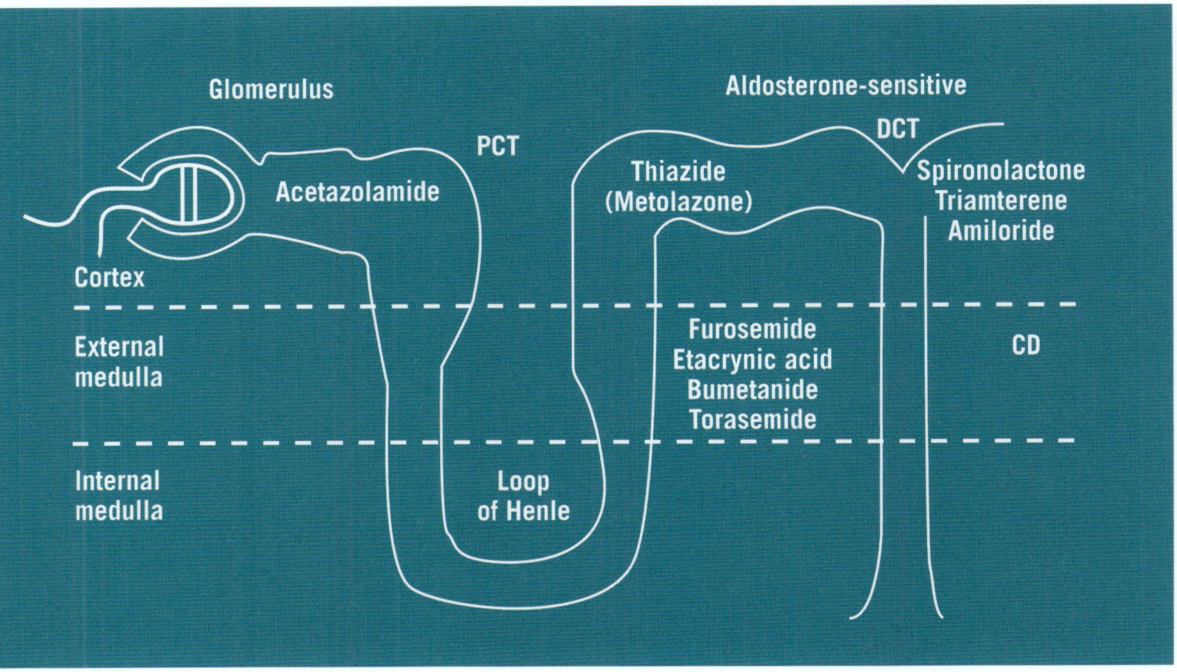

Figure 8.7 Sites of diuretics action in the tubule.
CD: collecting duct; DCT: distal convoluted tubule; PCT: proximal convoluted tubule.

hormone, which is conserved in neurosecretory granules in the posterior pituitary gland from which, if necessary, it can be rapidly released into the circulation thanks to the vascular patency of these structures. The most important physiological activity is the renal one. The mechanism by which ADH promotes the permeability of the collecting duct is the insertion, in the apical membrane of duct cells, of water channels called aquaporins. The AQP1, which we have already seen to adjust the permeability to water in the proximal tubule, is not sensitive to antidiuretic hormone, unlike the typical canal of distal nephron, aquaporin 2 (AQP2).

ADH, by promoting the insertion of water channels (aquaporin 2) in the membrane of main cells of the collecting duct, increases their permeability, balancing it with the surrounding interstitial hypertonicity and thus favoring reabsorption of water with consequent concentration of the urine that can reach 1200 mOsm/Kg H_2O (**Figure 8.8**).

The stimulus for ADH secretion is the increase in osmolality of body fluids, represented by plasmatic osmolality. The threshold for hormone secretion is around 284 mOsm/Kg H_2O. However, osmolality is not the only stimulus for the secretion of the antidiuretic hormone. Another stimulus is the decrease of the circulating extracellular volume or arterial pressure; this is important both because it lowers the osmolar threshold, and above all because if the hypovolemia remains or progresses, the non-osmotic release of ADH persists and rather increases even if facing a decrease in osmolality and hyponatremia.

ADH is also sensitive to several other neurological stimuli such as pain, nausea, and immune stress: the increase in circulating ADH is therefore not uncommon during surgical procedures, predisposing to hyponatremia in post-operative period.

Finally, there is integration between ADH and thirst in the regulation of water balance.

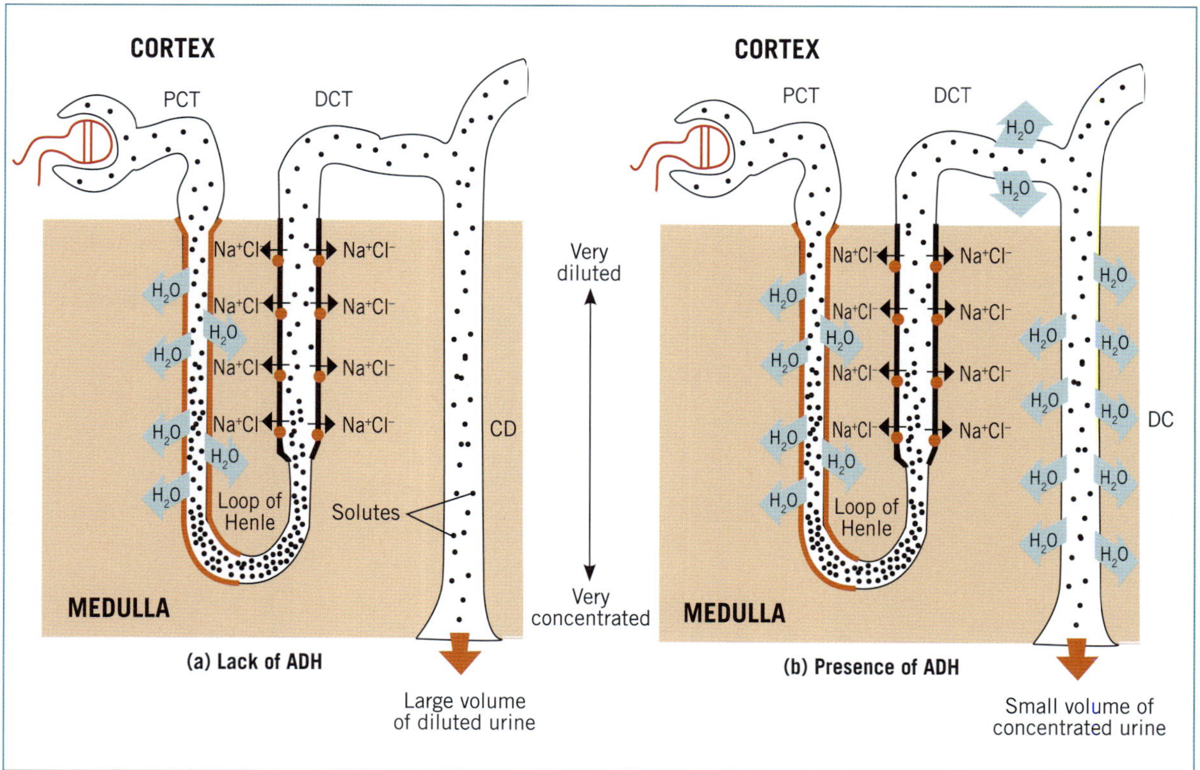

Figure 8.8 Physiological function of ADH at the collector duct level (modified from the web).

At plasma osmolality values around 295 mOsm/Kg the circulating ADH is 4-5 pmol/L and produces the maximum antidiuresis.

The additional defense against dehydration is entrusted to thirst, whose osmolar threshold is slightly higher than that for ADH, around 290 mOsm/Kg.

As we have seen, therefore, the homeostasis of body water and the osmolality of physiological fluids have very effective and sensitive regulatory mechanisms. Therefore, as we will see in the subsequent clinical chapters, a persistent water retention with consequent hyposmolality and hyponatremia can be observed, with rare exceptions, only if there is a serious incapacity of renal water elimination, as in the patient we presented at the beginning of this chapter, whose hyponatremia is due to the inability to adequately eliminate water due to the presence of compounds with antidiuretic activity produced by lung cancer (syndrome of inappropriate antidiuretic hormone secretion, SIADH). On the other hand, symptomatic hypernatremia may be due to alterations in the thirst mechanism or to the inability to access water. Therefore, as we have anticipated in the first pages of this chapter, the kidney has a wide capacity to regulate the body water balance and to maintain the organism's water compartments.

However, for this purpose it is also essential to regulate the metabolism of sodium and its anions.

Sodium regulation

As we have seen previously, total body sodium ($TBNa^+$) and extracellular compartment volume (ECF) are closely related. Since total sodium is the product of the sodium concentration in the ECF to the extracellular volume, and since natremia is regulated within very narrow limits, the signal for homeostatic regulation of sodium is the ECF, and the effector of this regulation is the urinary elimination of sodium.

However, it should be pointed out that in this regulation the ECF acts not with its overall volume, but with the part known as ECBV (effective circulating blood volume), an entity not easily definable in anatomical terms but rather understood in physiological terms as the part that perfuse the tissues, mainly identifiable with the intravascular part of the ECF.

The maintenance of the ECF is regulated by a variety and multiplicity of sensors that detect its volume changes: low and high pressure baroreceptors are distributed mainly in vascular structures and thoracic organs, but also in kidney, brain and liver (**Figure 8.9**).

No less rich is the set of effector processes that contribute to regulation of the ECF. At least four are the important effectors that contribute to renal regulation of sodium metabolism.

The most important and specific is the renin-angiotensin-aldosterone system (RAAS).

This mineralocorticoid acts at the level of the main cells of the nephron collecting duct, by binding to a specific cytoplasmic receptor, reducing the elimination of sodium and chloride, and increasing the excretion of potassium and ammonium.

Also of hormonal nature is the activity of ADH, which in addition to the main activity in the regulation of water, also acts by promoting sodium reabsorption both at the level of the loop of Henle where it stimulates the $Na^+K^+Cl^-$ co-transporter contributing to the interstitial hypertonicity, and at the level of the collecting duct, increasing the opening of the sodium channels in the apical membrane; of no less importance is the contribution of the atrial natriuretic peptide (ANP), whose natriuretic activity is distinguished from that of the other two hormones, which instead favor the renal reabsorption of sodium. These multiple hormonal activities are also accompanied by the activity of the sympathetic nervous system.

Water and sodium regulate ECF	
Sensors	Carotid sinus Atria Renal afferent arterioles
Effectors	Renin-angiotensin-aldosterone system (RAAS) Sympathetic nervous system Atrial natriuretic peptide and ADH
Action	Urinary sodium excretion

Figure 8.9 Water-sodium balance.

Other, less important and recently acquired factors demonstrate natriuretic activity. The recently acquired endogenous ATP inhibitor is an endogenous steroid that inhibits the Na^+/K^+ pump in a wide variety of cells and increases following a salt load and in patients with hypertension. It is thought that, in the presence of a salt load, this inhibitor acts preferentially in the collecting duct, favoring the elimination of sodium.

Furthermore prostaglandins, bradykinin and dopamine, produced locally in the kidney, act through the protein kinase C inhibiting sodium reabsorption, probably through phosphorylation of sodium and potassium channels. In conclusion, homeostasis of osmolality and of body fluids volume is entrusted to very effective and sensitive regulatory mechanisms, aware of the risks that alterations of both these properties can cause. The knowledge of these mechanisms of physiological regulation is imperative for correct treatment of salt-water balance disorders.

References

- Agrawal V, Agarwal M, Joshi SR et al. Hyponatremia and hypernatremia: disorders of water balance. J Assoc Physicians India. 2008;56:956-64.
- Alleva K, Chara O, Amodeo G. Aquaporins: another piece in the osmotic puzzle. FEBS Lett. 2012;586(19):2991-9.
- Bankir L, Bichet DG, Morgenthaler NG. Vasopressin: physiology, assessment and osmosensation. J Intern Med. 2017; 2824):284-97.
- Bhave G, Neilson EG. Body fluid dynamics: back to the future. J Am Soc Nephrol. 2011;22(12):2166-81.
- Eladari D, Chambrey R, Peti-Peterdi J: A new look at electrolyte transport in the distal tubule. Annu Rev Physiol 2012;74:325-49.
- Esposito P, Piotti G, Bianzina S et al. The syndrome of inappropriate antidiuresis: pathophysiology, clinical management and new therapeutic options. Nephron Clin Pract. 2011;119(1):c62-73.
- Frame AA, Wainford RD. Renal sodium handling and sodium sensitivity. Kidney Res Clin Pract. 2017;36(2):117-31.
- Frøkiaer J, Nielsen S, Knepper MA. Molecular physiology of renal aquaporins and sodium transporters: exciting approaches to understand regulation of renal water handling. J Am Soc Nephrol. 2005;16(10): 2827-9.
- Giebisch G, Windhager E. Urine concentration and dilution. In: Boron WF, Boulpaep EL. Medical Physiology. Elsevier Saunders 2005; Ch 37, 828.
- Giebisch G, Windhager E. Integration of salt and water balance. In: Boron WF, Boulpaep EL. Medical Physiology. Elsevier Saunders 2005; Ch 39, 861.
- Goldberg M. Hiponatremia. Med Clin North Am. 1981;65 (2):251-69.
- Hellerstein S. Fluids and electrolytes: Physiology. Pediatr Rev. 1993;14(2):70-9.
- Hoffert JD, Chou CL, Knepper MA. Aquaporin-2 in the "-omics" era. J Biol Chem. 2009;284(22):14683-7.
- Klein J, Blount MA, Sands JM. Pflügers Archives 2012; 464(6):561-72.
- Knepper MA, Kwon TH, Nielsen S. Molecular physiology of water balance. N Eng J Med. 2015;372(14): 1349-58.
- Loudon KW, Fry AC. The renal channelopathies. Ann Clin Biochem. 2014;51(Pt 4):441-58.
- Palmer BF, Alpern RJ. Integrated renal response to abnprmalities in tonicity. In: Seldin DW, Giebisch G (eds). Clinical Disorders of Water Metabolism. Raven Press 1993.
- Pfortmueller CA, Uehlinger D, von Haeling S, Schefold JC. Serum chloride levels in critical illness-the hidden story. Intensive Care Med Exp. 2018;6(1):10.
- Rahman SS, Boesen EI: Outside the mainstream: novel collecting duct proteins regulating water balance. Am J Physiol Renal Physiol. 2016;311(6):F1341-F1345.
- Ramin S, Iraj F. Understanding Hypernatremia. Am J Nephrol. 2012;36:97-104.
- Rose BD. The Regulation of plasma osmolality. In: Rose BD. Clinical physiology of acid-base and electrolyte disorders. 4th Ed. McGraw Hill 1994; Ch 9, 261.
- Rossier BC, Baker ME, Studer RA. Epithelial sodium transport and its control by aldosterone: the story of our internal environment revisited. Physiol Rev 2015;95(1):297-340.
- Roumelioti ME, Glew RH, Khitan ZJ et al. Fluid balance concepts in medicine: Principles and Practice. World J Nephrol. 2018;7(1):1-28.
- Sinke AP, Deen PM. The physiological implication of novel proteins in systemic osmoregulation. FASEB J. 2011; 25(10):3279-89.
- Stanhewicz AE, Kenney WL. Determinants of water and sodium intake and output. Nutr Rev. 2015;73 Suppl. 2:73-82.
- Wall SM. Renal intercalated cells and bood pressure regulation. Kidney Res Clin Pract. 2017;36(4):305-17.
- Weiner ID, Verlander JW. Recent advances in understanding renal ammonia metabolism and transport. Curr Opin Nephrol Hypertens. 2016;25(5):436-43.
- Zacchia M, Capolongo G, Rinaldi L et al. The importance of the thick ascending limb of Henle's loop in renal physiology and pathophysiology. Int J Nephrol Renovasc Dis. 2018;11:81-92.

Hyponatremia

Ivo Casagranda

Introduction to plasma sodium concentration disorders

The disorders that affect plasma sodium concentration are very frequent.

Hyponatremia is present in 15-20% of critically ill patients arriving in the emergency department and up to 30% of those hospitalized. It manifests itself at all ages and its causes are many. Hypernatremia is instead less frequent than hyponatremia and occurs mainly in young children and in elderly subjects, often due to difficult access to water or to a reduced perception of thirst. Before facing up to the study of natremia alterations, it is essential to read Chapter 8 on the physiology of salt and water. Of that chapter we would like to recall some contents that are essential for dealing with hypo- and hypernatremia.

1) Natremia

$$\text{plasma } [Na^+] = \frac{\text{total body sodium } (Na^+_e + K^+_e)}{\text{total body water}}$$

The equation explains that natremia is given by the ratio between total exchangeable body sodium and total body water. The exchangeable potassium is included in the equation because there may be a sodium shift, in the case of potassium reduction in the intracellular space. When we evaluate the pathological changes in natremia (hypo- or hypernatremia), we must consider them starting from denominator. They therefore depend on changes in total body water (TBW), regardless of total body sodium. As written in Chapter 8, alterations in sodium may be seen through the lens of water.

2) Cellular volume

Osmotic variations generally occur in the ECF and are determined by variations in sodium concentration which, in turn, since the cell membrane is semi-permeable, influences osmotic pressure of the ICF. It can therefore be said that the concentration of sodium in the ECF determines osmotic pressure in the ICF and therefore the cell volume.

3) Extracellular volume

Loss of sodium from the ECF (i.e., via the kidney) results in a reduction in the total body sodium and consequently a reduction in the total body water lost by the ECF together with sodium. The reduction of total body sodium is evidenced by the clinical and instrumental signs of hypovolemia (we will see how this will be important in the diagnosis of hyponatremia causes) and not by the values of natremia that can be normal, increased or decreased.

Definition

The term hyponatremia refers to the reduction of plasma sodium concentration $[Na^+]_p < 135$ mEq/L. The reduction is considered severe for values < 125 mEq/L, moderate for values between 125 and 129 mEq/L and slight between 130 and 135 mEq/L.

Pathophysiology

As previously stated, when referring to plasma sodium disorders, these must be seen through the lens of water. Hyponatremia is always due to an excess of total body water compared to the exchangeable total sodium which can be reduced, normal or even increased. For further explanations see Chapter 8 on the physiology of salt and water. Individual insights will be made by treating the specific disorder.

Classification

There are several classifications in literature based on the severity of hyponatremia, onset rate or symptoms. In this chapter a pathophysiological classification will be used (**Table 9.1**). Expressions such as "dilution hyponatremia" (which suggests excess water as one of the causes, while it is the cause in all cases of hyponatremia) are to be advised against "true hyponatremia" the only from sodium loss (which would suggest that "true" is the only one related to the loss of sodium), which only generate confusion.

Pseudohyponatremia

Pseudohyponatremia is due to a laboratory error in the determination of $[Na^+]_p$. In routine the analyzers for the determination of the electrolytes dilute the plasma samples in a test tube, all with the same amount of diluent. Normally the plasma consists of a 7% solid phase, essentially due to proteins, and an aqueous phase containing sodium and other electrolytes. The volume of diluent introduced by the analyzer is based on these concentrations. If a paraprotein (myeloma) or severe hypertriglyceridemia is present, the solid phase increases and the aqueous phase is reduced. Even in these cases the analyzer dilutes the aqueous part with the same volume, causing excessive dilution and thus causing a reduction in the electrolyte concentration, which is not real. The electrodes of the blood gas analyzers are exempt from this error since they determine electrolytes on whole (undiluted) blood. In the presence of hyperproteinemia, sodium can be corrected by 0.7 mEq/L for each g/dL of total protein increase.

Hypertonic hyponatremia

Hypertonic hyponatremia occurs when low molecular weight solutes accumulate in the ECF, as in the course of severe hyperglycemia in which there is a shift of water from the ICF to the ECF with dilution of all the solutes contained therein, including sodium.
There may be an apparent reduction in $[Na^+]_p$ of 1.6 mEq/L for every 100 mg/dL increase in blood glucose. The correction of sodium may be done with the following formula: [0.016 (blood glucose – 100)] + measured Na^+. Some Authors consider a correction index of 2.4 mEq/L more accurate, in particular for blood glucose levels above 400 mg/dL. Effective osmolality can be calculated as follows: effective osmolality (tonicity) (mOsm/Kg) = 2 × Na^+ (mEq/L) + K (mEq/L) + blood glucose (mg/dL)/18. In hypertonic hyponatremia, hypertonicity is due to excess glucose.

Isotonic hyponatremia

Isotonic hyponatremia is due to the presence of osmoles which can cause the shift of water from the from ICF to ECF. This occurs for example with the use of isotonic mannitol washing solutions in gynecological or urological interventions. In other cases the use of

TABLE 9.1 Hyponatremia classification.

Pathophysiological classification	Cause
Pseudohyponatremia	Laboratory error, it does not occur with the use of blood gas analyzers
Hypertonic hyponatremia	Accumulation of low molecular weight solutes (in the course of severe hyperglycemia)
Isotonic hyponatremia	The presence of osmoles that recalling water, determine hyponatremia; the fluid remains isotonic
Osmostatic hyponatremia	Reset of natremia physiological regulations point
Hypotonic hyponatremia	Kidney inability to eliminate water: • reduced ECF • normal ECF • increased ECF Excessive introduction of free water: normal or slightly increased ECF

solution with glycine and sorbitol can lower the serum sodium by increasing the extracellular fluid volume because of absorption of large quantity of fluid. In these cases there is hyponatremia with normal osmotic pressure values. Glycine and sorbitol, unlike mannitol, are then rapidly metabolized, resulting in hypotonicity, even severe, if utilization has been high.

Osmostatic hyponatremia

The osmostatic hyponatremia (or reset osmostat syndrome) is characterized by chronic hyponatremia due to a mechanism that determines a lower setting level of osmoceptors, which respond to lower than normal plasma osmolality levels. Since the capacity of the kidney to eliminate water is maintained, the sodium values are stable over time and are usually between 125 and 130 mEq/L. The causes of this syndrome are different: pregnancy, hypovolemic states, quadriplegia, psychosis, debilitating diseases and malnutrition, tuberculosis, encephalitis and malignant neoplasm.

Hypotonic hyponatremia (from inability of the kidney to eliminate water)

It is the most frequent type of hyponatremia and we will deal with it in detail. Water retention reflects in most cases the presence of causes that prevent the kidney from eliminating water, thus creating an excess of total body water, compared to the total body sodium that can be increased (expanded ECF), decreased (reduced ECF) or normal (unchanged ECF) (**Figure 9.1**).

Hypotonic hyponatremia (from excessive introduction of free water)

In this case the kidney is able to eliminate water, but the excessive introduction of free water exceeds the capacity of the kidney to eliminate it in sufficient quantities. These are cases that are not very frequent and are often also associated with difficult conditions of the kidney to eliminate water for the simultaneous intake of drugs that cause a syndrome of inappropriate antidiuresis (SIAD).

Clinical and laboratory approach in hypotonic hyponatremia

Contrary to what is normally done in texts, the clinical-laboratory approach precedes the description of the causes. This happens because some clinical cases of hypotonic hyponatremia will be presented for educational purposes, in the paragraphs where the causes will be illustrated and discussed, so it is necessary to precede the method that will be used for the diagnosis.

The clinical approach, with the signs and symptoms, is fundamental to stratify the severity of hyponatremia and to understand if the ECF is normal, increased or decreased, a very important element for the diagnosis. Furthermore, laboratory tests on plasma and urine are essential to understand the cause of hyponatremia.

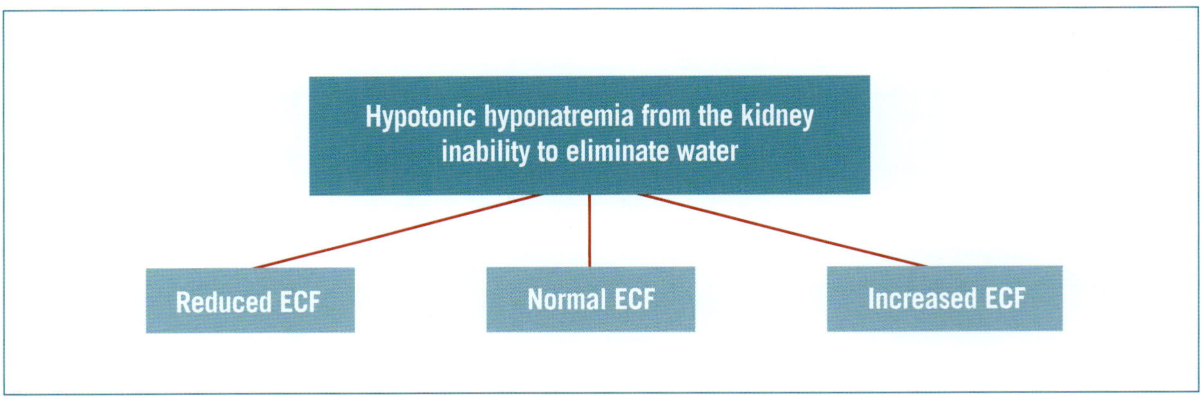

Figure 9.1 Hypotonic hyponatremia, kidney difficulty in eliminating water and ECF modifications.

Symptoms and signs of hypotonic hyponatremia

The symptoms and signs of hyponatremia may be the manifestation of two conditions (**Tables 9.2 and 9.3**):
1) the involvement of the central nervous system (CNS) and muscle cells due to edema caused by the passage of water from ECF to ICF (**Tables 9.2 B and 9.3 B**);
2) hypovolemia due to reduction of ECF that occurs in those conditions characterized by sodium and water loss through the renal or extra renal route and followed by appropriate ADH secretion (**Table 9.3 A**).

The symptoms and signs of involvement of the central nervous system depend on the extent of plasma sodium reduction but above all on the rapidity with which it is established.

Patients may present with modest symptoms such as a headache and asthenia or more severe manifestations such as seizures or coma and all indicate the presence of cerebral edema encephalopathy. In the case of normal ECF only neurological and muscular signs and symptoms may be present. If the reduction of natremia occurs very slowly so as to allow the adaptation of the brain cells to the conditions of hyposmolality of the ECF, the symptoms may be blurred or absent and the presence of random hyponatremia is detected. This occurs with some frequency in patients taking antidepressant drugs that inhibit serotonin reuptake (SSRIs) and are often implicated in SIAD. In the case of hypotonic hyponatremia accompanied by ECF reduction, in addition to symptoms related to cerebral and muscular involvement there may be signs and symptoms related to hypovolemia.

Sometimes these are not so obvious and you have to know how to look for them. Their highlighting is important because it allows you to orient yourself in defining the causes that led to hyponatremia.

In the suspicion of reduced ECF with symptoms and clinical signs that do not guide in a certain way it is appropriate to consider the central venous pressure. In these cases its measurement with the invasive classical method is not indicated but instead the calculation of

TABLE 9.2 Signs and symptoms of hypotonic hyponatremia with normal or increased ECF (A) and from CNS and muscle cell involvement (B).

Normal or increased ECF (A)	CNS and muscle cell involvement (B)
Absence of orthostatism Wet skin and mucous membranes Skin edema (in increased ECF) Normal or visible external jugular veins Normal or increased CVP	Headache Cerebral vomiting Seizure Coma Increased neuromuscular excitability Hyporeflexia and muscle flaccidity

TABLE 9.3 Signs and symptoms in the course of hypotonic hyponatremia with reduced ECF (A) and from CNS and muscle cell involvement (B).

Reduced ECF (A)	CNS and muscle cell involvement (B)
Presence of orthostatism Dehydrated skin and mucous membranes Thirst Flat external jugular veins Reduced CVP	Headache Cerebral vomiting Seizure Coma Increased neuromuscular excitability Hyporeflexia and muscle flaccidity

the caval index (inferior vena cava) is recommended by means of an ultrasound probe that can provide, in a very short time, useful indications. An index > 50% or a caval diameter < 10 mm at the end of expiration, in the presence of particular clinical-anamnestic conditions, can be used in the diagnosis of hypovolemic hyponatremia.

Laboratory tests

Laboratory tests are important for the diagnosis and management of hypotonic hyponatremia and **Table 9.4** shows those needed to be performed on serum and urine. The result of these tests allows us to construct a very useful algorithm for diagnostic purposes, where urinary osmolality or the specific gravity are fundamental in distinguishing the two groups of patients with hyponatremia, those with normal ability to eliminate water from the kidney (**Figure 9.2 A**) and those with reduced capacity (**Figure 9.2 B**). In the second group it is then the value of urinary sodium that allows to retrace the cause of the disorder.

NOTE

One way to convert the specific gravity into mOsm/Kg is to multiply the last two digits of the specific gravity (SG) by 32 (for example, SG 1012 = 32 × 12 = 384 mOsm/Kg). The result is reasonably approximate.

When the value of urinary osmolality is < 100 mOsm/Kg or the urinary specific gravity is ≤ 1,003 it means that the kidney is able to eliminate the water and therefore the reasons that have caused its excessive introduction or conditions that change receptor setting alteration of plasmatic osmolality (homeostatic reset syndrome) must be sought.

In cases (much more frequent) with a urinary osmolality > 100 mOsm/Kg or with a urinary specific gravity > 1,003, the kidney is not able to eliminate water due to the presence of ADH secreted in an appropriate or inappropriate manner.

In these situations the determination of urinary sodium is fundamental to trace the cause of hyponatremia.

If urinary sodium, which can be measured on an urine specimen (spot), is less than 20 mEq/L, the cause is due to hypovolemia or a reduction in effective arterial blood volume. When urinary sodium is higher than 40 mEq/L it is probable that there is a SIAD or a renal loss of sodium (*renal salt wasting*: RSW).

For the differential diagnosis, the anamnesis (pharmacological in particular), the clinical examination and the evaluation of the hematic volume (for example with the measurement of the vena cava diameter) are fundamental. If the urinary sodium is between 20-40 mEq/L and the clinical and instrumental components are lacking for a correct diagnostic orientation it is useful to administer two liters of normal saline solution in 48 hours. If natremia does not increase it is likely that there is a

TABLE 9.4 Blood and urine tests to be performed during hypotonic hyponatremia.

Serum tests	Urine tests (even spot)
Sodium Osmolality Urea Creatinine Urea/Creatinine ratio* Uric acid TSH (in selected cases) Cortisol (in selected cases)	Sodium Osmolality or specific gravity

* Reference values of U/Cr 12-20 (ratio between concentrations in mg). The decision values are < 10 and > 20. U/Cr > 20: prerenal failure (heart failure, dehydration, etc.); U/Cr < 10 : SIAD.

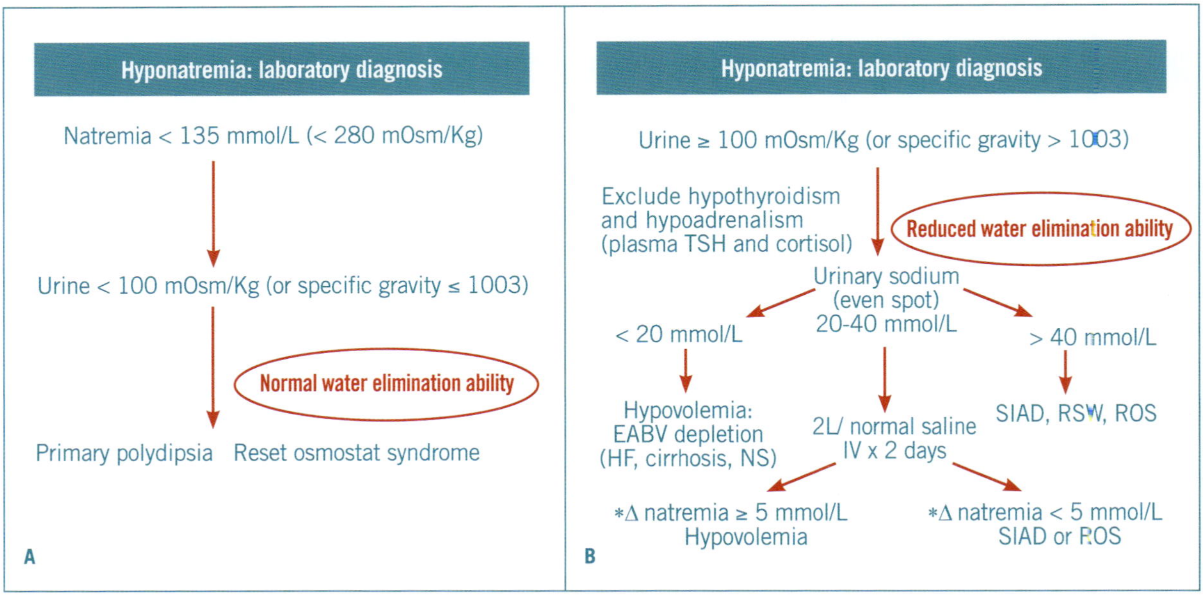

Figure 9.2 A, B Decision algorithm in determining the causes of hyponatremia (from Millionis et al., modified).
EABV: effective arterial blood volume; HF: heart failure; NS: nephrotic syndrome; ROS: reset osmostat syndrome; RSW: renal salt wasting; SIAD: syndrome of inappropriate antidiuresis.

SIAD, otherwise if it increases beyond 5 mEq/L it means that we are in the presence of causes that had led to a loss of volume (often via the kidney). Finally, if the differential diagnosis is not yet clear, the determination of plasma TSH and/or plasma cortisol may be useful.

NOTE

The increase in $[Na^+]_p$ after normal saline infusion is not due to the sodium administration (154 mEq/L) but to fluid volume contribution that causes an inhibition of the appropriate ADH secretion. In the case of SIAD the ability to eliminate sodium remains unchanged, not that of eliminating water due to the secretion of ADH that continues despite the increase in fluid volume (inappropriate secretion).
Therefore, when we administer a normal saline, water is eliminated with difficulty and this determines the lack of increase in sodium.

Causes of hypotonic hyponatremia

As previously written, hyponatremia is characterized by an excess of water in relation to the total sodium which can be reduced, normal or increased.
In some cases the cause is due to the difficulty of the kidney to eliminate free water, in others to an excessive ingestion of water with a normal renal excretory capacity.

Hyponatremia from kidney inability to eliminate water and its causes

The causes can be divided according to the changes provoked in ECF (**Figure 9.3**).
Some cause its decrease due to loss of fluids (Na^+ and H_2O) from the kidney or from another extra-renal site (i.e., bowel or third space), others lead to its increase and finally there are causes that do not provoke any change in ECF.

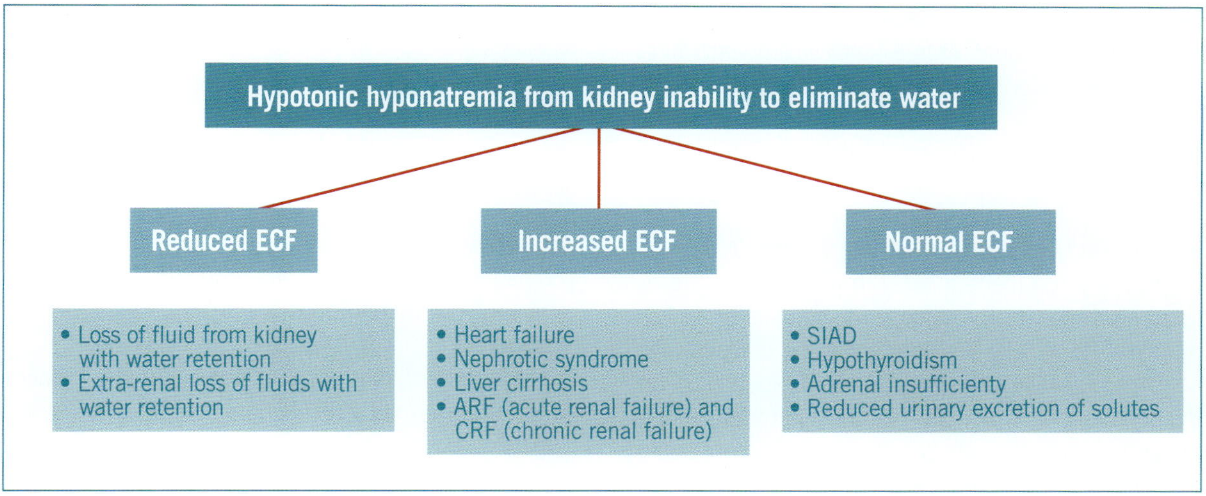

Figure 9.3. Causes of hypotonic hyponatremia and ECF status.

TABLE 9.5 Causes of hypotonic hyponatremia with reduced ECF.

Hypotonic hyponatremia from extra-renal fluid loss
Loss of gastrointestinal fluids (diarrhea, vomiting)
Loss of fluids in the "third space" (pancreatitis, peritonitis, ileus, muscle trauma)
Burns, bleeding
Excessive sweating. Exercise-associated hyponatremia (i.e., marathon runners)
Hypotonic hyponatremia due to renal fluid loss
Use of diuretics (especially thiazides)
Bicarbonate in urine (renal tubular acidosis and during vomiting)
Nephropathy with salt loss
Cerebral salt wasting syndrome (CSWS)
Adrenal insufficiency (mineralocorticoid deficiency)

Hypotonic hyponatremia with reduced ECF

The causes that determine hypotonic hyponatremia with reduced ECF are shown in **Table 9.5**.

The characteristic of this type of hyponatremia is the reduction of the total body sodium that determines a reduction of the ECF, but where in any case the water is in excess with respect to total body sodium.

Hypotonic hyponatremia due to extra renal fluid loss

In this case two situations can occur: the loss of hypotonic liquids (more water than sodium) and the loss of isotonic liquids compared to plasma. In both cases, the introduction of water electrolyte-free is necessary to show hypotonic hyponatremia. The loss of fluids containing sodium leads to a reduction in the extracellular volume with activation of the system that leads to the secretion of ADH. The secretion of ADH results in a greater reabsorption of free water which leads to excessive water retention in relation to total body sodium.

Hypotonic hyponatremia due to renal fluid loss

Hypotonic hyponatremia from diuretics

There are three mechanisms, in addition to water intake, attributed to the genesis of hyponatremia from diuretics (especially thiazides): volume depletion with activation of ADH secretion, potassium depletion and the consequent intracellular sodium shift and direct inhibition of urine dilution by reduced NaCl reabsorption at the loop of Henle and distal tubule.

It also appears that there may be a direct action on the release of ADH as well as it appears that diuretics increase the response of collecting ducts to ADH. Hypotonic hyponatremia due to diuretics concerns in particular older women taking thiazides.

NOTE

Loop diuretics (furosemide) rarely cause hyponatremia. If it is found in patients who are taking diuretics of this class, it is appropriate to exclude other causes before considering them responsible for hyponatremia (see Chapter 8, page 161).

Clinical case 1 A 75-year-old woman suffering from high blood pressure arrives in the emergency department because in the morning she had a pre-syncope while getting out of bed. For three weeks she has been suffering from weakness, muscle cramps and postural vertigo. For two months she has been taking hydrochlorothiazide 25 mg, which she had stopped taking for four days.

Vital signs BP 165/95 mmHg in supine position and 120/90 mmHg orthostatic, HR 102 bpm, RR 25 bpm, T 36.2 °C, GCS 15.

On physical examination, flat external jugular veins, dry skin and moderate dehydration of the mucous membranes.

Laboratory tests

Plasma: osmolality 252 mOsm/Kg, Na^+ 119 mEq/L, Cl^- 71 mEq/L, K^+ 2.1 mEq/L, HCO_3^- 34 mEq/L, U/Cr 50, uricemia 6.8 mg/dL;

Urine spot: osmolality 340 mOsm/Kg, Na^+ 4 mEq/L, K^+ 60 mEq/L.

Reasoned comment

The patient has severe hyponatremia. Plasma osmolality is very low, therefore we are dealing with hypotonic hyponatremia.

The osmolality of urine is > 100 mOsm/Kg, which means that the kidney has difficulty in eliminating free water. Urinary sodium is greatly reduced as it happens in the conditions of hypovolemia (left side of the algorithm, Figure 9.2 B). Clinically, the dehydrated skin and mucous membranes, the reduced jugular turgor and the orthostatic fall of pressure, point towards hypovolemia. This is secondary to thiazide diuretic use and urinary sodium is not high because the diuretic has been suspended for four days. From a pathophysiological point of view the administration of thiazides involves the loss of sodium and volume, which causes the stimulation (appropriate) of ADH with water retention and therefore hyponatremia. To this picture it also contributes the loss of K^+ which causes an intracellular shift of sodium. Furthermore, as is known, thiazide diuretics cause hyponatremia more frequently in elderly women.

Final diagnosis

Hypotonic hyponatremia with reduced ECF due to thiazide diuretics use.

Clinical case 2 A 74-year-old woman suffering from arterial hypertension arrives in the emergency room for ataxia and vertiginous syndrome that has ongoing for two days. For about a year she has been taking delapril 30 mg to which indapamide 2.5 mg has been associated for a month. The morning before arrival in the emergency department she took the antihypertensive therapy as usual. Vital signs BP 140/85 mmHg in supine position and 110/90 mmHg orthostatic, HR 98 bpm, RR 24 bpm, T 36.4 °C, GCS 14. On physical examination: confused but co-operative, dry skin, dry tongue with longitudinal furrows.

Laboratory tests

Plasma: osmolality 230 mOsm/Kg, Na^+ 115 mEq/L, Cl^- 77 mEq/L, K^+ 2.8 mEq/L, blood glucose 134 mg/dL, U/Cr 35; ABG: pH 7.49, $PaCO_2$ 36 mmHg, HCO_3^- 28 mEq/L; Urine spot: osmolality 450 mOsm/Kg, Na^+ 147 mEq/L, Cl^- 159 mEq/L, K^+ 65 mEq/L.

Reasoned comment

Very severe hyponatremia is present with reduced plasma osmolality which indicates hypotonic hyponatremia. The value of urine osmolality > 100 mOsm/L leads to an inability of the kidney to dilute the urine and urinary sodium of 147 mg/dL (the woman is taking a thiazide) suggests for RSW (right part of the algorithm, Figure 9.2 B). Since the physical examination suggests a condition of hypovolemia (reduced ECF) this is the most likely hypothesis.

Final diagnosis

Hypotonic hyponatremia from intake of a thiazide diuretic in an elderly woman.

NOTE

The two clinical cases are quite clear in their clinical and laboratory development. We wanted to show what happens from a laboratory point of view in the case of a suspended diuretic or diuretic intake and how the position in the algorithm varies.

Cerebral salt wasting syndrome

An interesting condition, although often underestimated, is the cerebral salt wasting syndrome (CSWS), due to inflammatory, vascular, tumor or traumatic cerebral lesions.

It was first described in 1950. These lesions determine the secretion of mediators (ANP, BNP) and also reduce α-adrenergic activity on juxtaglomerular cells and on the proximal convoluted tubule, whose final effect is sodium loss from the kidney without potassium loss. In fact, characteristically, in CSWS, blood potassium is normal.

Often the CSWS is confused with the syndrome of inappropriate antidiuresis (SIAD). Its identification is important because the therapeutic approach is different from that of the SIAD as in this the ECF is normal while in the CSWS it is reduced.

Clinical case 3 A 53-year-old man is taken to the emergency department for headache, vomiting and consciousness impairment. Two weeks earlier tubercular meningitis was diagnosed based on clinical data and on CSF and therefore started anti-tubercular therapy. Vital signs BP 135/75 mmHg, HR 105 bpm, RR 26 bpm, T 37.2 °C, GCS 13. On physical examination, dehydrated skin and mucous membranes and flat external jugular veins. Laboratory tests show Na^+ 118 mEq/L and blood creatinine 2.5 mg/dL. Considering dehydration, he is subjected to fluid replacement with normal saline solution, followed by an improvement in creatinine which goes to 1.0 mg/dL and natremia to 132 mEq/L. Diuresis 1900 mL/day.

After a few days the patient is discharged with hydrated skin and mucous membranes.

20 days later, new admittance to the emergency room for headache, vomiting and reduced consciousness level. Clinically, he still shows signs of dehydration in the presence of abundant diuresis (3 L/day).

BP 100/70 mmHg, HR 110 bpm, RR 32 bpm, T 37.4 °C, GCS 13.

Laboratory tests

Plasma: osmolality 250 mOsm/Kg, Na^+ 120 mEq/L, Cl^- 80 mEq/L, K^+ 4.2 mEq/L, creatinine 1.3 mg/dL, uricemia 3 mg/dL;

Urine: osmolality 260 mOsm/Kg, Na^+ 114 mEq/L.

Reasoned comment

The patient is on therapy for an infectious cerebral form. He arrives in the emergency department for important neurological symptoms with evidence of severe hyponatremia and kidney failure, for which he is hospitalized. During the first access, the therapy is aimed at restoring the fluid volume without following a thorough clinical reasoning: the volume, the dehydration and plasma sodium improve sufficiently to be discharged.

After 20 days he returns with symptoms and a clinical picture similar to the previous admittance. At this point the case is investigated in-depth. We are faced with a hypotonic hyponatremia with urine osmolality > 100 mOsm/Kg and a high urinary sodium (right side of the algorithm, Figure 9.2B).

The differential diagnosis is between SIAD and RSWS: the clinical picture of hypovolemia points toward RSWS. Considering the fact that the patient does not take diuretics and there is no obvious tubular damage, but he suffers from CNS disease, the CSWS hypothesis is the most probable.

Final diagnosis

***Cerebral salt wasting syndrome* in a patient with tubercular meningitis.**

Acute adrenal failure

Hyponatremia is present during adrenal failure. In the chronic form this is generally not serious and is often the only sign of the disease, while in the acute form it tends to be severe.

The cause is due to primary hypoaldosteronism that causes sodium loss, reduced ECF and hyponatremia with increased secretion of ADH. This form of presentation is the one requiring urgent treatment.

Clinical case 4 A 24-year-old man arrives in the emergency department in coma and in shock. Parents report being affected by chronic adrenal failure in replacement therapy. In the previous days he had fever, involvement of the upper airways, vomiting and diarrhea. Over the course of a few hours he had a rapid deterioration of the cognitive functions.

Vital signs. BP 70/? mmHg, HR 125 bpm, RR 32 bpm, T 38.4 °C, GCS 8. On physical examination dehydrated skin and mucous membranes, flat external jugular veins.

Laboratory tests

Plasma: osmolality 220 mOsm/Kg, Na^+ 107 mEq/L, Cl^- 74 mEq/L, K^+ 6.6 mEq/L, blood glucose 61 mg/dL, U/Cr 38;
Urine: osmolality 350 mOsm/Kg, Na^+ 130 mEq/L.

Reasoned comment

The clinical picture is quite clear. The man suffers from chronic adrenal failure in replacement treatment.

An infectious form, probably viral, was the "stress" cause leading to acute adrenal failure.

The significant decrease in plasma sodium was the cause of coma to which was added the circulatory shock due to significant ECF reduction.

Etiopathogenesis is confirmed by hypotonic hyponatremia and hyperkalemia.

Urinary osmolality is the mirror of sodium loss due to hypoaldosteronism and kidney failure to eliminate free water from the increase in ADH secretion.

Final diagnosis

Hypotonic hyponatremia due to acute adrenal failure (addisonian crisis).

TABLE 9.6 Causes of hypotonic hyponatremia with increased ECF.

Hyponatremia from EABV reduction
Congestive heart failure
Liver cirrhosis
Nephrotic syndrome
Hyponatremia due to acute or chronic renal failure
Acute tubular necrosis, acute glomerulonephritis, acute interstitial, vascular and obstructive forms
Chronic renal failure with or without salt loss
Hyponatremia in pregnancy (complex pathogenesis)

Hypotonic hyponatremia with increased ECF

This is a condition that occurs if there is a reduction in the effective arterial blood volume (EABV) or when renal function is severely compromised (**Table 9.6**).

In the case of EABV reduction due to both vasodilation and the shift of fluids from the vascular compartment to the extravascular compartment, caused by reduction of oncotic pressure (as happens in liver cirrhosis and in the nephrotic syndrome) or due to an increase in hydrostatic pressure (as in course of heart failure) there is an activation of the secretion of ADH. This determines an increased reabsorption of free water that causes an alteration of the sodium/water ratio and consequent hyponatremia.

In the case of alteration of the renal function there is an inability of the kidney to eliminate free water and this retention causes hyponatremia.

In pregnancy there can be different factors involved both related to water and sodium retention and others determining vasodilation with ECF reduction.

Hypotonic hyponatremia with normal ECF

This condition is characterized by situations in which the kidney is able to eliminate sodium but not free water (**Table 9.7**).

Syndrome of inappropriate antidiuresis

The syndrome of inappropriate antidiuresis (SIAD) or inappropriate ADH secretion (SIADH) is the most frequent condition of hypotonic hyponatremia. The syndrome is due to inappropriate and continuous secretion of ADH, centrally from the pituitary gland or from another ectopic site and/or a continuous action of the hormone on the receptors, despite osmolality or circulating blood volume being normal.

Some Authors prefer to use the acronym SIAD instead of the more common one of SIADH because numerous studies indicate that there is not always an increase in ADH secretion in correlation to plasmatic osmolality. We have used and will use the acronym SIAD because it seems more correct.

The causes of SIAD are numerous and can act by stimulating the pituitary secretion of ADH (brain lesions, drugs) or causing its ectopic production (cancer) or with strengthening effects on tubular receptors (drugs) (**Table 9.8**).

Many brain injuries can determine both CSWS and SIAD. The differential diagnosis is important (**Table 9.9**) because therapy is totally different: fluid replacement in the first case, water restriction in the second.

Clinical case 5 A 61-year-old man with diabetes is taken to the emergency department for generalized malaise, a growing confusion, and seizure. According to his wife, for several days the patient has

TABLE 9.7 Causes of hyponatremia with normal ECF.

SIAD or SIADH (syndrome of inappropriate antidiuresis or inappropriate ADH secretion)
Neoplastic diseases
Lung diseases
Alterations of the central nervous system
Drugs
Miscellaneous
Hypothyroidism
Hypoadrenalism
Low solute diet

TABLE 9.8. Most common causes of SIAD.

Neoplasm	Lung diseases	Drugs	Neurological diseases	Miscellaneous
• Pulmonary Small cells Mesothelioma • Cerebral • Gastrointestinal Oropharynx Stomach Duodenum Pancreas • Genitourinary Prostate Bladder Endometrium • Lymphomas	Cystic fibrosis Pneumonia (viral and bacterial) Parenchymal abscess Tuberculosis Aspergillosis COPD Respiratory failure with positive pressure ventilation	• Antipsychotic Phenothiazine Butyrophenone • Antidepressants SSRIs Tricyclic MAO inhibitors Venlafaxine • Antiepileptics Carbamazepine Sodium valproate Lamotrigine • Anticancer Vinca alkaloids Platinum compounds Ifosfamide Melphalan Cyclophosphamide Methotrexate Pentostatin • Analogues of the vasopressin • Miscellaneous ACE-inhibitors Chlorpropamide Proton pump inhibitors Interferon NSAIDs Clofibrate Nicotine Amiodarone Amphetamines and derivatives	Encephalitis Meningitis Intracranial hemorrhage Head trauma Abscess Guillain-Barré syndrome Multiple sclerosis HIV infections	Pain Stress Post-surgical Idiopathic Acute intermittent porphyria

TABLE 9.9 Differential diagnosis between CSWS and SIAD.

	CSWS	SIAD
ECF	Reduced	Normal
Potassium	Normal or increased	Normal
Uric acid	Normal or reduced	Reduced
Treatment	Normal saline solution	Water restriction

become increasingly confused, sleepy and unable to perform even the simplest tasks.
Medication history: metformin 500 mg twice a day and glyburide 2.5 mg/day. For 35 days he has been on antidepressant therapy with citalopram 20 mg, which he takes in the evening. Vital sign. BP 135/80 mmHg in clinostatism (orthostatic evaluation is not possible), HR 76 bpm, RR 18 bpm, T 36.4 °C, GCS 13.
Physical examination: normally hydrated skin and mucous membranes, normal external jugular veins, absence of edema.
Neurological examination: consciousness reduction, no focal neurological deficit but reduced strength in the lower extremities. Normal head CT and EEG.
Lower vena cava diameter: normal.

Laboratory tests

Plasma: osmolality 263 mOsm/Kg, Na^+ 120 mEq/L, Cl^- 86 mEq/L, K^+ 3.2 mEq/L, blood glucose 125 mg/dL, U/Cr 9, uric acid 3.5 mg/dL;
Urine: osmlality 450 mOsm/Kg, Na^+ 141 mEq/L.

Reasoned comment

The patient presents with severe hypotonic hyponatremia, in a neurological framework consistent with the water-electrolyte balance alteration. Urinary osmolality > 100 mOsm/Kg indicates a kidney with reduced ability to eliminate free water. High urinary sodium places the patient on the right side of the algorithm (differential diagnosis between SIAD and RSW). The clinical picture characterized by normal body fluid volume (normally hydrated mucous membranes, normal external jugular veins and normal vena cava diameter) points toward SIAD, also considering that the symptoms started after the beginning of citalopram therapy, whose ability is known to cause, as an adverse effect, an inappropriate antidiuresis.

Final diagnosis

SIAD caused by citalopram intake.

Clinical case 6 A 46-year-old woman with cerebral paralysis arrives in the emergency department for persistent fever. Her doctor had prescribed levofloxacin, considering probable an infection of the urinary tract. Despite this the temperature remained high (38.6 °C).
The patient has been nourished for nearly a year almost exclusively through a J-tube, to prevent aspiration complications. She is also affected by hypothyroidism treated with levothyroxine.
Neurological alterations have been present for some time and consist of spastic movements and a posture characterized by dystonia.
Family members report that the patient was hospitalized several times due to fever and that the tests were always negative.
Hyponatremia has been present for about 5 years. Occasionally she takes NSAIDs.
Vital signs BP 135/80 mmHg, HR 76 bpm, RR 18 bpm, T 37.4 °C, GCS 14. On physical examination, normally hydrated skin and mucous membranes, normal external jugular veins, there is no skin edema.

Laboratory tests

Plasma: osmolality 263 mOsm/Kg, Na^+ 129 mEq/L, Cl^- 90 mEq/L, K^+ 4.1 mEq/L, blood glucose 89 mg/dL, U/Cr 28, uric acid 5.6 mg/dL, normal TSH and thyroid hormones;
Urine: osmolality 550 mOsm/Kg, Na^+ 120 mEq/L.

Following the finding of hyponatremia that dates back many years, SIAD is suspected. To confirm this diagnostic doubt the patient is subjected to water restriction, but after two days a natremia check still shows 131 mEq/L. At this point a plasma cortisol dosage is required which turns out normal.
Drug review does not lead to any association between these and SIAD. The hypothesis of reset osmostat syndrome therefore arises. A water load test is programmed.
One liter of this is administered in over thirty minutes through the J-tube, followed by a decrease in urine osmolality (< 100 mOsm/Kg) and sodium (20 mEq/L) after 30 and 90 minutes with repositioning of osmolality to the starting values after 24 hours.
The test demonstrates the ability to maximally dilute the urine with ADH suppression. Thus the diagnosis of ROS (reset osmostat syndrome) is confirmed.

Reasoned comment

The woman presents hypotonic hyponatremia in a complex neurological picture. Urinary osmolality is high and so is urinary sodium.

This places the patient on to the right side of the algorithm in differential diagnosis with SIAD, RSW and ROS. RSW is to be excluded because there are no signs of dehydration/hypovolemia.

The whole picture might suggest SIAD also in consideration of the neurological pathology.

Since the prolonged water restriction did not cause any change in natremia, it was thought of ROS. The per os water load test showed that the kidney is able to dilute the urine (which is not the case in SIAD), confirming the suspected diagnosis.

Final diagnosis

Reset osmostat syndrome in a patient with cerebral paralysis.

Hypothyroidism

The pathogenesis of hypotonic hyponatremia in hypothyroidism is unclear. Since cardiac output and GFR are often reduced in these patients, there may be an increase in ADH secretion, together with an alteration of the osmotic gradient at the kidney medulla with a reduction in free water production. Furthermore, it is believed that cortisol control over ADH secretion is deficient. Hyponatremia during isolated hypothyroidism, in the absence of other comorbidities, is very rare. In cases where the cause of hypotonic hyponatremia with normal volume cannot be defined, the dosage of TSH is indicated. In these patients hormonal therapy is resolutive.

Hypoadrenalism (adrenal failure)

Hyponatremia is a frequent complication of hypoadrenalism to which two main factors contribute: hypoaldosteronism which causes renal sodium loss and cortisol deficiency which causes an increase in ADH secretion and water retention according to the following mechanism: ADH stimulates ACTH secretion and is co-secreted with CRH (corticotropin releasing hormone); cortisol causes negative feedback on the release of ADH and CRH and when this is deficient the inhibition exercised lowers and consequently increases the secretion of ADH. Beyond the forms of acute adrenal failure of which we have spoken above, the chronic forms are usually paucisymptomatic and suspected just because of hyponatremia.

Low solute diet

A particular condition that can be observed is hyponatremia in patients, especially the elderly, who follow a low solute diet (tea and toast diet) or in heavy beer drinkers who introduce large quantities of fluids with low solute content. Since the kidney requires solutes to eliminate water, if these are deficient, as in the situations described above, the elimination of free water is made difficult.

Hyponatremia due to excessive introduction of free water and its causes

In these cases the kidney is functionally normal and water intake voluntary or involuntary is excessive (**Figure 9.4**).

The most frequent disorder is primary polydipsia characterized by a compulsive water intake.

Normally in these patients the values of natremia are moderately reduced, but they can decrease significantly following the intake of large quantities of water, in a short period of time. In these conditions the osmolality of the urine is < 100 mOsm/Kg.

Psychotic patients with polydipsia have a greater risk of hyponatremia because they often take antipsychotic drugs that can cause SIAD.

The increased water ingestion added to the difficulty in its elimination easily causes hypotonic hyponatremia, often severe. In these cases the urine could have an osmolality > 100 mOsm/Kg.

Clinical case 7 A 32-year-old woman, suffering from a severe psychotic illness, arrives in the emergency department due to confusion and alternating periods of delirium. From the history it results that the woman is in chronic treatment with short-acting

Referred to specific causes

- Aviram A, Pfau A, Czaczkes JW et al. Hyperosmolality with hyponatremia, caused by inappropriate administration of mannitol. Am J Med. 1967;42(4):648-50.
- Brimioulle S, Orellana-Jimenez C, Aminian A et al. Hyponatremia in neurological patients: cerebral salt wasting versus inappropriate antidiuretic hormone secretion. Intensive Care Med. 2008;34(1):125-31.
- Budisavljevic MN, Stewart L, Sahn SA et al. Hyponatremia associated with 3,4-methylenedioxymethylamphetamine ("Ecstasy") abuse. Am J Med Sci. 2003;326(2):89-93.
- Chow KM, Kwan BC, Szeto CC. Clinical studies of thiazide-induced hyponatremia. J Natl Med Assoc. 2004;96(10):1305-8.
- Clark BA, Shannon RP, Rosa RM et al. Increased susceptibility to thiazide-induced hyponatremia in the elderly. J Am Soc Nephrol. 1994;5(4):1106-11.
- Goldman MB, Luchins DJ, Robertson GL. Mechanisms of altered water metabolism in psychotic patients with polydipsia and hyponatremia. N Engl J Med. 1988;318(7):397-403.
- Goldman MB, Robertson GL, Luchins DJ et al. The influence of polydipsia on water excretion in hyponatremic, polydipsic, schizophrenic patients. J Clin Endocrinol Metab. 1996;81(4):1465-70.
- Gowrishankar M, Lin SH, Mallie JP et al. Acute hyponatremia in the perioperative period: insights into its pathophysiology and recommendations for management. Clin Nephrol. 1998;50(6):352-60.
- Hanna FW, Scanlon MF. Hyponatraemia, hypothyroidism, and role of arginine-vasopressin. Lancet. 1997;350(9080):755-6.
- Hariprasad MK, Eisinger RP, Nadler IM et al. Hyponatremia in psychogenic polydipsia. Arch Intern Med. 1980;140 (12):1639-42.
- Hill AR, Uribarri J, Mann J et al. Altered water metabolism in tuberculosis: role of vasopressin. Am J Med. 1990; 88(4): 357-64.
- Kahn T. Reset osmostat and salt and water retention in the course of severe hyponatremia. Medicine (Baltimore). 2003;82(3):170-6.
- Liamis G, Milionis H, Elisaf M. A review of drug-induced hyponatremia. Am J Kidney Dis. 2008;52(1):144-53.
- Olchovsky D, Ezra D, Vered I et al. Symptomatic hyponatremia as a presenting sign of hypothalamic-pituitary disease: a syndrome of inappropriate secretion of antidiuretic hormone (SIADH)-like glucocorticosteroid responsive condition. J Endocrinol Invest. 2005;28(2):151-6.
- Ramos-Levi AM, Duran Rodriguez-Hervada A, Mendez-Bailon M et al. Drug-induced hyponatremia: an updated review. Minerva Endocrinol. 2014;39(1):1-12.
- Rodenburg EM, Hoorn EJ, Ruiter R et al. Thiazide-associated hyponatremia: a population-based study. Am J Kidney Dis. 2013;62(1):67-72.
- Smith JP, Burren C, Cherinet Y. Extreme hyponatraemia with intact neurological outcome in a young child with Addison's disease. BMJ Case Rep. 2011.
- Sørensen JB, Andersen MK, Hansen HH. Syndrome of inappropriate secretion of antidiuretic hormone (SIADH) in malignant disease. J Intern Med. 1995;238(2):97-110.
- Sterns RH, Silver SM. Cerebral salt wasting versus SIADH: what difference? J Am Soc Nephrol. 2008;19(2):194-6.
- Thaler SM, Teitelbaum I, Berl T. "Beer potomania" in non-beer drinkers: effect of low dietary solute intake. Am J Kidney Dis. 1998;31(6):1028-31.

Refered to treatment

- Angeli P, Wong F, Watson H et al. Hyponatremia in cirrhosis: Results of a patient population survey. Hepatology. 2006;44(6):1535-42.
- Bajaj JS, Tandon P, O'Leary JG et al. The Impact of Albumin Use on Resolution of Hyponatremia in Hospitalized Patients With Cirrhosis. Am J Gastroenterol. 2018;113(9):1339.
- Gerbes AL, Gülberg V, Ginès P et al. Therapy of hyponatremia in cirrhosis with a vasopressin receptor antagonist: a randomized double-blind multicenter trial. Gastroenterology. 2003;124(4):933-9.
- Ginès P, Guevara M. Hyponatremia in cirrhosis: pathogenesis, clinical significance, and management. Hepatology. 2008;48(3):1002-10.
- Konstam MA, Gheorghiade M, Burnett JC Jr et al. Effects of oral tolvaptan in patients hospitalized for worsening heart failure: the EVEREST Outcome Trial. JAMA. 2007;297(12):1319-31.
- Lee WH, Packer M. Prognostic importance of serum sodium concentration and its modification by converting-enzyme inhibition in patients with severe chronic heart failure. Circulation. 1986;73(2):257-67.
- Lin SH, Chau T, Wu CC et al. Osmotic demyelination syndrome after correction of chronic hyponatremia with normal saline. Am J Med Sci. 2002;323(5):259-62.
- Patel S, Nguyen DS, Rastogi A et al. Treatment of Cirrhosis-Associated Hyponatremia with Midodrine and Octreotide. Front Med (Lausanne). 2017;4:17.
- Rozen-Zvi B, Yahav D, Gheorghiade M et al. Vasopressin receptor antagonists for the treatment of hyponatremia: systematic review and meta-analysis. Am J Kidney Dis. 2010;56(2):325-37.
- Schuster M, Diekmann S, Klingebiel R et al. Central pontine myelinolysis despite slow sodium rise in a case of severe community-acquired hyponatraemia. Anaesthesia Intensive Care. 2009;37(1):117-20.
- Snell DM, Bartley C. Osmotic demyelination syndrome following rapid correction of hyponatraemia. Anaesthesia. 2008;63(1):92-5.
- Sterns RH, Nigwekar SU, Hix JK. The treatment of hyponatremia. Semin Nephrol. 2009;29(3):282-99.
- Verbalis JG, Goldsmith SR, Greenberg A et al. Hyponatremia treatment guidelines 2007: expert panel recommendations. Am J Med. 2007;120(11 Suppl 1):S1-21.
- Verbalis JG, Greenberg A, Burst V et al. Diagnosing and Treating the Syndrome of Inappropriate Antidiuretic Hormone Secretion. Am J Med. 2016;129(5):537.e9-537.e23.

CHAPTER 10

Hypernatremia

Ivo Casagranda

Definition

Hypernatremia is, an electrolyte disorder characterized by a plasma sodium concentration $[Na^+]_p > 145$ mEq/L.
In the western countries, this disorder mainly affects the elderly and in some cases the pediatric population.

Pathophysiology

As already highlighted in Chapters 8 and 9, when referring to plasma sodium disorders, these must be seen through the "lens" of water. In fact, hypernatremia is in almost all cases due to a relative deficit of free water in the body (reduction of total body water) and almost never to an excess of sodium.
It can therefore be said that hypernatremia is not a problem of sodium homeostasis, but a problem of water deficit. During hypernatremia there is a passage of water from the ICF to the ECF clinically evidenced by the signs of dehydration.

NOTE

Often the terms dehydration and hypovolemia are used interchangeably.
In fact dehydration means a water deficit compared to the total body sodium that causes hypernatremia which is followed by a water deficit in the ICF while hypovolemia is a reduction of fluids in the ECF and in the vascular spaces due to loss of water and sodium (or blood)
Frequently the two disorders coexist.

Classification

Hypernatremia can be classified into hypernatremia due to lack of water introduction, loss of free water or hypotonic fluids and salt overload (**Figure 10.1**):

- *Hypernatremia due to lack of water introduction.* This is a very frequent condition and concerns in particular the elderly population or patients with mental disorders, with an altered perception of the sense of thirst. Another cause may be the difficulty in procuring water despite having a normal perception of thirst and this concerns people who are bedridden, in particular the elderly or infants.
- *Hypernatremia due to fluid loss.* The loss can consist of water without electrolytes (free water) or with electrolytes (sodium and potassium) at a lower concentration than that of plasma (hypotonic fluids). The route of elimination can be renal or extra-renal. Failure to replace losses leads to hypernatremia.
- *Hypernatremia due to salt overload.* It is due to the introduction of excess salt into the body, either through enteral or parenteral administration.

Causes of hypernatremia

The causes of hypernatremia are shown in **Table 10.1**. They are divided according to the classification just seen. Whatever the cause, it is the inadequate supply of water that is crucial in the development and subsequent maintenance of hypernatremia.

Lack of water intake

This condition, which we repeat is quite frequent and may also be associated to the use of diuretics, to insensible or sensible losses of water, has been defined above.

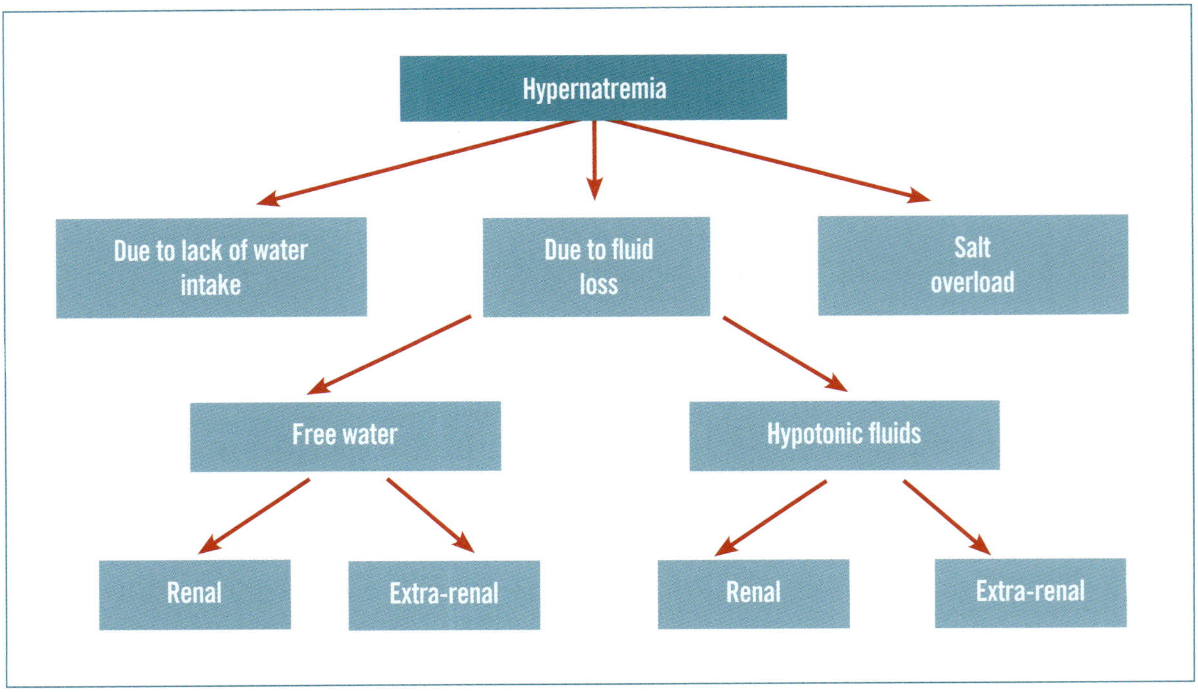

Figure 10.1. Classification of hypernatremia.

TABLE 10.1 Causes of hypernatremia.

Lack of water intake	Loss of free water	Loss of hypotonic fluids	Sodium overload	Rare causes due to water intracellular shift
Hypodipsia of the elderly Guests in a nursing home Inpatients at the hospital	*Renal route* • Central diabetes insipidus • Nephrogenic diabetes insipidus • Pregnancy • Adipsic diabetes insipidus	*Renal route* • Use of loop diuretics • Polyuria during restoration of renal function • Osmotic diuresis	• Administration of hypertonic saline solutions • Sodium intake per os for an emetic purpose • Primary hyperaldosteronism • Cushing syndrome	• Generalized seizure • Intense physical exercise • Rhabdomyolysis
	Extra-renal route • Insensible losses (fever, closed environments with high temperatures) • Burns	*Extra-renal route* • Excessive sweating • Osmotic diarrhea • Vomiting • Use of lactulose for cathartic purposes		

Renal loss of free water

Diabetes insipidus

It is caused by a decreased release of ADH (central diabetes insipidus) or by a resistance of the renal tubule to the action of ADH (nephrogenic diabetes insipidus). The value of $[Na^+]_p$ depends on the replacement capacity for lost water: in some cases it may be normal, in others it may be high and it reaches the highest values in the case of patients with concomitant alteration of the mechanism of thirst and with inability to release ADH (adipsic diabetes insipidus).

Hypernatremia in pregnancy

It occurs in the second half of pregnancy, in women with increased activity of placental vasopressinase or with central diabetes insipidus or subclinical nephrogenic that is evident during pregnancy.

Extra-renal loss of free water

Insensible losses

They are caused by water loss due to transepithelial diffusion with the mechanism of evaporation and not with that of sweating.

Water loss can be significant and if not supported by adequate introduction of water it causes significant hypernatremia. This does not happen with the elimination of water by the respiratory route because this is equal to the quantity produced by the final metabolism of carbohydrates and fatty acids (CO_2 + H_2O). Often there is concomitance of water loss through the transepthelial route and the glandular route with sweat (sensible loss).

Renal loss of hypotonic fluids

Diuretics use

Loop diuretics cause the loss of hypotonic urine. Hypernatremia from loop diuretics is relatively rare and may occur in elderly patients with multiple diseases who do not drink enough water.

Osmotic diuresis

It is caused by the presence of non-reabsorbable solutes as is the case of glucose in diabetic ketoacidosis or hyperosmolar hyperglycemic syndrome or following the administration of parenteral mannitol or urea during the period of uremia resolution. In these cases, there is a loss of fluids with a lower electrolyte concentration than plasma (hypotonic fluids).

Polyuria due to restoration of renal function

It occurs during the restoration phase of a tubular damage (i.e., from hypokalemia). At this stage there can be an important loss of water, sodium and potassium. The mechanism is due to a delayed restoration of tubular cellular function.

Extra-renal loss of hypotonic fluids

Sweating

Sweat is hypotonic compared to plasma (Na^+ ~ 40 mEq/L and K^+ 5 mEq/L). During abundant and prolonged sweating $[Na^+]_p$ increases. As for the other cases, hypernatremia occurs when adequate water intake is lacking.

Diarrhea

Hypernatremia can occur in osmotic diarrhea (i.e. malabsorption pathologies) where there is a loss of hypotonic fluids, while it does not occur in the secretory ones (i.e., cholera, VIPoma) where lost fluids are isotonic compared to plasma.

Use of lactulose

The use of lactulose for cathartic purposes, in particular if in large quantities and not followed by water intake, can lead to a considerable loss of water from the intestine, mainly with an osmotic type mechanism.

Sodium overload

These are infrequent situations due to particularly high sodium intake as can occur as a result of infusion of a sodium bicarbonate hypertonic solution in children or by oral administration, more often accidental, of sodium chloride in newborns. Even more rarely it can happen in adults as a result of incorrect administration of hypertonic saline solutions or by ingestion of hypertonic saline solutions for emetic purposes or gargling. In these cases the patients have an increase in ECF and intravascular volume, a urine osmolality > 600 mOsm/Kg and a urinary sodium > 100 mEq/L.

Rare causes

Intracellular water shift

It is very likely due to an increase in intracellular osmolality, as can occur during a generalized epileptic seizure or following intense exercise or, more rarely, during rhabdomyolysis.

Clinical and laboratory approach to hypernatremia

Symptoms and signs of hypernatremia

The symptoms and signs are primarily linked to the involvement of the central nervous system. Following the onset of hypernatremia there is loss of water from the brain with a reduction in the volume of brain cells and consequent suffering of the same with the appearance of functional alterations (**Table 10.2**). Furthermore, the loss of water from ICF determines a high concentration of potassium which causes symptoms such as fatigue, muscle flaccidity, tendon hyporeflexia. In addition to the described symptoms and signs there are those related to salt and water depletion (**Table 10.3**).

NOTE

Brain volume reduction can cause brain vein rupture, subarachnoid hemorrhage, the consequences of which can be serious. The examination of the cerebrospinal fluid can show, in these cases, the presence of blood.

The symptoms and signs of salt and water depletion are related to water loss from the ICF and the ECF. In the event of only free water loss (i.e. insensible losses) the signs of hypovolemia appear late, because in these cases about two thirds of the water comes from the ICF.

TABLE 10.2 Signs and symptoms of CNS involvement caused by hypernatremia.

Mild	Moderate	Severe
Irritability Restlessness Mental state alteration	Disorientation Confusion	Stupor state Comitial seizure Coma Death

TABLE 10.3 Signs and symptoms of water-saline depletion.

Water-saline depletion	Mild	Moderate	Severe
Signs and symptoms			
Pulse	Normal	Tachycardia	Tachycardia
Systolic arterial pressure	Normal	Normal or moderately reduced	Reduced > 20 mmHg
Postural hypotension	No	Yes/No	Yes
External jugular veins	Normal	Normal	Flat
Dry tongue and mucous membranes	No	Moderate	Severe
Skin turgor	Normal	Discrete	Very reduced
Tension of the eyeballs	Normal	Slightly reduced	Reduced
Thirst	Not increased	Increased	Very increased

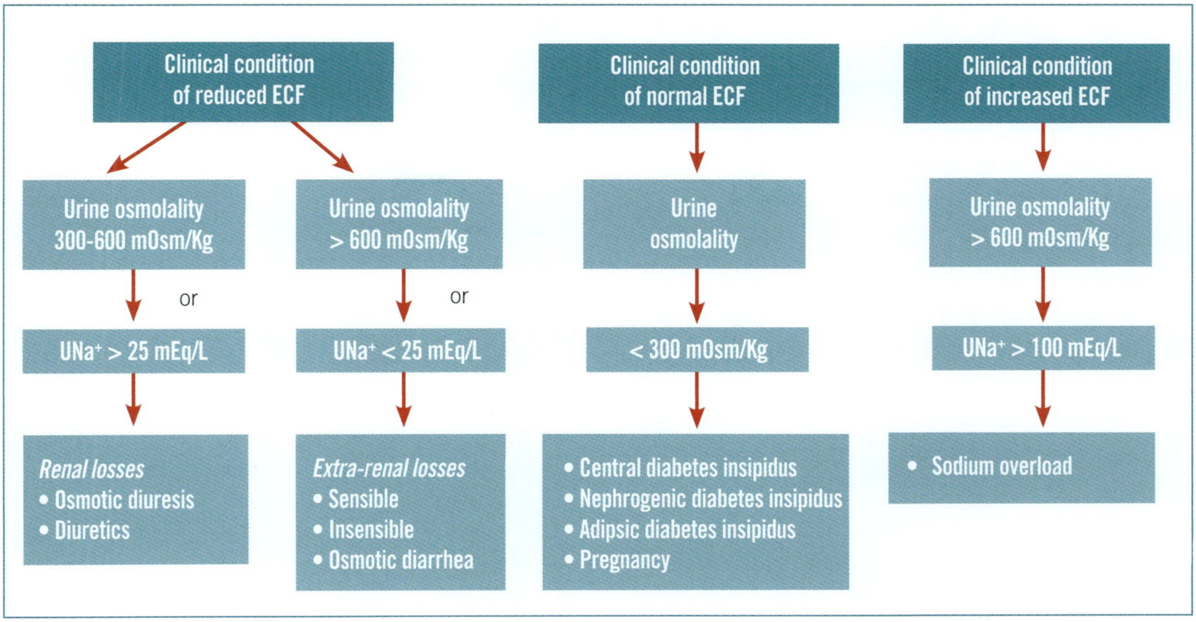

Figure 10.2 Useful algorithm for the diagnostic orientation of the causes of hypernatremia.

Laboratory tests

Some laboratory tests are fundamental both for the diagnosis and the etiology of hypernatremia and to set up the treatment. Beyond the $[Na^+]_p$, it is important to determine plasma osmolality, urinary sodium and urine osmolality. In addition, plasma potassium, creatinine, urea, urea/creatinine ratio and blood glucose are fundamental tests.

Diagnosis and differential diagnosis

The diagnosis of hypernatremia mainly relies on clinical findings and laboratory tests. The clinical presentation very often allows a fairly clear orientation in detecting the conditions of dehydration and hypovolemia. A correct request for laboratory tests, along with their interpretation, allows us to confirm the clinical suspicion and can direct us towards the cause that led to the event.

The use of the following algorithm allows a rational use of the laboratory tests and permits to reach the correct diagnosis in most cases (**Figure 10.2**).

Clinical cases

Two commented clinical cases follow showing how to apply the concepts expressed above. The same cases will then be used to discuss the treatment.

Clinical case 1 An 84-year-old woman in a nursing home suffers from chronic cognitive deficit and Parkinson's disease. For about four days, her general condition has worsened with an increase in cognitive impairment and confusion. For about 30 days she has had a fever of unclear origin for which she has taken antibiotic therapy. She feeds with difficulty and tends to refuse water intake.

Over the past two days she has had several episodes of diarrhea and a couple of episodes of vomiting. Following this, she is sent to the local emergency department. On physical examination dehydrated mucous membranes, reduction of skin turgor, flat jugular veins. Estimated body weight 50 Kg. Vital signs BP 105/88 mmHg, HR 102 bpm, RR 26 bpm, T 37.6 °C, SpO_2 94% on room air, GCS 13. The ultrasound examination shows a reduction in the diameter of the inferior vena cava. Research is required on the *C. difficile* toxin which will result negative later.

Laboratory tests

Plasma: osmolality 330 mOsm/Kg, Na^+ 165 mEq/L, Cl^- 122 mEq/L, K^+ 4.4 mEq/L, U/Cr 26;
Urine spot: osmolality 612 mOsm/Kg, Na^+ 21 mEq/L.

Reasoned comment

The patient represents a classic case of transepithelial free water loss with lack of fluid replacement.
The physical examination directs towards a severe reduction of the ICF with reduction also of the ECF probably secondary to diarrhea and vomiting. Laboratory tests show a high plasma osmolarity due to severe hypernatremia, a high urine osmolality with urinary sodium of just under 25 mEq/L. The reduced urinary sodium confirms the volume deficit.

Final diagnosis

Hypernatremia secondary to "insensible" extra-renal loss of water to which is probably added the loss of hypotonic fluids from diarrhea and vomiting.

Clinical case 2 A 68-year-old man is taken to the emergency department due to confusion that has worsened in the recent days.
The patient has been on therapy for at least 6 years with lithium for a chronic bipolar disorder with the indication to maintain a serum concentration of 0.8-1.2 mmol/L. Relatives affirm the presence of abundant diuresis and "watery" urine.
On physical examination modest reduction of skin turgor, dehydrated mucous membranes and moderately filled jugular veins. Estimated body weight 70 Kg. Vital signs BP 130/75 mmHg, HR 96 bpm, RR 29 bpm, T 36 °C, SpO_2 96% on room air, GCS 13. Dosage of blood lithium is requested, which resulted then 1.4 mmol/L.

Laboratory tests

Plasma: osmolality 330 mOsm/Kg, Na^+ 168 mEq/L, Cl^- 122 mEq/L, K^+ 3.6 mEq/L, blood glucose 98 mg/dL, U/Cr 18.
Urine spot: osmolality 98 mOsm/Kg, Na^+ 58 mEq/L.

Reasoned comment

The clinical picture shows a loss of water from the ICF with moderate maintenance of the ECF. Laboratory tests show a high plasma osmolality due to hypernatremia and a low urine osmolality with urinary sodium of 58 mEq/L. In consideration of the chronic intake of lithium (with values slightly above the therapeutic range), clinical data and laboratory examination, the diagnostic address is defined.

Final diagnosis

Hypernatremia caused by free water loss from the kidney (renal loss) in a patient with suspected nephrogenic diabetes insipidus due to lithium intake.

Treatment

The goal of therapy is to bring natremia back within the limits of normality by administering fluids and eliminating the causes that produced it. An important point to note is that this reduction must occur slowly (0.5 mEq/L/h) and must decrease to less than 12 mEq/L in the 24 hours. Rapid correction can cause cerebral edema with permanent damage, due to the rapid passage of water from the ECF to the brain cells. Rapid correction of natremia (1 mEq/L/h) is recommended in acute sodium overload. If there is a condition of symptomatic hypovolemia, this should be corrected first with normal saline solution.

NOTE

A recent (2019) analysis of the literature shows that a more rapid correction of hypernatremia is not associated with greater risk of mortality, convulsive episodes, alterations of consciousness and cerebral edema.

When hypernatremia is due to loss of free water, a 5% dextrose solution is administered. Glucose is rapidly metabolized and water remains for two thirds in the ICF one third in the ECF and 1/12 in the vascular space. The same result is obtained, in a more physiological way, with the administration of tap water per os, if the patient succeeds in drinking, or through a nasogastric tube in the opposite case.

During central or nephrogenic diabetes insipidus if hypernatremia is present, there must be a restoration of free water losses with the administration of 5% dextrose solution. In central diabetes insipidus, next to the restoration of water-electrolyte alterations, the administration of desmopressin is then indicated.

When hypernatremia is due to loss of hypotonic fluids, after correcting any symptomatic hypovolemia, the use of 0.45% NaCl saline solution is indicated. Also in this case natremia should decrease to less than 12 mEq/L in 24 hours.

NOTE

The 0.9% NaCl saline solution remains entirely in the ECF of which 1/4 in the blood vessels while as regards the 0.45% NaCl saline solution, 50% is place in ICF and the other 50% in ECF.

In the management of hypernatremia it is useful to calculate the total water deficit which gives an idea of the quantity of fluids that should be replaced. This calculation is obtained as follows:

$$\text{CBW} \times \frac{\text{(actual plasma sodium)}}{140} - 1 \quad (1)$$

where for CBW (current body water) is meant the total body water in liters, which in male is 60% of body weight, while in female it is about 50%. In the dehydrated person it is advisable to reduce this percentage by about 10%.

In clinical practice to use correctly the 5% dextrose solution or the 0.45% NaCl saline solution, so as to reduce the plasma sodium according to the needs and without incurring the risk of reducing it too quickly, it is used, as already written in the Chapter on hyponatremia, the formula proposed by Adrogué and Madias.

$$\Delta \text{Na}^+ = \frac{(\text{plasma Na}^+) - (\text{infused Na}^+)}{\text{TBW} + 1} \quad (2)$$

ΔNa^+ is the change in sodium concentration obtained with an infusion of a liter of the chosen solution. The (infused Na^+) is that contained in a liter of solution which in the case of the 5% dextrose solution will be 0 mEq, while for the 0.45% NaCl saline solution will be 77 mEq. TBW is the total body water.

The infusion rate is obtained with the following proportion:

1000 : ΔNa = X : desired reduction of PNa/mEq/L/h

where X stands for the infusion rate.

Clinical cases

As already mentioned above, at the end of the treatment section we will try to describe the management of the two cases described above.

The 84-year-old woman (*Clinical case 1*) had an "insensible" loss of free water and most likely also of hypotonic fluids from osmotic diarrhea secondary to the use of antibiotics and vomiting. The ICF is certainly reduced as well as the ECF even if the present hypovolemia is not symptomatic. Therefore, the most appropriate solution to use could be the 0.45% saline solution where 50% is available in the ECF and 50% in the ICF.

The water deficit is about:

$$0.40 \times 50 \text{ Kg} \times (165/140 - 1) = 3.57 \text{ L} \quad (1)$$

To correctly reduce hypernatremia we use the formula:

$$(165 - 77) / 26 = 3.36 \text{ mEq/L} \quad (2)$$

The infusion rate in mL per hour, if we want to reduce the natremia by 0.5 mEq/L/h will be:

1000 mL : 3.36 mEq/L = X : 0.5 mEq/L = 148 mL/h of 0.45% NaCl saline solution

It is always recommended to check the natremia at least every three hours.

The 62-year-old man (*Clinical case 2*), with probable nephrogenic diabetes insipidus due to lithium intake had a significant water loss through the kidney, with reduced ICF and good maintenance of the ECF. Therefore, having essentially lost free water, the 5% dextrose solution is indicated for the correction of sodium.

The presumed loss of water is:

$$0.50 \times 70 \text{ Kg} \times (168/140 - 1) = 7 \text{ L} \qquad (1)$$

To correctly reduce hypernatremia we use the formula:

$$(168 - 0) / 43 = 3 \text{ mEq/L} \qquad (2)$$

The infusion rate in mL/h, if we want to reduce the natremia by 0.5 mEq/L/h, will be:

1000 mL : 3.90 mEq/L = X : 0.5 mEq/L = 128 mL/h of 5% dextrose solution

The specific therapy and the suspension of lithium administration will follow.

References

- Adrogue HJ, Madias NE. Hypernatremia. N Engl J Med. 2000;342(20):1493-9.
- Ayus JC, Arieff AI. Abnormalities of water metabolism in the elderly. Semin Nephrol 1996;16(4):277-88.
- Chassagne P, Druesne L, Capet C et al. Clinical presentation of hypernatremia in elderly patients: a case control study. J Am Geriatr Soc. 2006;54(8):1225-30.
- Chauhan K, Pattharanitima P, Patel N. Rate of Correction of Hypernatremia and Health Outcomes in Critically Ill Patients. Clin J Am Soc Nephrol. 2019;14(5):656-63.
- Eisenberg Y, Frohman LA. Adipsic diabetes insipidus: A review. Endocr Pract. 2016;22(1):76-83.
- Emmett M. Dehydration versus volume depletion. Kidney Int. 2005;68(1):412-3.
- Gipstein RM, Boyle JD. Hypernatremia complicating prolonged mannitol diuresis. N Engl J Med. 1965;272:1116-7.
- Hawkins RC. Age and gender as risk factors for hyponatremia and hypernatremia. Clin Chim Acta. 2003. 337(1-2):169-72.
- Hughes F, Mythen M, Montgomery H. The sensitivity of the human thirst response to changes in plasma osmolality: a systematic review. Perioper Med (Lond). 2018;7:1.
- Kugler JP, Hustead T. Hyponatremia and Hypernatremia in the elderly. Am Fam Physician 2000;61(12):3623-30.
- Lameire N. The pathophysiology of acute renal failure. Crit Care Clin. 2005;21(2):197-210.
- Liamis G, Filippatos TD, Elisaf MS. Evaluation and treatment of hypernatremia: a practical guide for physicians. Postgrad Med. 2016;128(3):299-306.
- Liamis G, Tsimihodimos V, Doumas M et al. Clinical and laboratory characteristics of hypernatraemia in an internal medicine clinic. Nephrol Dial Transplant. 2008;23(1):136-43.
- Lindinger MI, Heigenhauser GJ, McKelvie RS et al. Blood ion regulation during repeated maximal exercise and recovery in humans. Am J Physiol. 1992;262(1 Pt 2):R126-36.
- Lindner G, Funk GC. Hypernatremia in critically ill patients. J Crit Care. 2013;28(2):216.e11-20.
- Mange K, Matsuura D, Cizman B et al. Language guiding therapy: the case of dehydration versus volume depletion. Ann Intern Med. 1997;127(9):848-53.
- Mavrakis AN, Tritos NA. Diabetes insipidus with deficient thirst: report of a patient and review of the literature. Am J Kidney Dis. 2008;51(5):851-9.
- Moder KG1, Hurley DL. Fatal hypernatremia from exogenous salt intake: report of a case and review of the literature. Mayo Clin Proc. 1990;65(12):1587-94.
- Muhsin SA, Mount DB. Diagnosis and treatment of hypernatremia. Best Pract Res Clin Endocrinol Metab. 2016;30 (2):189-203.
- Nanji AA, Lauener RW. Lactulose-induced hypernatremia. Drug Intell Clin Pharm. 1984;18(1):70-1.
- Nelson DC, McGrew WR Jr, Hoyumpa AM Jr. Hypernatremia and lactulose therapy. JAMA. 1983;249(10):1295-8.
- Palevsky PM. Hypernatremia. Semin Nephrol. 1998;18(1): 20-30.
- Palevsky PM, Bhagrath R, Greenberg A. Hypernatremia in hospitalized patients. Ann Intern Med. 1996;124(2):197-203.
- Pfennig CL, Slovis CM. Sodium disorders in the emergency department: a review of hyponatremia and hypernatremia. Emerg Med Pract. 2012;14(10):1-26.
- Phillips PA, Bretherton M, Johnston CI et al. Reduced osmotic thirst in healthy elderly men. Am J Physiol. 1991;261(1 Pt 2):R166-71.
- Rose BD, Post TW. Clinical Physiology of Acid-Base and Electrolyte Disorders. 5th ed. New York, McGraw-Hill 2001.
- Sands JM, Bichet DG; American College of Physicians; American Physiological Society. Nephrogenic diabetes insipidus. Ann Intern Med. 2006;144(3):186-94.
- Schwartz IL, Thaysen JH. Excretion of sodium and potassium in human sweat. J Clin Invest. 1956;35(1):114-20.
- Shah MK, Workeneh B, Taffet GE. Hypernatremia in the geriatric population. Clin Interv Aging. 2014;9:1987-92.
- Snyder NA, Feigal DW, Arieff AI. Hypernatremia in elderly patients. A heterogeneous, morbid, and iatrogenic entity. Ann Intern Med. 1987;107(3):309-19.
- Sterns RH. Disorders of plasma sodium--causes, consequences, and correction. N Engl J Med 2015;372(1):55-65.
- Sterns RH, Evidence for Managing Hypernatremia: Is It Just Hyponatremia in Reverse? Clin J Am Soc Nephrol. 2019;14(5):645-47.
- Zaworski J, Delannoy PY, Boussekey N et al. Lithium: one drug, five complications. J Intensive Care. 2017;5:70.

The use of fluids in clinical practice

Ivo Casagranda

Introduction

The use of fluids is a frequent practice in clinical medicine and in particular in emergency and critical care medicine. There are many types of solutions available that are often used without a particular rationale. In this chapter we will try to describe the main solutions available on market, the rationale for their use and indications. While dealing with some issues concerning emergency medicine, the hemodynamic aspects or the instrumental methods for their evaluation following the use of fluids will not be studied in depth, referring to specific texts or scientific articles.

Anatomy of body fluids and their composition

In Chapter 8 the anatomy of body fluids and their composition has already been described. These topics are summarized here to encourage greater understanding with reference to the use of fluids.

Water makes up about 60% of the adult male body weight and 50% of the female, tending to decrease with age.

Total body water (TBW) is divided into two main compartments: intracellular (ICF or intracellular fluid) and extracellular (ECF or extracellular fluid).

The latter is in turn divided into the interstitium, which constitutes the environment where cells live, and into the vascular space where the fluids circulate. In the ICF 2/3 of the water is found, while 1/3 will be in the ECF, of which 3/4 in the interstitium, while only 1/4 is circulating in the blood vessels (1/12 of the TBW).

As an example, a 70 Kg man will have an TBW of about 42 liters of which 28 will reside in the ICF and 14 in the ECF, of which about 3.5 in the vascular space (**Figure 11.1**).

The electrolytes are dissolved in body water, in different proportions between them and depending on whether they are in the ECF or in the ICF (**Table 11.1**). The main ions are sodium and potassium; the sodium content is almost entirely confined to the extracellular compartment, while potassium is prevalent in the intracellular volume. The ions present in the water, and in particular the sodium in the ECF and the potassium in the ICF, exert an equivalent osmotic pressure which, expressed as osmolality, is about 280 mOsm/Kg H_2O.

Since the cell membrane that separates the two compartments behaves like a semi-permeable membrane (permeable to water but not to solutes), the water is in equilibrium in the two systems. Since it is the extracellular compartment that can vary its own osmolality, it is clear that the cells are affected by these variations, increasing their volume if the surrounding environment is hypotonic or reducing it if it is hypertonic.

Glucose is also responsible for the osmolality of the ECF, but this varies only in the case of a substantial increase in glucose concentration.

Intracellular	**Extracellular**	
28 L	**Interstitium**	**Vessels**
	10.5 L	**3.5 L**

Figure 11.1. Water distribution in the ICF and ECF.

TABLE 11.1 Concentration of electrolytes in serum, in serum water and in interstitial and intracellular fluids.

Electrolytes (mEq/L)	Circulating fluid Serum	Serum water	Interstitial fluid	Intracellular fluid
Cations				
Sodium (Na^+)	142	152.7	145	10
Potassium (K^+)	4	4.3	4.1	160
Calcium (Ca^{++})	5	5.4	5	2
Magnesium (Mg^{++})	2	2.2	2	26
Total cations	153	164.6	156	198
Anions				
Chloride (Cl^-)	101	108.5	114	3
Bicarbonate (HCO_3^-)	27	29.3	31	10
Phosphate (HPO_4)	2	2.2	2	100
Sulfate (SO^4)	1	1	1	20
Organic acids	6	6.4	7	
Proteins	16	17.2	1	65
Total anions	153	164.6	156	198

The same is true for urea, which, however, being able to cross the membrane in both directions, does not actually contribute to the osmotic pressure of the ECF. Therefore the osmolality of the ECF can be expressed in this way:

$$(Na^+ \times 2) + \frac{\text{blood glucose}}{18} = 290 \text{ mOsm/Kg}$$

Since, as just written, the component related to urea is not considered, the osmolality thus expressed coincides with the tonicity which is the effective osmotic pressure. These notes of fluid anatomy and physiology are important to understand how the solutions that are introduced directly into the circulatory system can behave. In this regard, another element to keep in mind is vascular permeability (capillary).

In fact there is a continuous exchange of water, electrolytes and other molecules between the vascular space and the interstitial one, and this occurs at the level of the capillaries and post-capillary venules (so-called exchange vessels).

The mechanisms involved are hydrostatic pressure, oncotic pressure and permeability of the vessel wall, which is limited by the integrity of endothelial cells and glycocalyx.

As shown in **Figure 11.2**, there are two opposing hydrostatic forces: capillary hydrostatic pressure (Pc) and tissue interstitial pressure (Pi).

Since Pc is generally greater than Pi the fluids come out of the capillaries.

The other two opposing forces are the oncotic ones: the capillary oncotic pressure (ϖc) and the interstitial oncotic pressure (ϖi). Since $\varpi c > \varpi i$, liquids are reabsorbed from the interstitium into the capillary. Consequently, if fluids with high oncotic pressure are put into circulation, they will remain in the vascular tree for a long time. If vascular endothelium and glycocalyx were damaged (i.e., during severe sepsis or septic shock, major trauma, major surgical procedures and in diabetic ketoacidosis) the capillary oncotic pressure would play a minimal role because there would be a passage of an important quantity of protein-enriched plasma from the vessel into the interstitium, minimizing the oncotic pressure gradient, with fluid loss and interstitial edema, at constant hydrostatic pressure gradient.

Fluids used in clinical practice

Fluids have been used in critically ill patients for almost two centuries, particularly in the treatment of various types of shock. In the last few decades, several have appeared and much has been debated about which ones are most suitable for critically ill patients.

As shown in Table 11.1 a "physiological" solution, similar in composition to the aqueous component of the serum, should contain 153 mEq/L of Na^+, 109 mEq/L of Cl^-, 4.3 mEq/L of K^+, 5.4 mEq/L of Ca^{++} and 2.2 mEq/L of Mg^{++}. Checking the composition of the fluids that are commonly used in clinical practice, only few approach the composition of the aqueous part of the serum (**Table 11.2**).

In the market there are many types of solutions with indications for their use, not always based on efficacy studies. Beyond this, the solutions currently available to clinicians can refer to two large groups: crystalloids and colloids.

Crystalloids

The fluids that contain substances (electrolytes) capable of forming crystals are called crystalloids.

These substances pass easily through the vascular endothelium followed by water, redistributing between vessels and interstitium. The solutions may contain a variety of inorganic cations such as Na^+, K^+, Ca^{++}, Mg^{++}, inorganic anions such as Cl^- and organic anions such as lactate, acetate or bicarbonate. The normotonic crystalloids, once infused, are totally arranged in the ECF: 1/3 in the blood and 2/3 in the interstitium. If we infuse 1000 cc of 0.9% NaCl saline solution, 250 mL will remain intravascular and 750 will end up in the interstitium (**Figure 11.3**). Nothing will enter in the intracellular area.

Crystalloids are cheap, expand the extracellular compartment, restore interstitial fluids and determine a transient hemodynamic improvement (20-30 minutes). On the other hand, they often cause peripheral edemas and can cause pulmonary edema due to protein dilution and increase in pulmonary artery occlusion pressure.

The first-choice products are the 0.9% NaCl saline solution (so-called physiological) and the Ringer lactate (so-called balanced solution). Another well-balanced solution is the Plasma-Lyte 148®, although its use is not particularly widespread.

0.9% saline solution (normal saline)

It is the most prescribed crystalloid in clinical practice. It is slightly hypertonic with respect to plasma and due

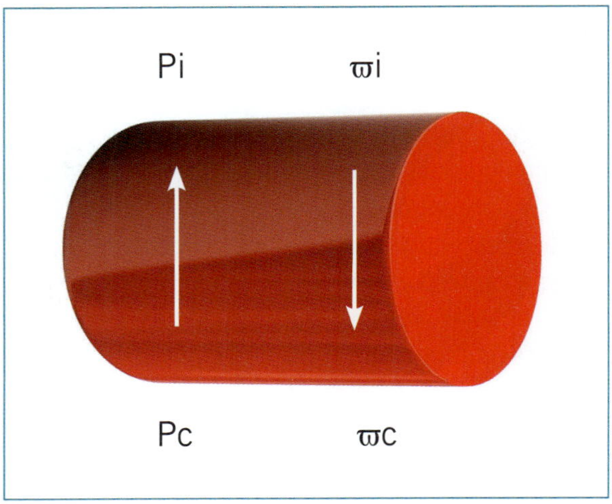

Figure 11.2 Pi interstitial hydrostatic pressure; Pc capillary hydrostatic pressure; ϖi interstitial oncotic pressure; ϖc capillary oncotic pressure.

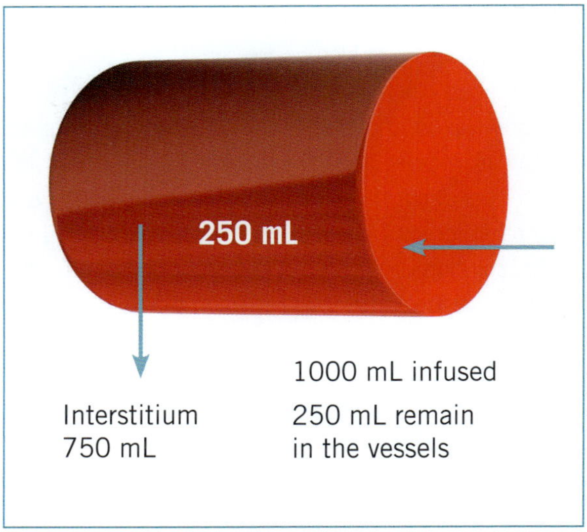

Figure 11.3 Infusion of 0.9% NaCl saline solution.

TABLE 11.2 Composition of the main solutions used in clinical practice.

	Plasma	Crystalloids			Colloids	
		NaCl 0.9%	**Ringer's lactate**	**Plasma-Lyte 148®**	**Voluven®**	**Haemaccel®**
Na^+ (mEq/L)	142	154	130	140	154	145
Cl^- (mEq/L)	103	154	109	98	154	145
K^+ (mEq/L)	4.5	0	4	5	0	5.1
Ca^{++} (mEq/L)	5.0	0	5.4	0	0	12.50
Mg^{++} (mEq/L)	2.5	0	0	3.0	0	0
Buffer (mEq/L)	24	0	28	27/23	0	0
Oncotic pressure (mmHg)	0	0	0	0	36	35-39
Osmolality (mOsmol/Kg)	288	286	254		N/A	
Osmolarity (mOsmol/L)	291	308	273	294	308	301
pH	7.4	5.0	6.5	7.4	4.0-5.5	7.3 ± 0.3

to its content it is not very "physiological" inclosing an excess of sodium but above all of chloride; moreover it is totally lacking in buffers and has a pH of 5.0. This solution initially called "indifferent", then "normal" and finally "physiological" derives from studies conducted by Hamburger on hemolysis in the years 1882-1883. Since in this solution the red blood cells lysis occurs less, led him to believe that the concentration of salts in human blood was 0.9%, instead of the actual one which is 0.6%.
If infused with high volumes it causes hyperchloremic metabolic acidosis, due, according to Stewart's theory, to the infusion of a "strong ion" such as chloride.
Chloride excess can also cause renal vasoconstriction with reduced glomerular filtration.
The survival in the circulation is short: studies on healthy volunteers have shown that after the infusion of two liters of normal saline in 1-2 hours, the intravascular retention was about 20%. After 6 hours only 13% of the solution remained in the intravascular space, with 60% of the same still present in the ECF.

Ringer's lactate

It is a balanced solution. In reality it is neither balanced nor isotonic, having an osmolality of 254 mOsm/Kg (hypotonic) and a concentration of sodium lower than plasma. This solution, like the other balanced ones, does not cause metabolic acidosis or renal vasoconstriction, thanks to a concentration of the chloride ion similar to plasma. Being a hypotonic solution with respect to the plasma it can determine both the passage of water in the brain and an increase in diuresis, thus reducing the survival time in the ECF. Theoretically reduced tonicity could create problems in some types of critically ill patients (i.e., with head trauma).

Plasma-Lyte 148®

This solution that has an osmolarity, a concentration of Na^+ and Cl^- and a pH that can be superimposed to those of the plasma could obviate the problems reported above. Recent studies (2016) seem to confirm this hypothesis.

Hypertonic saline solution

Hypertonic solution is defined as any saline solution with salt concentration > 0.9%.
The theoretical advantages of its use concern the hemodynamic response in shock conditions with the infusion of small volumes, the reduction of intracranial pressure, improvement of microcirculation and immunomodulation.
These advantages, along with some disadvantages, are described in **Table 11.3**. This type of solution has been proved effective in the treatment of patients with head trauma, in those with hemorrhagic shock and during hyponatremia with neurological symptoms. In the treat-

TABLE 11.3 Advantages and disadvantages of hypertonic saline solution.

Advantages	Disadvantages
• Reduces intracranial pressure • Improves cerebral perfusion pressure • Improves hemodynamics in shock with small volumes • Improves microcirculation • Immunomodulatory activity • Vasoregulation activity • Low cost	• Theoretical risk of osmotic demyelination • Rebound increase in intracranial pressure • Increase of mean arterial pressure and bleeding worsening in patients with uncontrolled bleeding

ment of the first two conditions small volumes (250 mL or 4 mL/Kg) of NaCl 7.5% solution (2400 mOsmol/L) are infused alone or in combination with dextran (**Figure 11.4**).

While showing effective action in the two conditions described, in the case of head trauma, a meta-analysis published in 2011 by Tan highlighted how the use of hypertonic solution has not been shown to be superior compared to the normal saline in terms of mortality and neurological outcomes.

Regarding hemorrhagic shock, this solution rapidly improves the hemodynamic conditions but there is no sufficiently strong evidence to indicate its routine use in patients with hemorrhagic trauma shock.

In the case of hyponatremia with neurological symptoms, the most commonly infused hypertonic solution is the 3%. For indications on its use and infusion methods, see Chapter 9.

Hypotonic solutions

They are solutions with a lower tonicity than plasma. The most used is the 0.45% NaCl saline solution, which is distributed 50% in the ECF and 50% in the ICF. The 5% dextrose solution (**Figure 11.5**) is an isotonic solution that becomes hypotonic once the glucose is metabolized when released into the circulation. For this reason its infusion is equivalent to the infusion of free water and therefore the distribution of one liter

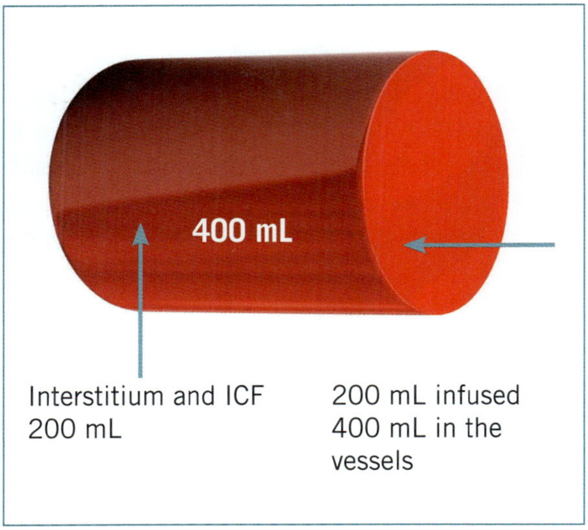

Figure 11.4 Infusion of 7.5% NaCl hypertonic saline solution.

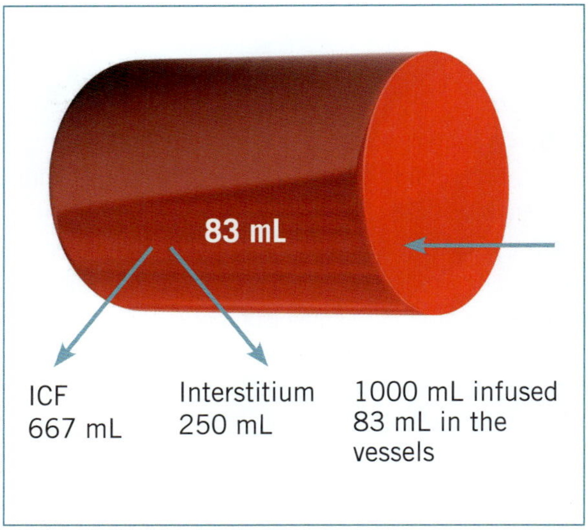

Figure 11.5. Infusion of 1000 mL of 5% dextrose solution.

of glucose solution will be 2/3 in the ICF and 1/3 in the ECF.

Therefore, its use is aimed at restoring intracellular water (i.e., in case of dehydration), while it has almost no influence on volume filling. If we administer 1 liter of 5% dextrose solution, 667 mL will go to the ICF and only 333 mL to the ECF, of which just 83 mL to the blood vessels (1/12).

Colloids

A colloidal solution is an aqueous solution containing both organic macromolecules and electrolytes. These macromolecules do not pass the endothelial membrane of the vessels and increase the oncotic pressure, thus leading to water retention in the intravascular space. The most used colloids are albumin, gelatin, dextran and hydroxyethyl starch (HES).

Human albumin

Human albumin is marketed at different concentrations (4-5-20-25%) in saline solution.

The concentration at 4 or 5% is considered the reference for colloidal solutions. An important limitation is given by the high cost.

The studies carried out (SAFE – 2014 and FEAST – 2011) did not show a superiority of albumin compared to normal saline in improving the hemodynamic aspects in patients, both adult and pediatric, who underwent resuscitation operations.

Gelatin

Solutions such as those based on polygeline (*Haemaccel®*) now find few indications in emergency and critical care medicine.

From the literature analysis (RCT and systematic reviews) and from the guidelines no clear elements emerged in favor of their use compared to that of other colloids available or even with regard to the use of one type of gelatin compared to another.

With some solutions containing gelatin, there may be interference in the determination of blood group, so it is advised to determine it before their administration. This would not concern solutions containing polygeline and gelatin lysate.

Dextran

Dextrans are branched glucose polymers of variable molecular weight produced by bacteria during the ethanol fermentation process. Even dextran-based solutions are now abandoned and there are no clear indications for their use in emergency and critical care medicine.

HES solutions (hydroxyethyl starch)

They are produced by replacing sorghum, corn and potato amylopectin, with ethyl hydroxide. This replacement determines a protection from the attack of some blood amylases, causing however the accumulation of this product in the endothelial reticulum system of the skin, liver and kidney as well as coagulation alterations. To reduce these side effects, the concentrations of hydroxyethyl starch (6%) and its molecular weight (130 KD) have been reduced.

The carrier solutions are made up of different types of crystalloids.

The most used are: HES 6% in solution with Na^+ 154 mEq/L and Cl^- 154 mEq/L with a pH between 4.0 and 5.5 and an osmolarity of 308 mOsm/L (*Voluven®*) or in solution with electrolyte concentrations similar to those of plasma (Na^+ 137 mmol/L, K^+ 4 mmol/L, Mg^{++} 1.5 mmol/L, Cl^- 110 mmol/L) with the addition of 34 mmol/L acetate with a pH 5.7-6.5 and an osmolarity of 286 mOsm/L (*Volulyte®*). Following the reporting of cases of acute nephropathy, particularly in patients with sepsis or septic shock, the EMA (European Medicines Agency), following the indications of the US FDA (Food and Drug Administration), proposed to limit the use of HES to the correction of hypovolemia due to acute hemorrhage, when crystalloids alone are not able to improve hemodynamic alterations; in any case, their use must not be extended beyond 24 hours.

HES should not be used in patients:

- with severe sepsis and septic shock and those hospitalized in ICU;
- with pre-existing modifications in renal function;

It is also recommended:

- treatment interruption at the first signs of coagulopathy;

SECTION III

ELECTROLYTES

CHAPTER 12

Hypokalemia

Michele Santoro

Potassium and its homeostasis

Potassium is the main intracellular electrolyte. Involved as a cofactor in various intermediate metabolism reactions, it plays a key role in the membrane potential (both at rest and action), for which it is involved in the correct functioning of nerve, cardiac and skeletal cells.

The potassium plasma concentration $[K^+]_p$ is normally 3.5-5.0 mEq/L.

In healthy adults the total body content (or total body pool) of potassium is approximately 3,000-4,000 mEq (about 50-55 mEq/Kg); this quantity is almost all, about 98%, confined to the ICF (intracellular volume or intracellular fluid), while only 2% is dissolved in the ECF (extracellular volume or extracellular fluid); considering that the plasma constitutes about 1/4 of the ECF the kalemia (blood potassium levels) that we usually measure and use in clinical practice is the expression of only a very small part of the total pool.

The different potassium distribution between ICF and ECF is due to the activity of the Na^+/K^+ pump (or Na^+/K^+-ATPase), which continuously moves two K^+ ions in the cells and extrudes three Na^+ ions; as known, the same mechanism explains why sodium is the main extracellular electrolyte.

Several factors can influence the activity of the Na^+/K^+ pump: in particular, it is stimulated by insulin and circulating catecholamines (epinephrine and norepinephrine), released in response to stress or administered for therapeutic purposes.

From a clinical-practical point of view, the biological effects of potassium depend on the ratio between extracellular K^+ and intracellular K^+ rather than on the absolute value of potassium; just think, for example, that if another 2% of K^+ went from ICF to the ECF the kalemia would double and reach the dangerous value of 8 mEq/L.

Potassium homeostasis (i.e. the set of mechanisms that maintain kalemia within the normal values of 3.5-5.0 mEq/L) is not only due to the Na^+/K^+ pump, but also to the balance between intake, elimination and reabsorption.

To carry out a correct diagnostic framework, and therefore an appropriate therapy, it is essential to know the physiological mechanisms that regulate kalemia (**Table 12.1**).

TABLE 12.1 Potassium homeostasis.

Intake	Distribution		Elimination	Reabsorption
• Per os • Intravenous (in the hospital)	98% ICF	2% ECF	• Renal (~ 90%) mainly regulated by aldosterone, which to the DCT reabsorbs Na^+ in exchange for K^+, which is excreted • Gastrointestinal • Sweat	• Renal At the level of the intercalated cells due to the effect of the H^+/K^+ ATP-dependent pump
	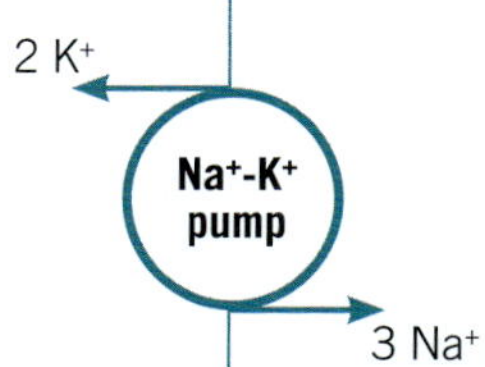 			

Normally potassium is introduced into the body through nutrition, while pharmacologically it can be taken orally or intravenously; it is first allocated inside the cells and subsequently, in order to keep the kalemia constant, it is mainly excreted (about 90%) through the urine and to a lesser extent through feces and sweat.

Thus, any alteration in any point of the aforementioned path can lead to the development of an alteration of the blood potassium levels, without forgetting, however, that the various causes may also be present simultaneously.

Renal function is particularly important both in terms of elimination and reabsorption. 50% of the potassium filtered at the glomerular level is reabsorbed at the level of the PCT (proximal convoluted tubule), while another 40% is reabsorbed at the level of the thick ascending limb of the loop of Henle.

At the DCT level (distal convoluted tubule) K^+ secretion occurs, under the action of aldosterone, whose plasma increase leads to an increase in K^+ excretion in exchange with Na^+, whose reabsorption is instead increased (**Figure 12.1**).

Aldosterone is the key hormone in potassium homeostasis. It is produced in the glomerular area of the adrenal gland, and its secretion is regulated not only directly by kalemia (hypokalemia inhibits, while hyperkalemia stimulates aldosterone secretion), but also from the so-called renin-angiotensin-aldosterone system (RAAS). It is activated in the course of hypovolemia, favoring the reabsorption of Na^+ (therefore of volume) at the expense of K^+, which is lost in the urine; at the level of the collecting ducts the main cells perform the fine regulation of potassium excretion.

The reabsorption, on the other hand, occurs by the intercalated cells through specific H^+/K^+ ATP-dependent pumps (not to be confused with the H^+/K^+ exchangers), which, in case of reduced intake, increase their activity by reabsorbing greater potassium in response to hypokalemia.

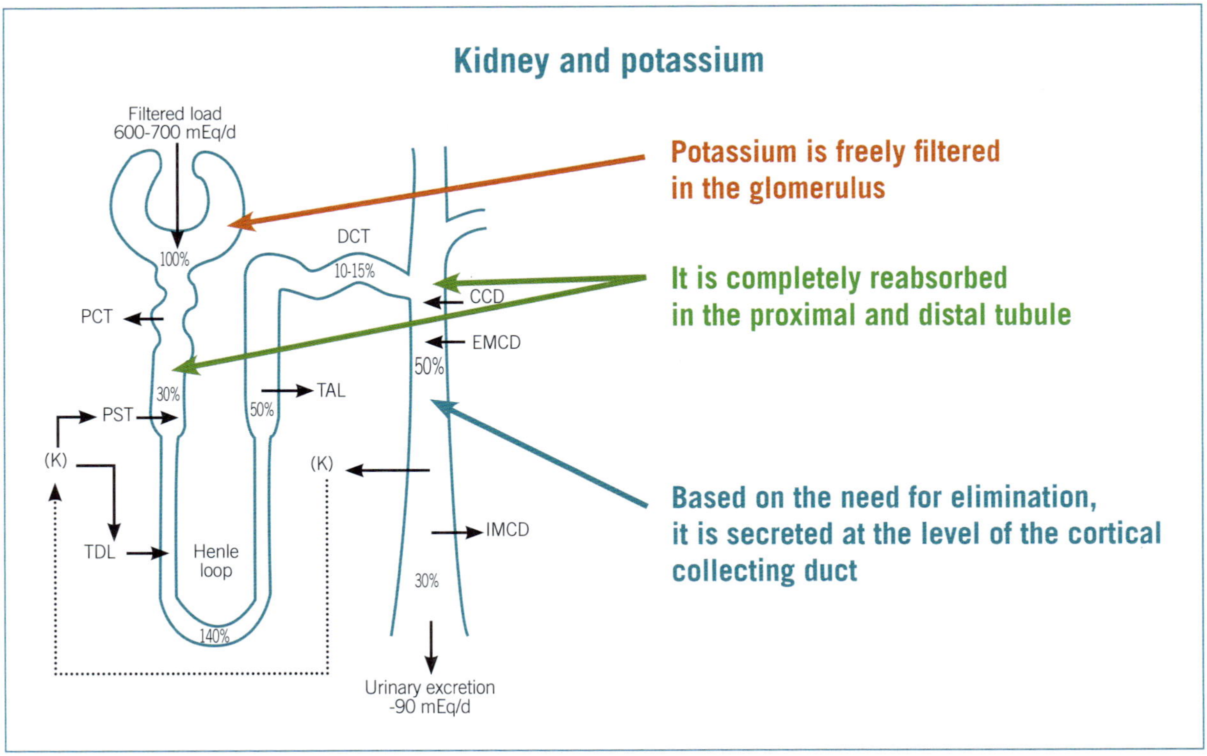

Figure 12.1 Kidney and potassium.
CCD: cortical collecting duct; DCT: distal convoluted tubule; EMCD: extramedullar collecting duct; IMCD: intramedullar collecting duct; PCT: proximal convoluted tubule; PST: proximal straight tubule; TAL: thick ascending limb; TDL: thin descending limb.

Although the main role is up to aldosterone, renal potassium excretion is influenced by other factors, such as the reabsorption of Na^+ and the transluminal gradient of K^+.

Since Na^+ is a positive charge, its reabsorption by DCT generates intraluminal electronegativity, which is fundamental for attracting K^+ ions, which are thus excreted in the urine. This mechanism explains the effect of potassium-sparing drugs on preserving potassium levels, such as amiloride and triamterene, which block the reabsorption of Na^+ to DCT.

However, the electronegativity generated by the reabsorption of Na^+ is not sufficient to guarantee the excretion of K^+: in fact this mechanism would soon reach saturation (due to intraluminal accumulation of K^+), Without an adequate distal flow which, through a "wash out" effect, it maintains a transluminal gradient favorable to accept new K^+. It follows that the renal excretion of K^+ is altered in all those conditions in which the reabsorption of sodium and water to DCT (diuretics, tubulopathies, etc.) is altered or the distal flow is altered.

Hypokalemia definition

Hypokalemia (or hypopotassemia) is defined as the detection of a plasma potassium concentration $[K^+]_p$ < 3.5 mEq/L; on the basis of value, more specifically, slight (3.5-3.0 mEq/L), moderate (2.9-2.5 mEq/L) and severe (<2.5 mEq/L) hypokalemia can be distinguished.

This is an electrolytiedisorder of frequent occurrence, according to some studies up to 20% of hospitalized patients and 2-3% of outpatients, especially if suffering from chronic diseases affecting the elderly, in which hypokalemia is often iatrogenic.

The term pseudohypokalemia refers to the finding of a false hypokalemia, generally due to pre-analytical conditions.

In fact, it is characteristic of blood samples left for a long time in inadequate environmental conditions: since the cells remain metabolically active for a certain period, they introduce K^+ so that the laboratory result shows a false $[K^+]_p$, that is less than the real. Pseudohypokalemia can be avoided by separating plasma and figurative elements or by keeping the sample at 4 °C.

As already illustrated, potassium is introduced in the body through nutrition, subsequently (for the Na^+/K^+ pump) 98% is allocated in the ICF and 2% in the ECF, finally it is excreted mainly through the urine (90%) and to a lesser extent through feces and sweat. The alteration of one or more of the aforementioned stages can cause a reduction in $[K^+]_p$ and it is for this reason that, based on the pathophysiological mechanism, in clinical practice the causes of hypokalemia are classically classified in one or more than three major "drawers":

1) reduced intake;

2) redistribution (shift) of potassium from the extracellular to the intracellular environment;

3) increased loss or elimination (**Table 12.2**).

Since the kidney plays the main role in the excretion of potassium, it is intuitive that hypokalemia with increased elimination (the third "drawer") is generally to be found in the context of tubular mechanisms, which can be primitively altered, as in the case of severe nephropathy in the course of systemic diseases, or secondarily altered, as occurs during diuretic therapy or in case of increased activity of RAAS.

In fact, many forms of hypokalemia have in common a clinical condition of hyperaldosteronism, often secondary to loss of volume (diuretics, laxatives, nasogastric suction, etc.), in which the metabolic alkalosis, inevitably present, becomes a mechanism for strengthening hypokalemia itself.

TABLE 12.2 General causes of hypokaliemia.

Hypokalemia causes
A) Potassium reduced intake
B) Redistribution (shift of potassium from the extracellular to the intracellular environment)
C) Increased loss or elimination of potassium

Hypokalemia and acid-base balance

Although for educational convenience they are treated separately, the acid-base and the water-electrolyte balance represent a unique entity so that, especially in moderate-severe forms, disorders of blood electrolytes are associated with acid-base alterations.

As a general rule it can be stated that hypokalemia and alkalemia are associated conditions, although – as described below – there are exceptions.

Being it of metabolic or respiratory origin, the alkalemia (pH > 7.45) is associated with hypokalemia: in the presence of a reduced plasma hydrogen ion concentration $[H^+]_p$, a special exchanger H^+/K^+ (not to be confused with the H^+/K^+ ATP-dependent pump of the intercalated cells), located on the cellular membrane and functioning by simple gradient, allows the passage of H^+ ions from the inside to the outside of the cell thus allowing to contribute to the buffering of high pH. However, to maintain electroneutrality, at the same time K^+ passes instead from the external environment (plasma and extracellular fluid) inside the cell, thus determining hypokalemia.

Hypokalemia plays an important role not only in the genesis but also in the maintenance of metabolic alkalosis, as happens, for example, in primary hyperaldosteronism. In fact, in this condition it can happen that, in addition to the metabolic alkalosis from hypokalemia (direct effect of aldosterone), there is also a metabolic alkalosis induced by the H^+/K^+ pumps of the intercalated cells, which in an attempt to reabsorb K^+, extrude H^+ ions which are then further lost in the urine. In this context, the so-called "paradoxical aciduria" appears, or rather that occurence in which, despite a condition of alkalemia, H^+ ions are excreted (in exchange with the K^+ reabsorbed in response to hypokalemia) thus leading to a vicious and clinically dangerous circle, in which hypokalemia and alkalemia mutually enhance one another. Such a condition is further worsened by the simultaneous presence of hypomagnesemia.

Next to the "consolidated" couple formed by alkalemia and hypokalemia, there are also clinical pictures characterized by the "strange" couple consisting of metabolic acidosis and hypokalemia.

Such a condition can be achieved during: potassium-losing nephropathies (salt-wasting nephropathies, described below), in which alongside metabolic acidosis due to renal failure we also find hypokalemia due to renal loss; profuse diarrhea, during which potassium is lost but also bicarbonate; more rare disorders such as tubular acidosis.

In the latter a genetic defect causes a reduced tubular reabsorption of $NaHCO_3^-$: the loss of HCO_3^- determines metabolic acidosis, while the loss of Na^+, which is accompanied by a loss of water (hence the volume), triggers the RAA system, which finally determines hypokalemia. In essence, hypokalemia occurs in tubular acidosis as the potassium lowering effect of hyperaldosteronism (secondary to the loss of volume) overcomes the potassium increasing effect of the H^+/K^+ exchange in the course of acidosis.

Hypokalemia causes

Divided according to the pathophysiological mechanism (read the 3 large "drawers"), the causes of hypokalemia will be described below, which are outlined also in **Table 12.3**. The drugs can cause hypokalemia both by favoring the intracellular shift and the renal excretion of K^+.

Hypokalemia from reduced potassium intake

A healthy adult takes about 60-100 mEq of potassium daily, of which 90% is excreted via the urine and the remaining 10% mainly via the fecal route, while only a very small amount is lost through sweat. In case of reduced intake, renal excretion is reduced from a minimum of 5 up to a maximum of 25 mEq/day (normal value of potassium in urine 30-120 mEq/day) both through a reduced secretion of aldosterone and through an increased reabsorption of K^+ at intercalated cells level, which are directly stimulated by hypokalemia.

TABLE 12.3 Causes of hypokalemia, divided into the three main "drawers".

Potassium reduced intake	Shift of potassium from the extracellular to the intracellular environment	Increased loss or elimination or elimination of potassium
• Anorexia • Malnutrition • Associated with other causes of ipokaliemia	• Alkalemia • Insulin • β-adrenergic activity • Drugs (chloroquine, theophylline) • Familial hypokalemic periodic paralysis • Other conditions – Thyrotoxic crisis – Hypothermia – Increased cellular K^+ uptake – Trauma	*Gastroenteric* • Vomit, diarrhea, sweating *Renal* • Nephropathy (kidney disease) – Renal failure and dialysis – Tubular-interstitial nephropathies – In systemic diseases • Loop diuretics and thiazides • Hypomagnesemia • Non-resorbable anions • Excess of mineralocorticoid hormones (licorice) • Rare disorders – Liddle syndrome – Bartter syndrome – Gitelman syndrome
	Drugs	

It is important to emphasize that drugs can cause hypokalemia with different mechanisms: through redistribution (insulin, β_2 agonists), through a direct effect on the kidney (diuretics), indirectly causing hypovolemia and, therefore, activation of the RAAS (diuretics, laxatives, antihypertensives).

Since potassium is widely present in all foods, particularly in fruit and vegetables, except for severe conditions such as anorexia or malnutrition, it is unlikely for hypokalemia to be caused only by reduced food intake, which instead becomes significant in the presence of other potassium lowering factors.

Redistribution hypokalemia (potassium shift from extra-to-intracellular environment)

The intracellular shift, that is the passage of potassium from the extracellular to the intracellular environment, can occur in different conditions, of which it is important to know the pathophysiology not only to prevent clinically relevant hypokalemia, but also to understand some principles of the potassium lowering therapy (shown in the appropriate section).

Alkalemia

As already described, alkalemia (pH > 7.45) is associated with hypokalemia due to the effect of a special exchanger H^+/K^+, located on the cell membrane and functioning by simple gradient; it, in the presence of a reduced concentration of hydrogen ions, allows the passage of H^+ from the inside to the outside of the cell thus allowing to buffer the high pH. For every reduction of the pH of 0.1 we expect a reduction of the kalemia of 0.3-0.6 mEq/L.

In the diagnostic approach to the patient with hypokalemia, it is therefore necessary to investigate possible causes of alkalemia, such as hypovolemia, followed by activation of the RAA system, therapy with diuretics or the administration of sodium bicarbonate. The latter, in addition to determining itself the metabolic alkalosis, causes hypokalemia also because it behaves like a non-resorbable anion: at the level of the DCT, in fact, while the Na^+ is reabsorbed, the HCO_3^- remains in the tubular lumen, thus generating an electronegative gradient favorable to the excretion of K^+. It is believed that this mechanism is not only the basis of hypokalemia induced by drugs containing non-resorbable anions, but also of hypokalemia that is observed after persistent vomiting or the placement of a long-term nasogastric tube: the loss of HCl determines alkalemia with increased HCO_3^-, which at the level of the DCT behaves like a non-resorbable anion, thus causing an increased secretion of potassium according to the mechanism illustrated above.

Insulin

Insulin promotes the entry of potassium into skeletal muscle cells through increased activity of the Na^+/K^+ pump. Once again it is an important event in both pathophysiological and therapeutic terms. In clinical practice, in fact, in the case of severe glycemic decompensation, which requires the infusion of high-dose insulin, it is important to check that the kalemia does not drop too much as the blood sugar level is lowered. In a mirror way we understand why glucose solutions containing insulin, also called "repolarization" or "buffered" glucose solutions, are used in the treatment of hyperkalemia.

Beta-adrenergic activity

Catecholamines favor the entry of potassium into the cells through interaction with the β_2-adrenergic receptors, which increase the activity of the Na^+/K^+ pump. It is important to keep in mind the potassium lowering effect of catecholamines substantially for two reasons:

1) in clinical practice, β_2 agonists (normally used in aerosol form in asthmatic attacks) can also be useful to correct hyperkalemia;

2) during therapy with vasopressor amines, such as norepinephrine in septic shock, or dobutamine in cardiogenic shock, hypokalemia may occur or – worse still – a hypokalemia already induced by a possible simultaneous use of diuretics may be exacerbated.

Drugs

In addition to insulin and β_2 agonists, intracellular shift hypokalemia may also be caused by other drugs, including theophylline, chloroquine, β-mimetic tocolytics.

Hypokalemic periodic paralysis

Hypokalemic periodic paralysis (HPP) is a rare disorder characterized by recurrent episodes of muscle weakness up to and including paralysis, which can be fatal if they involve the respiratory muscles. Hyper-, hypo- and normokalemic forms have been described, but the hypokalemic form often manifests as familial, autosomal and dominant, or acquired, as an effect of thyrotoxicosis (which probably increases receptor sensitivity to catecholamines). Both disorders can be triggered by exercise, a meal rich in carbohydrates, stress or following administration of insulin or epinephrine. The pathogenesis is not well clarified, but it is known that the attacks are associated with a sudden passage of potassium from the ECF to the ICF with consequent abrupt reduction of the kalemia up to 1.5-2.5 mEq/L. The diagnosis is based on the finding of severe hypokalemia during the attacks, for which the blood gas analysis becomes an important diagnostic tool also for the speed of performance.

Other conditions determining the entry of potassium into cells

A thyrotoxic crisis can reduce the plasma concentration of K^+ through an intracellular shift mechanism due to increased activity of Na^+/K^+ ATPase. Even hypothermia, accidental or induced, can determine hypokalemia through a mechanism that is not yet well clarified, which pushes K^+ to enter the cells; the correction of hypokalemia during hypothermia must be carried out with attention to the risk that once the normal temperature is re-established, a rebound hyperkalemia may occur.

An increase in intracellular K^+ uptake may result in hypokalemia (generally moderate), which can be observed, for example, when folic acid and vitamin B_{12} are administered to treat megaloblastic anemia.

Trauma is usually associated with hyperkalemia, since K^+ is released by damaged cells, however, probably due to increased blood levels of circulating catecho-

but in substance they are the expression of a greater electrical vulnerability of the myocardial cell, in turn due essentially to a delayed ventricular repolarization. With the reduction of kalemia, in order we manifest: for values of potassium between 3.5 and 3.0 mEq/L flattening or inversion of the T waves; for potassium values between 3.0 and 2.3 mEq/L prolongation of the QT (longer duration of the T wave), appearance of the U wave, moderate depression of the ST segment (0.5 mm), extraventricular systoles; for potassium values < 2.3 mEq/L torsade de pointes, ventricular fibrillation (**Figure 12.2 and 12.3**).

It should be noted that none of these alterations is strictly specific to hypokalemia, as similar alterations of the ST tract can also appear in the case of ischemia or digital therapy, while the prolongation of the QT can also be observed in cases of hypocalcemia, hypomagnesemia and in cases of therapy with class III antiarrhythmics (according to the Vaughan Williams classification).

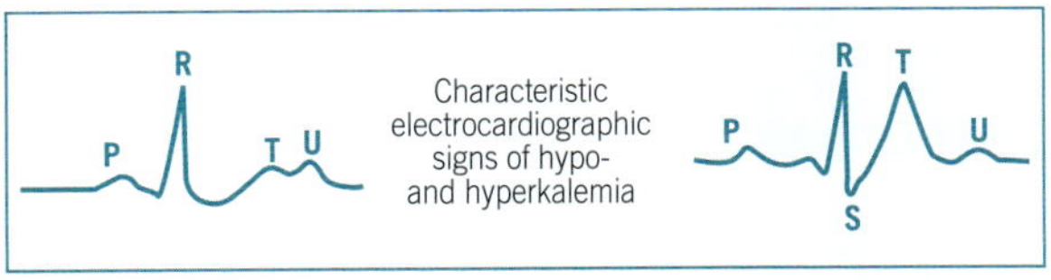

Figure 12.2 ECG changes during hypokalemia.

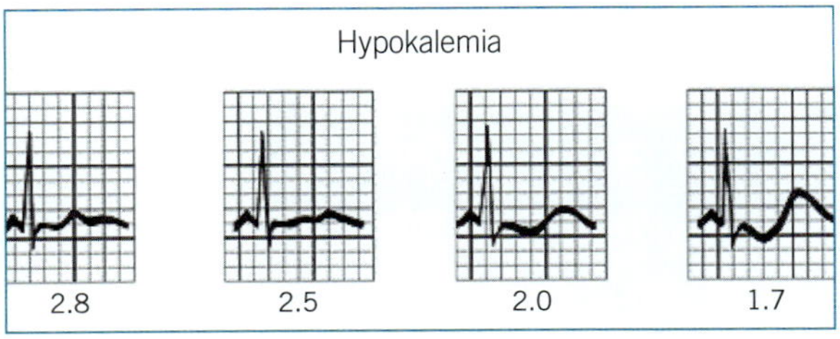

Figure 12.3 ECG changes during hypokalemia.

Alterations in renal function

During hypokalemia, various alterations in renal function may occur, such as impaired ability to concentrate urine, increased production of ammonium and acidification of the urine, reduced ability to reabsorb HCO_3^- up to proper renal failure. Normally such alterations regress by correcting $[K^+]_p$ provided that there is no co-present or previous nephropathy. In fact, while in the case of losses caused by a nephropathy, the urinary potassium excretion increases, in the case of hypokalemia due to extrarenal loss, the urinary potassium excretion usually falls below 25 mEq/day precisely because the kidney maintains its capacity to reabsorb potassium.

In addition, during hypokalemia we may verify:

1) the characteristic vacuolar lesions, localized at the level of the tubular epithelial cells, that generally regress after the correction of the kalemia;

2) rhabdomyolysis, the pathogenesis of which is not well understood, but the regulatory role of K^+ in regards to blood flow seems to be implicated, which decreases with consequent subsequent appearance of cramps, ischemia and rhabdomyolysis.

Diagnostic approach of hypokalemia

The cause of hypokalemia is generally identified through a good medical history, which allows rapid detection of the presence of a nephropathy and/or the use of diuretics (sometimes of different types of combination), that is the causes of hypokalemia most commonly found in clinical practice.

When the diagnosis is not immediate, there are usually underlying endocrinological diseases: in particular, an excess of mineralocorticoids should be suspected in any patient with hypokalemia associated with arterial hypertension; in these cases, in addition to the specific investigations related to the mineralocorticoid hormones (blood cortisol and urinary cortisol, blood aldosterone, plasma renin activity, etc.) the urinary K^+ dosage and the evaluation of the acid-base state are fundamental, because they allow to reveal more rare disorders such as tubular acidosis.

ECG

The electrocardiogram should always be performed, regardless of the presence or absence of clinically manifested arrhythmias. In severe hypokalemia, continuous monitoring is essential because it allows early identification and treatment of arrhythmogenic conditions, such as QT prolongation, and of major arrhythmias, such as torsade de pointes.

Urinary potassium excretion

Patients with hypokalemia due to extrarenal loss usually have a urinary concentration of $K^+ < 25$ mEq/L, expression of normal renal function, which appropriately reduces potassium excretion; on the contrary, a urinary potassium excretion above this value during hypokalemia suggests that, at least in part, hypokalemia is also caused by a renal loss. It should be pointed out that the measurement of the urinary excretion of potassium is more reliable if performed on urine collected in 24 hours compared to that on spot urine, to be preferred in emergency; moreover, it is good practice to confirm the measures of the urinary potassium excretion through several investigations; also depending on potassium intake, urinary potassium excretion can vary from 15 to 400 mEq/24h.

A reliable index of renal potassium excretion is the urinary potassium/urinary creatinine ratio (Uk/UCr) to be measured also on spot urine. When this ratio is < 1.5 hypokalemia may be due to intracellular shift, gastrointestinal losses, past use of diuretics, but if the ratio is > 1.5 hypokalemia is due to renal potassium losses (**Figure 12.4**).

NOTE

The Uk/UCr ratio should be expressed in mmol/L (mmol/mmol). Normally urinary creatinine is expressed in mg/dL. To transform the mg/dL into mmol/L the value in mg is multiplied by 88.5 obtaining the value in μmol/L, which divided by 1,000 gives us the value of the mmol/L. For example, if urinary creatinine is 150 mg/dL, 150 x 88.5 = 13.275 μmol/L which divided by 1,000 gives a urinary creatinine value of 13.275 mmol/L.

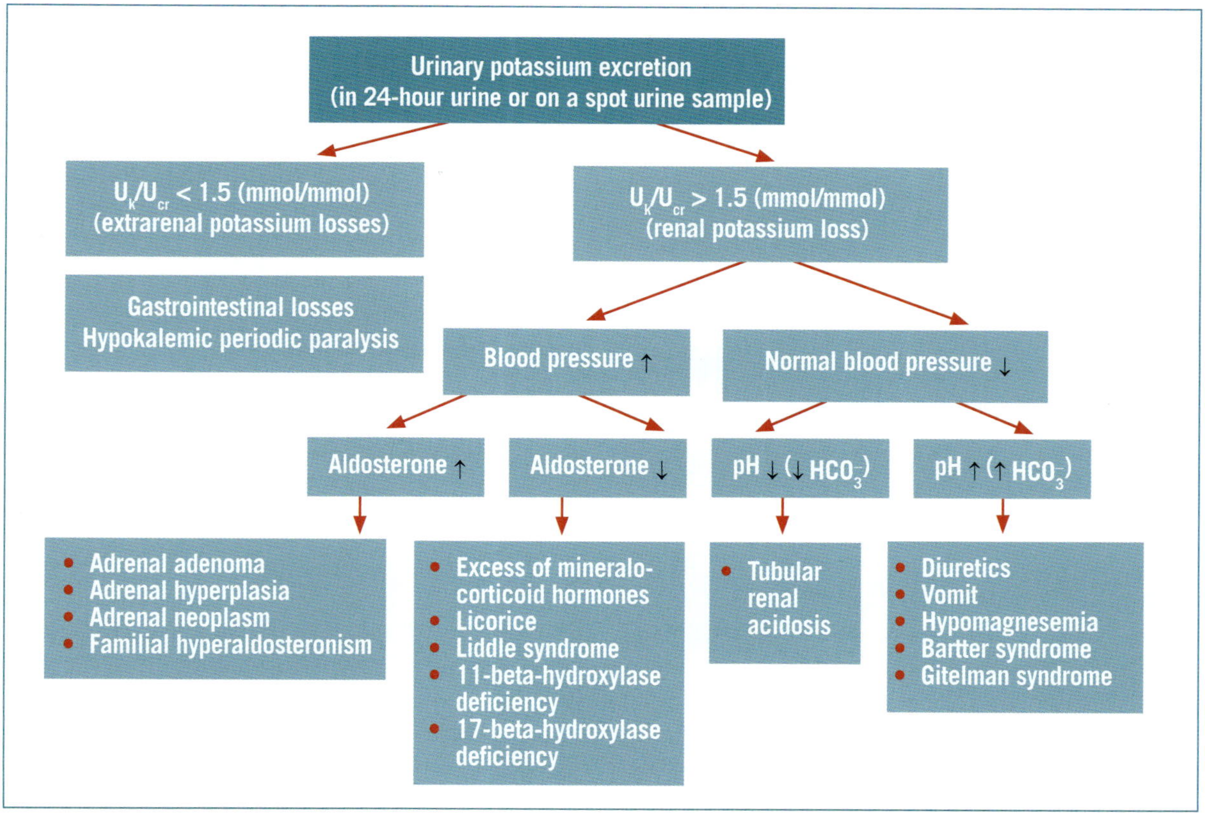

Figure 12.4 Hypokalemia. Diagnostic algorithm.

TABLE 12.5. During hypokalemia, blood pH can guide the diagnosis (modified by Rose BD, Post TW. Clinical Physiology of Acid-Base and Electrolyte Disorders, 5th edition. New York. McGraw-Hill 2001).

Hypokalemia associated with metabolic acidosis	Hypokalemia associated with metabolic alkalosis
Low intestinal losses (diarrhea, laxatives)	Diuretics
Ketoacidosis	Vomiting, nasogastric tube. Villous adenoma of the rectum
Renal tubular acidosis	Excess of mineralocorticoids
Salt-wasting nephropathies	Penicillin derivatives

TTKG (Trans-Tubular K^+ Gradient)

It is a parameter that is little used in clinical practice. TTKG is the ratio between the potassium concentration in the lumen of the cortical collecting duct and the potassium concentration within the peritubular capillaries (and therefore in the plasma, practically the kalemia); it can be calculated if the urinary osmolality is higher than the plasmatic osmolality through the following formula:

$$\text{TTKG} = (\text{urine } [K^+] \times \text{plasma osm} / \text{plasma } [K^+] \times \text{urine osm})$$

In the presence of hypokalemia, a high TTKG (greater than 7) indicates an inappropriate renal response to hypokalemia (so the kidney does not retain K^+ despite hypokalemia!), that indicates a renal loss of K^+ due to an increased distal secretion, as occurs in the conditions of hyperaldosteronism or in Liddle syndrome (disorder characterized by an aldosterone-like mechanism) or during diuretic therapy; the finding of a reduced TTKG (less than 3) during hypokalemia instead reflects an adequate renal response since in an appropriate manner the kidney retains K^+ (so that the trans-tubular gradient is reduced), so the cause of hypokalemia must be sought elsewhere and not at renal level (poor intake, gastrointestinal losses, previous use of diuretics, salt-losing nephropathies, etc).

The TTKG calculation is particularly useful in differentiating peripheral paralysis from secondary hypokalemia with total potassium pool deficit (non-HPP, not Hypokalemic Periodic Paralysis), from hypokalemia due to hypokalemic periodic paralysis (HPP, Hypokalemic Periodic Paralysis), in which it is less than 2.5; the finding of a TTKG < 2.5, together with the absence of acid-base disorders, suggests with high probability a HPP.

Blood pH

The evaluation of the acid-base status often allows a first diagnostic orientation. As already illustrated, some pictures of hypokalemia are characteristically associated with specific acid-base disorders (**Table 12.5**).

For example, the couple consisting of metabolic acidosis and urinary potassium loss suggests diseases such as diabetic ketoacidosis, renal tubular acidosis or salt-wasting nephropathy.

On the contrary, the association of metabolic alkalosis and hypokalemia usually occurs during diuretic therapy, vomiting, excess of mineralocorticoids; finally, rare genetic disorders (such as Liddle, Bartter or Gitelman syndrome) should be considered.

Clinical case 1 Mr. L.G., 32-years-old, shows up in the emergency department due to the appearance of some widespread muscle pain and motor deficit in the limbs and trunk; reports a meal rich in carbohydrates on the previous evening. For some years he has been suffering from similar episodes, which occur occasionally, so much so that four years earlier he had been admitted with a diagnosis of "hypokalemic myopathy" due to the finding of high total CPK (626 U/L) and hypokalemia (2.3 mEq/L); on that occasion the muscle biopsy showed a modest non-specific myogenic suffering, a lumbar CT showed a very modest disc protrusion L4-L5, while the EMG, thyroid hormones, blood cortisol and blood aldosterone were normal. The symptoms regressed after potassium supplementation. Returning to the latter entry into the emergency department: vital signs are normal (BP 125/80 mmHg, FC 90 bpm, SpO_2 98% on room air); the physical examination shows flaccid paralysis of the limbs mainly in the proximal and trunk areas, without sensitivity disturbances, with complete savings of the neck and head muscles, as well as the "usual" muscle pain. Blood tests show marked hypokalemia (2.5 mEq/L) and elevated CPK (1,442 U/L); arterial blood gas is normal (pH 7.39, $PaCO_2$ 40 mmHg, HCO_3^- 23.3 mEq/L, lactic acid 1.2 mmol/L), as well as the measurement of sodium (138 mEq/L), chloride (101 mEq/L), magnesium (1.9 mEq/L), blood glucose (110 mg/dL), creatinine 0.9 and blood urea 25 mg/dL; the ECG is within limits. Cortisol and ACTH dosages are also normal (at 8 am and at 4 pm), renin and aldosterone in the position of clino and orthostatism, thyroid function; urinary potassium excretion (spot) is equal to 9 mmol/L, urinary creatinine (spot) is 9.6 mmol/L and the Uk/Ucr ratio = 0.93. Plasma osmolality is 291 mOsm/Kg, the urinary osmolality 598 mOsm/Kg, the TTKG is equal to $(K^+_u \times osm_p)/(K^+_p \times osm_u)$ (9 x 291)/(2.5 x 598) = 2,619/1,495 = 1.75 (normal values 3-7).

Reasoned comment

In the case described the low value of urinary potassium excretion (9 mEq/L) and the ratio Uk/Ucr = 0.93, indicates that the cause of hypokalemia is not attributable to the kidney, which instead correctly reduces the excretion of potassium, while the normal hormone values exclude an endocrine pathology.

At this point it is important to establish whether hypokalemia is to be attributed to a shift mechanism or to a deficit in the total potassium pool, which can however be excluded since there is no clinical evidence of gastrointestinal or sweat loss.The value of TTKG < 3 (1.75 in this case), other than confirming an appropriate reduced potassium excretion by the kidney, points towards shift hypokalemia, an assumption also confirmed by the absence of acid-base alterations. From a clinical point of view and from the medical history, episodes of paralysis and muscle pain appear to be related to carbohydrate intake and disappear with the correction of hypokalemia; finally, considering the periodicity with which the disorder manifests itself and the regression of the symptoms with potassium supplementation, the picture shows the diagnosis of hypokalemic periodic paralysis (HPP).

Clinical case 2 Mr. C.D., 80-years-old, arrives in the emergency department due to the onset of increasing asthenia, which occurred the day before, first located in the upper limbs and then also in the lower limbs; subjected to left inguinal hernia repair three days before the onset of symptoms, from the day of discharge he reports diarrhea (6-8 episodes) without fever or other abdominal symptoms. For several years he has been suffering from Crohn's disease, treated with mesalazine, discontinued for a few months.

Upon arrival, the patient is alert, cooperative and oriented, GCS 15, vital signs are normal (BP 120/70 mmHg, FC 58 bpm, body temperature 36.7 °C, SpO_2 96% on room air); the neurological examination shows a complete paralysis in the upper limbs and almost complete in the lower limbs (weakly moving the right foot). The muscles of the head, neck and trunk show no deficit and the sensitivity is totally preserved; ECG shows sinus bradycardia (FC 58 bpm) with QRS at the upper limits of normality (0.12 sec), flattened T waves, U wave with increased QT interval. Arterial blood gas shows hyperchloremic metabolic acidosis (normal anion gap) and severe hypokalemia (pH 7.19, $PaCO_2$ 24.6 mmHg, 9.1 mEq/L, PaO_2 108 mmHg, AG 12 mEq/L, lactates 0.5 mmol/L, potassium 1.7 mEq/L, sodium 136 mEq/L, chloride 116 mEq/L).

Routine blood tests complete the picture showing hypomagnesemia (1.14 mg/dL), blood glucose 79 mg, as well as renal failure (creatinine 2.3 mg/dL, blood urea 111 mg/dL) with plasma osmolality equal to 278 mOsm/Kg; urinary potassium excretion (spot) is low (12 mmol/L), urinary creatinine (spot) is 14 mmol/L and Uk/Ucr = 0.85. Urinary osmolality is 520 mOsm/

Kg, TTKG is equal to $(K^+_u \times osm_p)/(K^+_p \times osm_u) = (12 \times 278)/(1.7 \times 520) = 3{,}336/884 = 3.7$. The neurological examination confirms tetraplegia (four limbs paralysis) with preserved cranial nerves and sensitivity; to exclude a Guillain-Barrè syndrome, a lumbar puncture is performed, with evidence of non-significant protein levels in the physical-chemical examination of cerebrospinal fluid, and also a normal cervical MRI, as well as an EMG, showing non-specific signs of diffuse axonal suffering.

Reasoned comment

In the context of a known inflammatory bowel disease (for some time untreated), probably exacerbated by the hernia repair, diarrhea (in the absence of fever and other abdominal symptoms) leads to hypokalemia due to gastrointestinal loss.

The low urinary potassium excretion and the Uk/Ucr ratio = 0.85, confirm that the loss is extrarenal; the value (3.7) of TTKG is at the lower limits (normal value 3-7), indicating that the kidney appropriately reduces the excretion of potassium, however it does not fall below 3, probably because the reduction in volume (from diarrhea) stimulates the production of aldosterone, thus favoring potassium excretion (and sodium reabsorption).

The increase in creatinine is related to a predominantly pre-renal acute renal failure (which, as will be seen later, responds to volume repletion).

Unlike the previous one, in this case the arterial blood gas reveals a hyperchloremic metabolic acidosis (or with normal AG), secondary to the loss of bicarbonate through diarrhea; in this context the "strange couple" consisting of metabolic acidosis and hypokalemia is realized.

The presence, in this case, of metabolic acidosis is important in differentiating hypokalemia secondary to potassium pool deficiency (non-HPP) from hypokalemia due to periodic hypokalemic paralysis (HPP), in which there are no alterations of the acid-base balance. Finally, it is worth emphasizing that hypomagnesemia which, as described, is associated with hypokalemia in about 50% of cases, helps explain the patient's asthenia.

Clinical case 3 Ms. S.M, 73-years-old, arrives in the emergency department for a motor deficit, present for two days and characterized by an inability to extend her right hand and the last three fingers. The patient has high blood pressure, treated with amlodipine 5 mg, benazepril 10 mg and hydrochlorothiazide 12.5 mg. Blood tests show: normal blood count, creatinine 0.6 mg/dL, blood urea 13 mg/dL, blood glucose 78 mg/dL, plasma osmolality 293 mOsm/Kg, CPK 1037 U/L, potassium 1.9 mEq/L, sodium 142 mEq/L, chloride 99 mEq/L, magnesium 1.7 mg/dL; TSH, FT_3 and FT_4 within the normal value. At arterial blood gas analysis: pH 7.54, $PaCO_2$ 40.9 mmHg, HCO_3^- 34.2 mEq/L, PaO_2 56.5 mmHg, calcium ion 1.22 mmol/L corrected for pH; urinalysis shows: potassium (spot) 45 mmol/L, urinary creatinine (spot) 10.2 mmol/L, Uk/Ucr ratio = 4.41. Urinary osmolarity 650 mOsm/Kg; the TTKG is equal to $(K^+_u \times osm_p)/(K^+_p \times osm_u) = (45 \times 293)/(1.9 \times 650) = 13{,}185/1{,}235 = 10.67$. At the ECG: regular sinus rhythm, narrow QRS, repolarization changes due to the presence of large U waves and a prolonged QT interval; Normal chest X-ray. A neurological examination attributes the deficit to an impairment of the carpal radial extensor; since brain CT scan is negative, a diagnosis of distal paralysis of the right upper limb by acute myopathy is made, caused by severe hypokalemia in a context of metabolic alkalosis associated with respiratory alkalosis (PCO_2 is lower than the expected adaptation for a value of HCO_3^- equal to 34.2 mEq/L).

Reasoned comment

The history is strongly decisive: the therapy with thiazide diuretic indicates that the hypokalemia is related to the renal loss; the assumption is confirmed by the high urinary potassium excretion (> 25 mEq/L) and by the Uk/Ucr = 04.41 ratio, while the high TTKG (> 7) indicates that the kidney inappropriately does not reabsorb potassium (indeed, it loses it), although in the presence of hypokalemia, as subjected to the pharmacological effect of hydrochlorothiazide; it is important to emphasize that also in this case there is associated hypomagnesemia. As in Case 2, the presence of metabolic alkalosis is important to differentiate between non-HPP hypokalemia and HPP hypokalemia.

Hypokalemia treatment

First of all it is necessary to frame the effects of the K^+ deficiency, remembering that clinical manifestations can vary and there is not always a close correlation between symptoms and level of kalemia. Therefore, the evaluation of the neuromuscular framework and above all of the ECG are fundamental. As with other plasma ion disorders even in hypokalemia it is important to correct the clinical symptom/sign rather than the kalemia itself, also to avoid the risk of an overtreatment that subsequently leads to hyperkalemia. It goes without saying that, where possible, the causes of hypokalemia must be corrected or removed. In those caused by shift the correction must be very cautious, to avoid rebound hyperkalemia.

A kalemia between 3.5 and 3.0 mEq/L is usually clinically well tolerated (except for patients who take digitalis): the treatment is not urgent and the correction is obtained by administering potassium chloride per os, starting from 60-80 mEq/day.

In pathological states characterized by a continuous loss of K^+ (i.e., primitive hyperaldosteronism or diuretics), a greater supplying is needed.

In symptomatic patients the administration should be carried out immediately; normally the kalemia rises by 1,0-1.5 mEq/L after administering 40-60 mEq of potassium chloride per os, or 2.0-2.5 mEq/L after 135-160 mEq per os.

The effect may be transient since the administered K^+ rapidly enters the cells to restore the total pool. In general it can be stated that a reduction in potassium from 4.0 to 3.0 implies a loss of about 200-400 mEq of K^+, while a further loss of the same amount can cause the kalemia to fall to 2.0 mEq/L. Furthermore, we must also consider factors that themselves cause $[K^+]$ alteration (such as metabolic acidosis or hyperglycemia), which, if corrected too quickly, can lead to hypokalemia.

Intravenous (IV) administration is effective but has a limit of 60 mEq per liter of solution, so it requires the infusion of large quantities of volume. Furthermore, unless severe hypoglycemia is also present, glucose solutions should not be used since, as described, they favor hypokalemia due to intracellular shift. Usually the maximum IV infusion rate is 10-20 mEq/h, although in highly symptomatic patients or those with dangerous arrhythmias it can reach 40-100 mEq/h. It is better to infuse in large caliber veins or through a central access if the potassium chloride concentration is high. The ECG monitoring is in any case indispensable when significant quantities are infused.

Type of potassium to be used

There are different preparations, in combination with different anions, such as chloride, gluconate, bicarbonate, phosphate.

As a rule KCl is preferred because, in addition to correcting the potassium deficiency, containing chloride also corrects the concomitant alkalosis.

$KHCO_3^-$ is preferred in particular situations such as hypokalemia in tubular acidosis, because, in addition to the correction of K^+ deficiency, bicarbonate acidosis is also corrected.

Calculation of potassium to be infused

It is possible to calculate the potassium deficit starting from known pathophysiological considerations. If, for example, we have an 80 Kg patient with 2.0 mEq/L of kalemia, how much potassium should we infuse? First of all, we need to understand the kalemia value we must reach.

Let's assume we want to go from 2.0 to 5.0 mEq/L of potassium. First we need to calculate the volume in which the K^+ will be distributed: we know that the TBW (Total Body Water) corresponds to about 60% of the total body weight in the male and 50% in the female, so, in the case of a male, 60% of 80 Kg is (0.6 x 80) = 48, that is TBW is equal to 48 L. We know that K^+ is distributed inside the cells (due to the Na^+/K^+ pump) and that the ICF (intracellular volume) is equal to 2/3 of the TBW, so the ICF is equal to 32 L (i.e. 2/3 of 48). Given that the ideal value to be reached is 5 mEq/L, the following calculation is performed: 5.0 (theoretical value in mEq/L to be reached) – 2.0 mEq/L (actual po-

Hyperkalemic form of family periodic paralysis

Alongside the hypokalemic periodic paralysis (HPP), described in the chapter on hypokalemia, there is also a hyperkalemic form: it is a rare familial disorder with an autosomal dominant transmission, characterized by recurrent attacks of muscle weakness or paralysis. The episodes are triggered by rest after intense exercise or by ingestion of K^+ and are associated with an increase in kalemia, usually moderate (< 5.5 mEq/L), although in some patients it may be > 7.0 mEq/L. It is believed that the cause is a defect in the cell membrane, which on the one hand favors extracellular shift and on the other does not allow K^+ to enter the cells.

The attacks are associated with a reduction in $[Na^+]_p$ and an increase in the concentration of plasma proteins, suggesting that Na^+ and H_2O enter the cell as soon as K^+ comes out.

Cell damage

This category includes all those conditions in which, due to increased cell lysis, large amounts of potassium can end up in the circulation. Severe trauma, rhabdomyolysis and crush syndrome are a classic example, but we must also consider other pathological conditions such as tumor cell lysis or massive hemolysis (from various causes).

Reduced urinary potassium excretion

Renal failure

As already described, in chronic renal failure the kalemia is maintained within the normal range since each of the still functioning nephrons increases the excretion of K^+; this adaptation mechanism is effective until the urinary flow is effective, i.e. until the patient becomes oliguric and the GFR does not fall below 30-20 mL/min.

When hyperkalemia develops in a patient suffering from chronic but not oliguric renal failure, this generally occurs because there are other conditions, such as an excessive intake of K^+, a therapy with K^+-sparing diuretics or a hypoaldosteronism. Furthermore, in renal failure, hyperkalemia is also secondary to a mechanism of altered distribution due to a reduced cellular uptake of K^+, due to both the present metabolic acidosis and the reduced activity of Na^+/K^+ ATPase caused by the uremic toxins.

Renal failure can be due not only to renal or tubular disease, but also to an EABV (effective arterial blood volume) reduction, which. Can occur in different conditions, such as: fluid loss, as in the case of diarrhea; the fluid sequester in the third space, as in the case of liver cirrhosis with ascites; reduced tissue perfusion, as occurs in heart failure. While on one hand hypokalemia is often present in these pathologies (secondary both to the loss of fluids containing K^+ and to any diuretic therapy), on the other hand it is also possible to find hyperkalemia.

In fact, the reduction of EABV results in reduced glomerular filtration, which in turn leads to reduced urinary K^+ excretion; this mechanism can be observed not only primitively in renal failure, but also in heart failure (read cardiorenal syndrome), or in liver cirrhosis (read hepatorenal syndrome), all conditions in which reduced renal perfusion can cause hyperkalemia, worsened by concomitant therapy with ACE inhibitors and/or anti-aldosteronic drugs.

Drugs

ACE inhibitors (captopril, enalapril, ramipril, perindopril, etc.) are widely used in the treatment of high blood pressure, chronic ischemic heart disease and heart failure; these drugs interfere with the RAA system by blocking the enzyme ACE (angiotensin converting enzyme), which transforms angiotensin I (in turn produced from the circulating angiotensinogen by renin) into angiotensin II, so, since the latter is a very powerful vasoconstrictor, hypotension is determined; however, angiotensin II stimulates aldosterone secretion, so ACE inhibitors also result in hypoaldosteronism with reduced K^+ excretion and subsequent hyperkalemia, which is enhanced by other potassium-increasing factors, especially renal failure.

Sartans also act by interfering with the RAAS, since they are angiotensin receptor antagonists; as for ACE inhibitors their potassium-increasing effect is enhanced by renal failure and/or heart failure. Although they are considered the cornerstone of the therapy of heart failure and diabetic nephropathy, due to their potassium-increasing effect in clinical practice they must be used with caution.

Potassium-sparing diuretics and anti-aldosteronic drugs include drugs such as: spironolactone and potassium canrenoate, which act by antagonizing the effect of aldosterone at the DCT level, thus reducing the excretion of K^+; the amiloride and triamterene, which act by blocking the Na^+ channels at the DCT level, thus preventing the generation of the electronegative gradient necessary to allow the excretion of K^+. With the same mechanism (for this mentioned here) also two antibiotics, the trimethoprim and the pentamide can determine hyperkalemia.

The NSAIDs (non-steroidal anti-inflammatory drugs) work by blocking the cyclooxygenase (COX), an enzyme that allows the transformation of arachidonic acid into prostaglandins (PG), thromboxanes (TX) and leukotrienes (TX). On the renal level, PGs are involved in the regulation of the vascular tone, therefore in the hemodynamics of the glomerulus, but also in the production of renin, which is stimulated by the PGs. It follows that NSAIDs can cause hyperkalemia due to reduced filtration by the glomerular vasoconstriction and reduced production of renin and therefore of aldosterone. Usually this effect is absent (or insignificant) in healthy individuals, but is accentuated in the presence of a nephropathy, heart failure or therapy with potassium-sparing diuretics.

Heparin reduces aldosterone secretion by acting directly on the adrenal gland through an unclear mechanism; hyperkalemia, however, occurs only if there are other overlapping conditions, such as kidney failure.

Hypoaldosteronism

It can be induced by various conditions, which interfere both with production and with the effects of aldosterone; the most common causes are "hyporeninemic hypoaldosteronism" and therapy with K^+-sparing diuretics in adults, while enzymatic deficits (especially 21-hydroxylase deficiency) are the main cause of hypoaldosteronism in children. From a pathophysiological point of view, hyperkalemia has a multifactorial pathogenesis, which may depend on several mechanisms: 1) the low levels of renin, which in itself cause reduction of angiotensin II with consequent reduced secretion of aldosterone; 2) an altered response to angiotensin II, secondary to a post-receptor defect in the glomerular part of the adrenal gland; 3) the presence of renal failure, especially considering that these are patients with diabetic nephropathy or chronic interstitial nephritis; 4) hypervolemia associated with renal disease, which leads to an increased release of ANP (atrial natriuretic peptide), a hormone capable of directly suppressing renin release.

Patients suffering from "primary adrenal failure" due to bilateral adrenal glands removal or autoimmune mechanisms (such as in AIDS), have a reduced production of glucocorticoid and mineralocorticoid hormones with consequent hyperkalemia.

Conversely, in the case of hypoadrenalism secondary to pituitary failure, the affected patients do not become hyperkalemic as ACTH plays a minor role in the regulation of aldosterone, whose secretion, as described, is essentially regulated by angiotensin II and directly from kalemia.

Pseudohypoaldosteronism

It is a condition due to an end-organ resistance to aldosterone, characterized by volume depletion, loss of Na^+, hyperkalemia, elevated levels of renin and aldosterone, i.e. finds similar to those found during therapy with K^+-sparing diuretics.

There are two types of pseudohypoaldosteronism: a) in an acquired form, with a limited clinical picture at the kidney level and observable in tubulointerstitial pathologies (such as chronic pyelonephritis, interstitial nephritis and amyloidosis); b) a genetically determined form, which is further distinguished as type

1 with an autosomal dominant and recessive transmission with a variable clinical picture, and in type 2 Gordon syndrome, characterized by an increase in sodium and chloride which results in hypokalemia which responds well to the treatment with thiazides.

Rare disorders

The type I (distal) tubular acidosis is a rare disorder, characterized at TCD level by an altered (reduced) H^+ secretion with consequent metabolic acidosis, which however, in the hyperkalemic form, also presents a reduced reabsorption of Na^+ with consequent reduced K^+ excretion (also in this case, therefore, due to lack of generation of the necessary electronegative gradient at endoluminal level).

The selective defect of potassium secretion is a rare disorder, characterized by an inappropriate reduced excretion of K^+, despite the normal levels of renin and aldosterone and although there is no loss of Na^+ .This condition, whose pathogenesis is not clear, is found in sickle cell anemia, in renal transplant rejection and in lupus nephritis.

Symptoms and signs

Since K^+ is involved in the genesis of the membrane potential, excitable cells are particularly sensitive to hyperkalemia, the effects of which are essentially expressed in the form of asthenia and muscle weakness (up to flaccid paralysis and hypoventilation), however the cardiac involvement is the most feared condition due to the risk of fatal arrhythmias. Generally patients become symptomatic when the $[K^+]_p$ exceeds the value of 6.5-7 mEq/L, but the onset of symptoms and signs – especially the ECG alterations – is determined by the speed with which the disorder is established rather than from the absolute value of potassium. Furthermore, it should not be forgotten that patients may also experience symptoms and signs related to the underlying pathology (i.e. renal failure), in addition to those related to hyperkalemia itself.

Muscle weakness

Muscle weakness is related to the altered neuromuscular conduction: the increase $[K^+]_p$ reduces the ratio between intra- and extracellular K^+, which leads to a reduction in the resting potential. Although we can expect an increase in membrane excitability (since even a minor stimulus could depolarize the cell), the opposite actually happens. In fact, the persistent depolarization inactivates the Na^+ channels, which results in a net decrease in membrane excitability, which clinically translates into muscle weakness up to paralysis. Generally, muscle weakness does not appear until kalemia exceeds 8 mEq/L; typically, it begins by involving the lower extremities, then spreading upwards to the trunk and upper extremities, while the respiratory muscles and cranial nerves are normally spared.

ECG alterations and cardiac arrhythmias

In the presence of hyperkalemia, electrocardiographic monitoring is essential because it allows the early identification of characteristic alterations, which lead to the development of dangerous arrhythmias. The most serious consequence of acute hyperkalemia is the slowing down and blocking of intra-cardiac conduction. Generally, ECG alterations occur when kalemia is > 6 mEq/L: the earliest changes are the peaking and narrowing of the T wave with a short QT interval, which reflect the altered repolarization; the T wave alterations due to to hyperkalemia can be confused with high T-waves characteristic of myocardial ischemia, but in the latter case the QT is generally normal or prolonged.

Usually we identify progressive ECG alterations, which depend not only on the absolute value of kalemia but also on the speed with which the disorder is established. Specifically, as the potassium increases: for values between 5.0 and 6.0 mEq/L, the appearance of high and peaked T-waves in the form of a “tent”, the shortening of the QT interval and the depression of the ST segment occurs; for values between 6.0 and 7.0 mEq/L we observe the reduction of the amplitude of the P wave, thewidening of the PR interval, the initial widening of the QRS complexes; for kalemia val-

ues > 7.0 mEq/L the amplitudes of the QRS is further increased with "fusion" of the S wave with the T wave and formation of a sinusoidal wave (sine wave pattern); a low frequency idioventricular rhythm may also arise, with subsequent evolution in ventricular fibrillation and, finally, in PEA/asystole.
The relationship, described in **Figure 13.1**, between the value of hyperkalemia and electrocardiographic changes may be variable (in rare cases the ECG may even be normal or almost normal despite the high value of plasma K^+) because it is influenced by others factors, such as the concomitant alterations of the electrolytes and of the acid-base state; in particular, the toxicity of hyperkalemia is accentuated by hypocalcemia, hyponatremia and acidemia.

Diagnosis

The hyperkalemic patient is a potentially life-threatening patient, particularly due to the feared cardio-circulatory complications.
The measurement of kalemia is mandatory in the unstable patient (if not already in cardiac arrest), but it is desirable to suspect hyperkalemia already on the basis of anamnestic data, even before obtaining the laboratory value. For this reason the initial evaluation of a hyperkalemic patient – or presumed such – must include: a complete medical history (diet, history of kidney disease, diabetes, diuretics, recurrent episodes of muscle weakness), physical examination (signs of muscle weakness, volume depletion, edema), ECG, ABG, laboratory tests (especially those related to the renal function). These informations make it possible to identify the cause of hyperkalemia, classifying it in one (or more) of the 3 "drawers" (increased intake, extracellular shift, reduced excretion). However, since the priority is to evaluate the possible need for a life-saving treatment, the first tests to be performed are undoubtedly the ECG and the ABG.
Once a pseudohyperkalemia (for example from a venous puncture) is excluded, since – as described – a simply increased intake is hardly the cause of hyperkalemia, the clinical and pharmacological history easily allow to identify a hyperkalemia from extracellular shift or reduced renal excretion. Since kidney failure is the main cause of hyperkalemia, especially when associated with other potassium-increasing factors (oral K^+ supplements, ACE inhibitors, K^+-sparing diuretics, digitalis, etc.), other causes of hyperkalemia such as depletion of effective EABV, liver cirrhosis or heart failure, can be rapidly identified by anamnesis (clinical history, vomiting, diarrhea, etc.) and physical examination (reduced or increased jugular vein distension, ascites, swelling edema in legs and feet, etc.).
In the absence of the aforementioned pathological conditions, if hyperkalemia persists, an endocrinological disorder can be suspected, in particular hypoaldosteronism through more specific tests such as hormonal dosages (renin, aldosterone) and enzymatic tests (for example the 21-hydroxylase in children) and instrumental investigations (for example, an ultrasound or a CT scan in the suspicion of adrenal adenoma). It is also important to consider the patient's age: hyporeninemic hypoaldosteronism and primary adrenal failure are more common in adults, while in children enzyme deficiencies and type 1 pseudohypoaldosteronism are more common.
The measurement of urinary K^+ concentration on spot urine can provide some information: the finding of a high kaliuria (> 20 mEq/L) indicates an extrarenal cause, due to an increased intake (rare) or an extracellular shift of K^+ (hemolysis, ketoacidosis, rhabdomyolysis, drugs), while a reduced kaliuria (< 10 mEq/L) indicates a renal cause (end stage renal failure, adrenal failure, drugs).

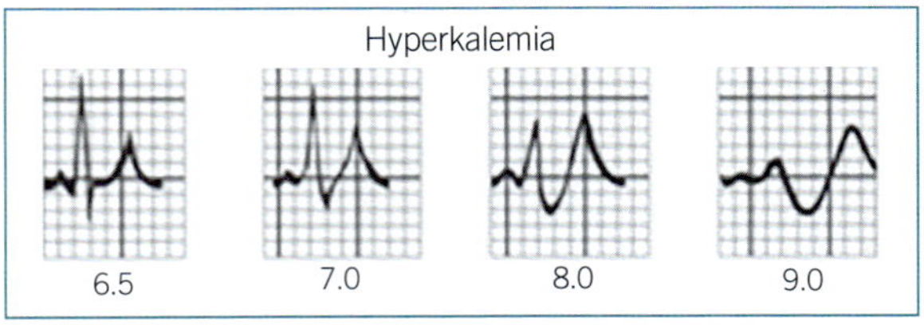

Figure 13.1. Electrocardiographic changes in relation to increasing values of hyperkalemia.

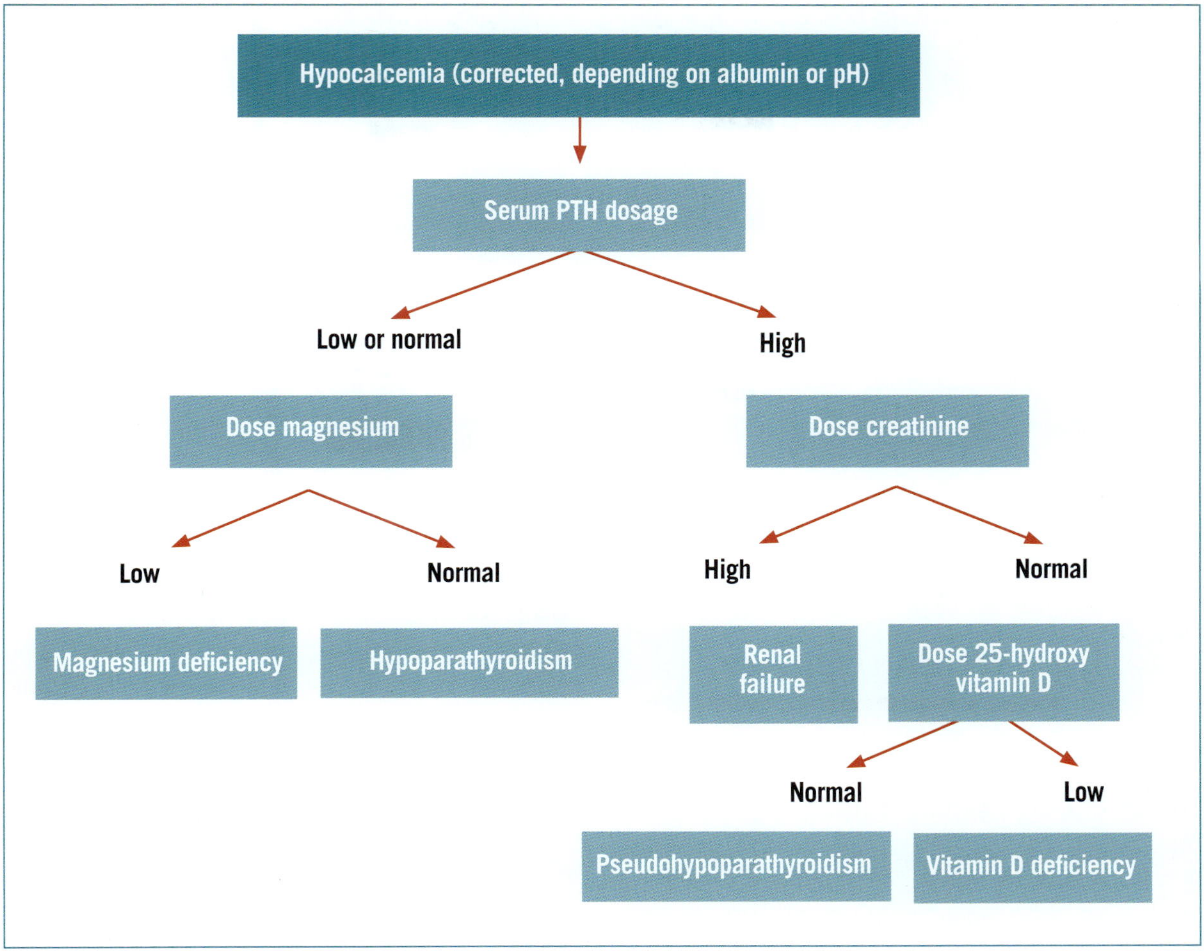

Figure 14.1 Diagnostic algorithm of hypocalcemia.

Clinical case A 58-year-old man arrives in the emergency department complaining of general malaise, epigastric pain, weakness, tingling in the lips, mental confusion, symptoms that occurred after a gastroenteritis, which occurred two, three days before, characterized by 3-4 diarrheal discharges per day, non bloody and not associated with fever or abdominal pain, self-limited after the doctor had prescribed lactic ferments. In the anamnesis, he reports that he has COPD, secondary to smoking, gastroesophageal reflux (in the last four years he underwent two gastroscopies) and dyslipidemia; in addition, he is a chronic drinker (over 1 ½ liters of wine a day for about 10 years). Regularly he takes pantoprazole 40 mg/day (which doubles for about 30 days at seasonal changes), atorvastatin 10 mg/day, aerosol cycles with steroids and β_2-agonists during bronchitis exacerbations.

Vital signs: BP 155/85 mmHg, HR 105 bpm, SpO_2 94% on room air, body temperature 36.8 °C; on physical examination: dry skin and mucous membranes, strong and rhythmic heart tones, free pauses, mild tachycardia; on the pulmonary examination harsh vesicular murmurs at the bases; the abdomen is normal. The ECG confirms sinus tachycardia (105-110 bpm), but there is a prolonged QTc interval (530 msec). After being admitted to the short observation unit, the patient is subjected to ECG monitoring which shows some brief ventricular tachycardia runs. The blood gas analysis with electrolytes shows normal parameters except ionized calcium which is 0.6 mmol/L (2.6 mg/dL); blood tests show a slight increase in creatinine (1.3 mg/dL), the total plasma calcium level is 5.7 mg/dL (albumin 3.8 mg/dL). Following the detection of hypocalcemia, the dosage of PTH is required, which results to be reduced as it is reduced serum magnesium (1.1 mg/dL – nv 1.8-2.3mg/dL).

Reasoned comment

The patient is hospitalized with the diagnosis of "malaise in dehydration and diarrhea" and monitored due to the prolonged QTc.

The history (chronic intake of pantoprazole and chronic alcohol abuse) and laboratory data (reduced serum PTH and hypomagnesaemia) lead to a diagnosis of hypocalcemia secondary to hypomagnesemia (see also Table 14.3). In addition the recent gastroenteritis, creating a condition of acute malabsorption, has revealed a chronic situation making the symptoms of hypocalcemia evident.

Treatment of hypocalcemia

Symptomatic patients ([Ca] < 2-2.5 mg/dL or < 1.0 mmol/L) should be treated with calcium chloride (10 mL 10%) or calcium gluconate (30 mL 10%), preferably with electrocardiographic monitoring; at the same dosage CaCl is three times more effective than calcium gluconate and should preferably be administered using a central venous route. Hypokalemia, hypomagnesaemia and/or alkalemia, if coexisting, should be corrected because they increase the arrhythmogenic risk; drugs that promote calcium excretion, such as loop diuretics, should be discontinued, while thiazides that reduce urinary calcium may be useful.

Since the effect of calcium tends to disappear in 20-30 minutes, it is generally recommended to start by practicing a slow infusion at the rate of 0.2-0.5 mg/kg/h for 12-24 hours; the infusion rate should then be modulated based on the plasma calcium values obtained. If the infusion alone is insufficient, vitamin D supplements are added in an active form. If patients are treated with digitalis therapy, special caution is needed as any transient hypercalcemia can cause arrhythmias. In the case of tetany due to hypocalcemia, calcium gluconate is administered 1-2 grams at slow bolus in 2-5 minutes or CaCl 0.5-1.0 gram in 10-20 minutes; administrations can be repeated every 4-6 hours until symptomatic remission is obtained. Chronic hypocalcemia is treated with oral calcium supplements, often in formulations associated with vitamin D, starting with 600 mg 1 or 2 times a day, avoiding exceeding 2,000 mg/day due to the risk of kidney stones.

Clinical case

Therapy

The patient is subjected to ECG monitoring and placed on therapy with NaCl 0.9% saline solution at 80 mL, potassium chloride 600 mg 1 capsule x 2/day, calcium gluconate 10% 10 mL IV x 3/day. The altered values of ionized calcium and electrocardiographic abnormalities still persisted after 24 hours of therapy. Assuming that hypocalcemia is secondary to hypomagnesemia, therapy with PPI is suspended (replaced with anti-H2 type of gastro-protectors), and a therapy with magnesium sulfate intravenously is established (10 grams in the first 24 hours, subsequently 4 g/day until the normalization of magnesium). After about 4 days the normalization of plasma magnesium and calcium (total and ionized) values is obtained, the QT interval length is normalized with disappearance of the previously reported ventricular tachycardia runs. On a clinical level, the patient becomes asymptomatic from the second day.

References

- Ahn C, Kang JH. Calcium Homeostasis in Diabetes Mellitus. J Vet Sci. 2017;18(3):261-66.
- Aishah AB, Foo YN. A retrospective study of serum calcium levels in a hospital population in Malaysia. Med J Malaysia. 1995;50(3):246-49.
- Akirov A, Gorshtein A, Shraga-Slutzky I et al. Calcium levels on admission and before discharge are associated with mortality risk in hospitalized patients. Endocrine. 2017;57(2):344-51.

Index

Page numbers followed by *f* indicate figures, *t* tables.

I

T

U

V

W